LIFE, PURPOSE, AND VISION

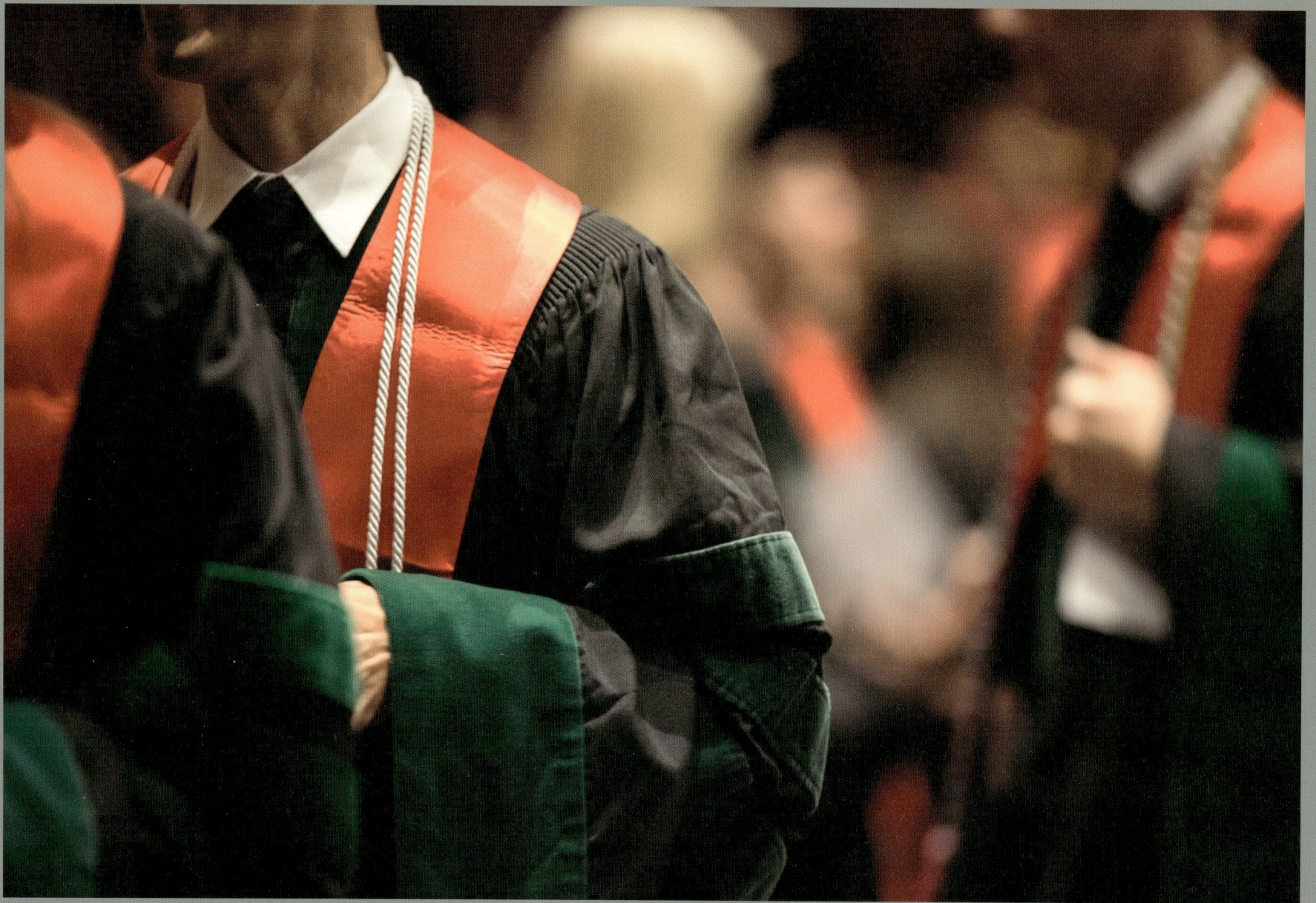

LIFE, PURPOSE, AND VISION

A Fiftieth Anniversary History of the
Texas Tech University Health Sciences Center

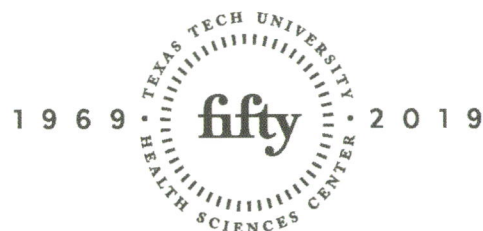

1969 · **fifty** · 2019
TEXAS TECH UNIVERSITY HEALTH SCIENCES CENTER

EDITED BY

Margaret Vugrin, MSLS, AHIP, MPH, MPA

Thomas F. McGovern, EdD

Richard Nollan, PhD, MLS, AHIP

TEXAS TECH UNIVERSITY PRESS
TEXAS TECH UNIVERSITY HEALTH SCIENCES CENTER

This book is typeset in Garamond Premier Pro. The paper used in this book
meets the minimum requirements of ANSI/NISO Z39.48–1992 (R1997). ∞

Designed by April Leidig

Library of Congress Control Number: 2019934083
ISBN: 978-1-68283-043-7

Printed in the United States of America

19 20 21 22 23 24 25 26 27 | 9 8 7 6 5 4 3 2 1

Texas Tech University Press
Box 41037
Lubbock, Texas 79409–1037 USA
800.832.4042
ttup@ttu.edu
www.ttupress.org

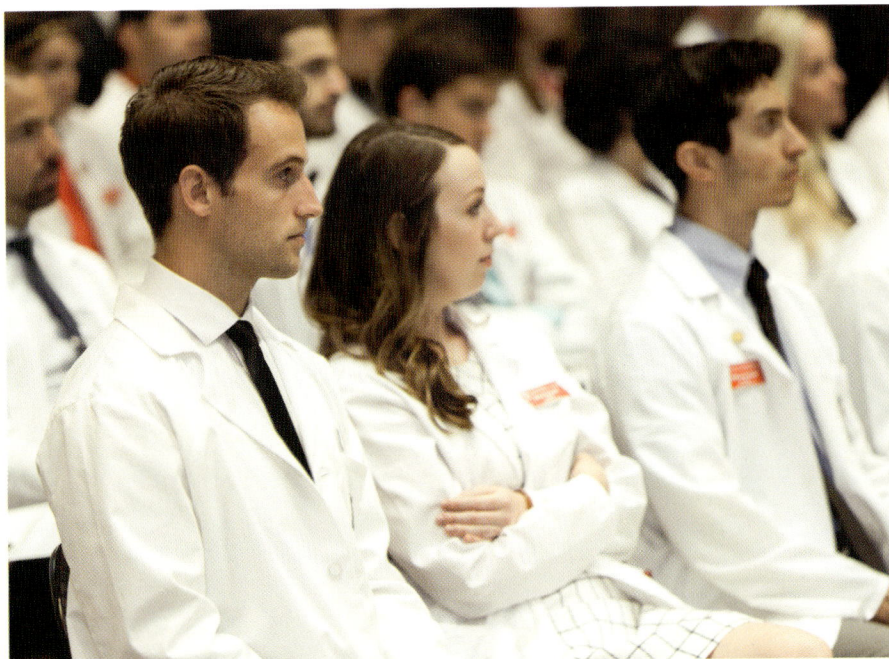

The editors dedicate this book to the faculty, alumni, staff, and students of Texas Tech University Health Sciences Center past, present, and future and to the patients and families we are privileged to serve.

It is also dedicated to the environment that has nurtured us and helped us grow. We were able to support the health and well-being of the communities and people surrounding us. Only with all of us working together have we become successful in our mission: to educate health practitioners for West Texans.

CONTENTS

FOREWORD

Although the story of the Health Sciences Center officially began in 1969, its roots were planted long before—back in 1901, when a young physician from Kentucky named Marvin Overton made Lubbock his home and endeavored to make the town the medical hub for the region. At the time Overton moved here, there was no easy way to get to Lubbock. It was small, not particularly impressive, and had only a few hundred residents. It had no railroad (Amarillo had been running passenger trains since 1888), no navigable river, no notable industry, no college, and no hospital. When Texans of the early twentieth century were considering the future of their state, I'm sure most did not consider Lubbock to be vital. And even for the West Texans of the time, I'm sure few could have seen the critical role that it would play with Dr. Overton's arrival and vision.

Over the course of his lifetime, Dr. Overton worked tirelessly to recruit physicians, families, and industry to the town he called home. In addition to establishing the first hospital, he also purchased the county's first automobile, which he used to travel to neighboring communities to see patients. Upon recruiting new physicians, Dr. Overton encouraged them to continue this form of emissary service. Over time, thanks in large part to his good reputation and the continued recruitment of physicians (there were 59 doctors in Lubbock by 1940), the city developed into the epicenter of medical care for the region, sowing the seeds for the future of Texas Tech University Health Sciences Center.

Fast forward to the 1960s. A Texan is in the White House, space exploration is anchored in Houston, Dallas has emerged as one of the nation's leading commercial centers, and oil has become the state's economic identity. Indeed, things are looking up for Texas. Here in West Texas, Lubbock is now home to Texas Technological College (established in 1923), the Panhandle boasts preeminence in the nation's cattle business, the South Plains in agriculture (cotton, wheat, corn, peanuts), and the Permian Basin in energy production. Yet despite the good fortune, a troubling trend has occurred in the western half of the state—too few doctors to support those people who support everyone else. In spite of the work done by Dr. Overton, the Hub City alone is inadequate for maintaining the health needs of the region and of West Texas. A similar though not as dire trend has occurred statewide as more and more youngsters raised in rural areas choose to move to the city. This urbanization leaves West Texas in an increasingly difficult bind. Conversations and political machinations take place in the capital as legislators wrestle over how best to address the problem. While it is clear that the state will need more doctors, it is not clear which institution should be in charge of producing them and where that university should reside. At the time, the only public university system in the state with medical components was the University of Texas. Naturally, there were many who felt that any new school should be under the UT banner and placed in the state's largest city (Houston). West Texans, however, were dubious of the impact such a plan would have on the needs of those living west of Fort Worth. After years of wrangling and horse trading, two schools of medicine were established during the sixty-first legislative session in 1969; one belonging to the University of Texas (headquartered in Houston) and the other belonging to Texas Tech (headquartered in Lubbock). This legislation was signed into law by Governor Preston Smith. The rest, as they say, is history.

At this anniversary, one can only look back over the past 50 years with a sense of awe at what's been accomplished. From humble beginnings as a small school of medicine with campuses in Lubbock, Amarillo, and El Paso to a comprehensive health university with Schools of Medicine (1969), Nursing (1979), Health Professions (1979),

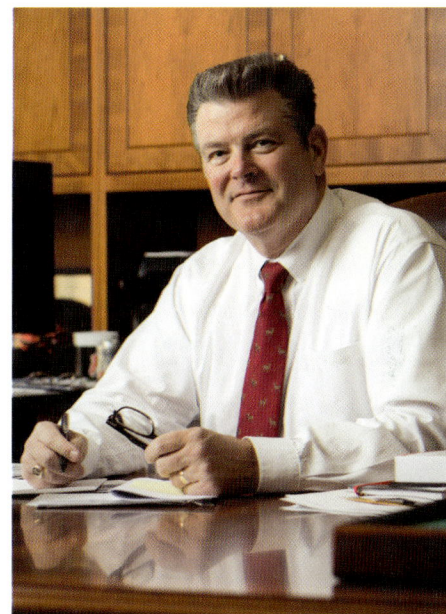

Tedd Mitchell, MD, President, TTUHSC and Chancellor, Texas Tech University System.

Pharmacy (1993), and Graduate Biomedical Sciences (1994) with campuses in Lubbock, Amarillo, Abilene, Midland, Odessa, and Dallas. The university is also proud to have established the Paul L. Foster School of Medicine in El Paso (2003) as well as the Gayle Greve Hunt School of Nursing in El Paso (2011), two schools that would eventually become the Texas Tech University Health Sciences Center at El Paso (2013), a new university within the Texas Tech University System.

Our university's history is as colorful as the West Texas sky. Our traditions are rooted in the pioneering spirit of our predecessors, those like Dr. Overton whose combination of a "can do" attitude and hard work built the region and solidified our role as the premier medical hub for West Texas and beyond. Times have not always been easy on the journey, but that never dissuaded the men and women who came before us—folks who understood the greater good, the need for perseverance, and the expectation of a brighter tomorrow. Finally, and perhaps most importantly, our historical purpose is a noble one—to care for those who provide the food, fiber, and fuel to our state, our nation, and our world. I believe young Dr. Overton felt this instinctively the moment he stepped off a carriage and scanned a dusty little town called Lubbock.

Today, our faculty, staff, students, and alumni are busy creating the next chapter for Texas Tech University Health Sciences Center. Our impact today reaches far beyond West Texas. Indeed, our folks are literally impacting lives around the globe. It is my hope that this book will serve many functions: a stroll down memory lane for those who studied, worked, taught, or performed research here; a reminder of our great accomplishments in modern health care for any who have been treated in one of our facilities; and an illustrative tale of Texas tenacity for all who seek to understand our heritage. Our past is exceptional, our future is bright. Sir Winston Churchill said, "History will be kind to me, for I intend to write it." Well, out here in West Texas we feel the same way—we will continue to write our own story and make our own future, because so much depends on us.

Tedd L. Mitchell, MD
President, TTUHSC, and Chancellor, TTU System

INTRODUCTION

In 1969, the Sixty-first Texas Legislature passed Texas House Bill 498, creating the Texas Tech University School of Medicine, which was then quickly signed by Governor Preston Smith. Dr. John Buessler became the founding dean in 1970, and an affiliation agreement was approved with Lubbock County Hospital District sponsoring a new hospital, which is now University Medical Center. Other agreements were developed with both Methodist Hospital of Lubbock and St. Mary's Hospital, later becoming Covenant Health System in Lubbock. The Board of Regents approved the establishment of the School of Allied Health in 1972, the School of Nursing in 1975, and the School of Pharmacy in 1974.

The establishment of the health sciences center was not without its challenges and controversies. The academic establishment, including the deans of other medical schools in Texas, did not think it wise to develop a medical school in West Texas without the usual big city resources, dense populations, and established hospitals. A new medical center formed by the Lubbock County Hospital District had political support, but the complexities of an affiliation agreement with the medical school were, and are to this day, important topics of negotiation. At the start, Methodist Hospital of Lubbock was a willing participant in the founding of the school but only as a temporary partner, not as a future teaching hospital.

Some, but not all, of the original mission survived the colorful history of the school. The school was established to meet the healthcare requirements of the diverse population of West Texas, spread over 131,000 square miles, and specifically to address the need for primary care doctors. While research would be an important component of the school and health sciences center, the first priorities were clearly patient care and clinical instruction. Producing family physicians for the surrounding area would be a priority but the method of instruction was of some debate.

There was more interest in bringing rural patients to Lubbock than bringing physicians to the rural areas, and it was assumed initially that those who would train family physicians needed to be specialists—internists, obstetricians, and surgeons—not family physicians themselves.

Those early pioneers who saw the need to train primary care and family physicians would be proud of the 50 years of progress. The School of Medicine now has the most innovative primary care program in the United States—the Family Medicine Accelerated Track (FMAT). It is a program currently being copied by 11 schools of medicine, many of which have a special interest in rural health. Due in part to this track, Texas Tech ranks twelfth in the country in the percentage of students entering a family medicine residency program. Texas Tech ranks among the top five schools in the United States for the percentage of students who stay in their home state. The ratio of physicians to patient population in West Texas has also been greatly increased. More than 20 percent of physicians practicing in the whole of West Texas are graduates of the Texas Tech School of Medicine.

From the very beginning the plan for the medical school was to have campuses in Amarillo, El Paso, Midland, and Odessa (Permian Basin) with some interest in Wichita Falls as well. While the regional campus idea was not unique, even in the 1970s, few of the founding leaders of the health science center could have predicted the blossoming and sophistication of these campuses to their current state. While the Association of American Medical Colleges sponsors a national group on regional campuses, few of the campuses represented display the level of autonomy, interprofessional education, and collaboration that currently exists on the TTUHSC campuses. Today, physicians in Lubbock and its other campuses combine to provide more than 500,000 clinical visits as part of the largest practice group in West Texas called Texas Tech

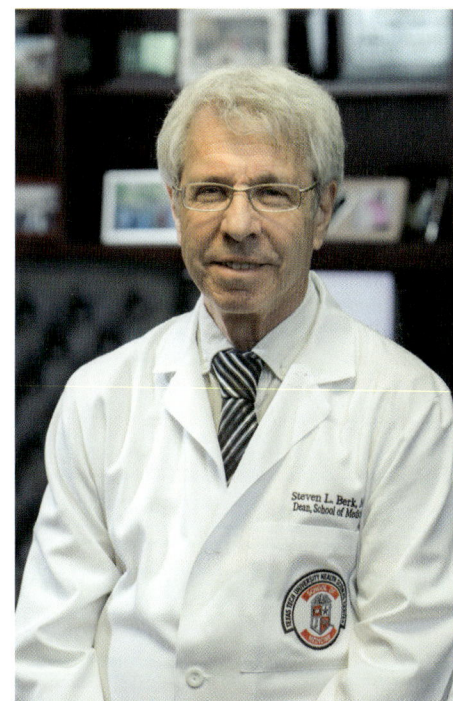

Steven L. Berk, MD, Dean and Provost, TTUHSC

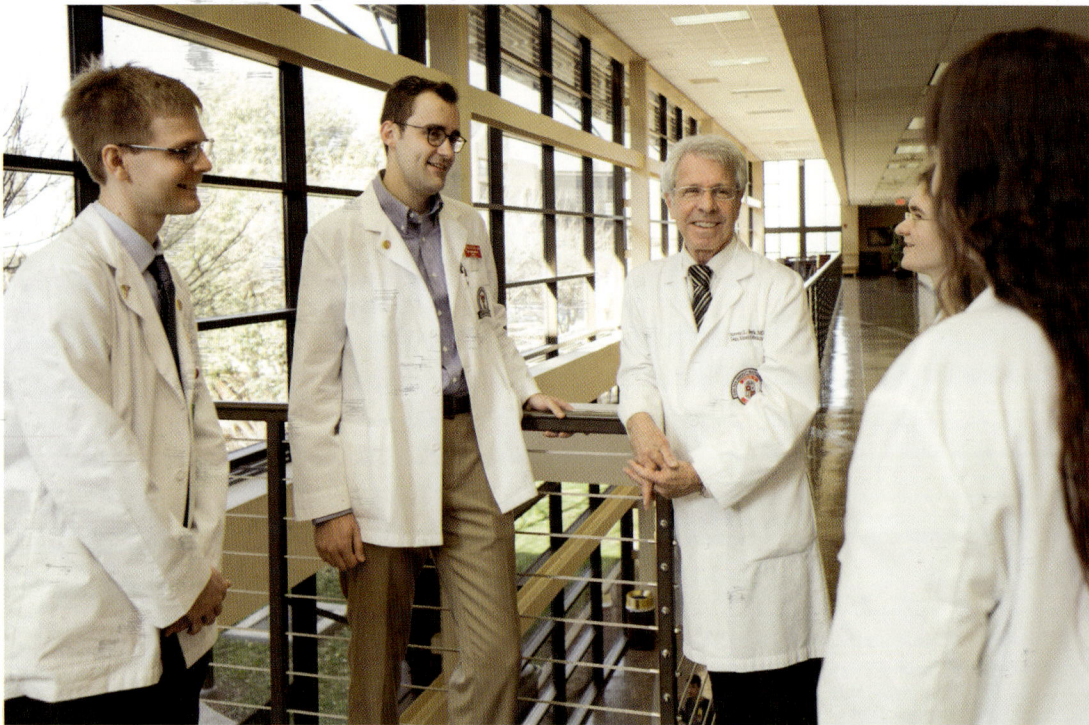

Dean Berk and Students

cessful and generous split of resources to develop the Paul L. Foster School of Medicine, a separate four-year medical school, and the separate and distinct Texas Tech University Health Sciences Center El Paso.

Dr. Buessler and the original associate deans proposed a unique plan to have the first two years of the medical school curriculum taught in the Department of Biology and Chemistry. While this plan was quickly found to be unrealistic, the Texas Tech University Health Sciences Center and Texas Tech University have explored numerous possible opportunities to work together throughout the decades. Currently TTUHSC, in association with TTU, has a combined MD/MBA program for medical students and a PharmD/MBA for pharmacy students that emphasizes health organization management. TTUHSC also has one of only about a dozen MD/JD programs and the only MPH/MPA (Public Administration) program in the state of Texas. There is an increasing emphasis on collaborative research between TTU and TTUHSC, which was also a dream of the original planners.

In 1974, The Liaison Committee on Medical Education (LCME) first accredited the School of Medicine following two site visits. However, a cautionary note was sounded and because of "many concerns," the medical school was given only one year of approval. In the 2017 LCME site visit, the school was commended by the LCME: "The school has effectively integrated a complex, multi-track educational program, . . . maintains a positive learning environment in a complex, multi-campus, multi-health system environment, . . . has negotiated the political and financial complexity of a competitive, health care environment to create a rich and diverse clinical learning program, . . . and has students who consistently comment on the warm, inclusive, supportive environment within the School of Medicine" (Liaison Committee on Medical Education, Site Visit Team Report, March 2016).

The TTUHSC affiliation with the University Medical Center (UMC) has likely surpassed all expectations. The two institutions share a 55-million-dollar contract agreement. UMC funds residents and fellows beyond expectations. The hospital provides funding for 11 endowed chairs and grants for research under the auspices of the Laura W. Bush Institute for Women's Health. The School of Health Professions provides services for audiology. The former Methodist Hospital (now Covenant Health System), which supported the early days of the school but was hesitant to become a permanent teaching hospital, is now

Physicians. With over 34 million dollars in uncompensated care, 27 clinical departments, 35 residency and fellowship programs, and 487 total residents, Texas Tech Physicians is a leading healthcare provider.

The School of Nursing's Combest Center has become a major center for indigent and Medicaid patients. Clinics in physical therapy, speech and hearing, many pharmacy affiliates, and a pharmacy anticoagulation clinic add to the spectrum of care provided at the health sciences center.

The School of Health Professions has expanded educational offerings to 20 different professional programs. Graduates from their Physician Assistant Studies program serve as primary care providers in communities around the state, many of whom work with Texas Tech Physicians. The School of Pharmacy now has campuses in Amarillo, Abilene, and Dallas. The Graduate School of Biomedical Sciences has opened a new Department of Public Health with classes in Lubbock and Abilene and offers an MPH degree program for concomitantly enrolled students from other TTUHSC schools. The School of Nursing has become a leading provider in the state for desperately needed nursing graduates, which also includes those with a doctor of nursing degree.

The amazing growth of the Texas Tech University Health Sciences Center does not include a uniquely suc-

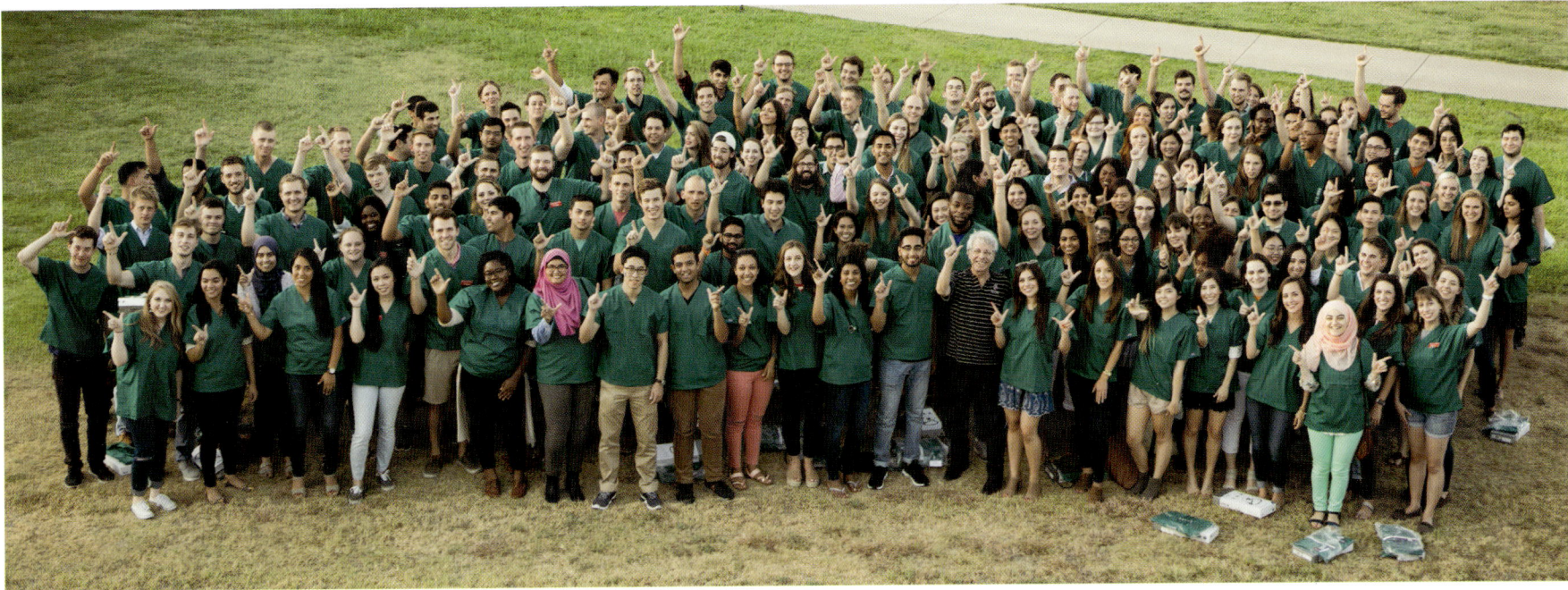

the home of a branch campus where third- and fourth-year students receive their clerkship training. Covenant Health System, too, provides three endowed chairs for the School of Medicine and one for the School of Nursing.

In R. McCartor and G. Tyner's 1986 book, *The Eye of the Storm*, the beginnings of the School of Medicine and the Texas Tech University Health Sciences Center are described. "The Eye of the Storm" was chosen as the title because, despite all the political and financial turmoil of establishing a new medical school, students were safe to learn and intellectually progress in the presumably peaceful "eye" of the storm. In a poetic sense, there will always be special challenges with the continued growth of a health sciences center in West Texas, now graduating more students than any other health sciences center in the state. However, students will continue to receive the best training possible with interprofessional experiences, state-of-the-art equipment, simulation, and personal guidance in compassionate care—even if it may sometimes appear to be in the eye of a storm.

Steven Berk MD

Steven L. Berk, MD, Dean, School of Medicine,
Executive Vice President and Provost, TTUHSC

ACKNOWLEDGMENTS

Any book that covers the length and breadth of an institution like the Texas Tech University Health Sciences Center was accomplished only with the input of over a hundred individuals from virtually every corner of the TTUHSC community. Some wrote about their specialty or their school while others contributed their memories.

Those who gave us their memories in the form of oral interviews included Teddy Langford Jones, Alexia Green, Rudy Arredondo, Steven Berk, Elmo Cavin, Manual de la Rosa, J. Ted Hartman, Richard Jordan, Robert and Marcie Lawless, Lorenz O. Lutherer, Terry McMahon, Tedd Mitchell, Bernhard Mittemeyer, Robert J. Salem, David Smith, Surendra Varma, Richard Weddige, and Tim Hayes. The interviews with these people would not have been successfully completed without the energy and foresight of Tom McGovern, who witnessed over 40 years of the HSC's growth. His dedication to preserving the accomplishments that he observed over this time motivated him to capture these memories as part of an ongoing initiative to preserve an oral archived history of our community. These recordings and transcriptions will be preserved in the Preston Smith Library Rare Book Room.

This history was the product of many writers from across the system. More people than we can recount here contributed their talents to create as complete and detailed a story as we could manage. Apart from the editors, contributors included Tedd L. Mitchell, Steven Berk, Michael Ragain, Richard Parks, Ryan Henry, Justin L. White, Didit Martinez, Smiley Garcia, Lori Rice-Spearman, Rial Rolfe, Robert Salem, Bob Goodwin, Billy Breedlove, Danette Baker, Betsy Jones, Simon Williams, Patrick Reynolds, Susan Bergeson, Pamela Johnson, Brandt Schneider, Margaret Burnett, Carol Daugherty, Edward Yeomans, Dale Dunn, Terry McMahon, Sharmila Dissanaike, Joe Cordero, Allan Haynes, Julie Cordero, Suzanna Cisneros, Volker Neugebauer, Kevin Halliburton, Mike Ragain, Dean Brannon, Catherine Hudson, Billy Philips, Scott Phillips, Gary Ventolini, Mark Funderburk, Wendell Davis, Debbie Milam, Cloyce Stetson, John C. De Toledo, Christy Meriwether, Ashley Hamm, Kendra Burris, Guillermo Altenberg, John Pelley, Alan Peiris, Josie Martinez, John Russell, Cathy Lovett, Keino McWhinney, Bill Sessions, Sharon Decker, Jason Cooper, Barbara Sawyer, Barbara Pence, Doug Stocco, Mark Hendricks, Yondell Masten, Kathy Sridaromont, Steven Urban, Cheryl Erwin, Thomas Tenner, Hemachandra Reddy, Quentin Smith, Vince Fell, Jim Hutson, Chip Shaw, Kate Serralde, Theresa Byrd, Lisaann Gittner, Allison Kerin, Patti Patterson, Sally Murray, Ryan Schmidt, Kiko Zavala, Renee Price, Deborah Conn, Norma Rincon, Denise DeShields, Gary L. Tonniges, Sr., Tommie Morelos, Rita Tecmire, Will Rodriguez, Sr., Rachael Paida, Paul Arrington, Terry Greenberg, Charles Family, Christy Fagan, David McCartney, Erik Wilkinson, Mubariz Naqvi, Joe Fralick, Sam Prien, Luke Reeger, Rick Richeda, Surendra Varma, Natalia Schlabritz-Lutsevich, Larry Starr, Matthew Grisham, Herb Janssen, Lorenz O. Lutherer, Michelle Ensminger, Lindsay Johnson, Jon McGough, Michael Mueller, Paul Landers, Cynthia Jumper, and Pam Brink. This list is certainly not exhaustive, many others supported this project in their own way, but it gives some idea of the many people who contributed to this narrative.

The illustrations used in this text are derived from a variety of sources. Foremost among them were those provided through the talents of medical photographer Neal Hinkle. In addition, Margaret Vugrin photographed and supplemented these with many of her own images. We would likewise thank Artie Limmer for allowing us to use some of his images. Others contributed images of their special areas. Together their work helps to visualize the broad themes and activities of TTUHSC. Where images were needed for chapter 1, we relied heavily on the photographic archives of the Texas Tech University Southwest Collection. Terry Greenberg's invaluable assistance pulled all the many textual pieces together and Pam Brink concentrated on crafting the history narrative. Many thanks to all!

We tried to capture the essence and spirit of a dynamic and growing institution. We wish we could have honored the invaluable contributions of so many over the past 50 years, but we could not. We have tried to present an overview that tells our story from 1969 to 2019.

This book was made possible through support provided by our president and chancellor, Tedd L. Mitchell, MD.

With all of the effort put forth by all of the contributors, the errors are the responsibility of the editors.

In addition, on a personal note, I want to acknowledge my husband's support.

Davor Vugrin, MD, brought me to Lubbock, "just for three to five years," some 30 years ago. Our move here gave both of us the opportunity to work with so many of the incredible people found in this book. The creation of this volume has been a labor of love. Thank you!

Margaret Vugrin, Co-Editor

LIFE, PURPOSE, AND VISION

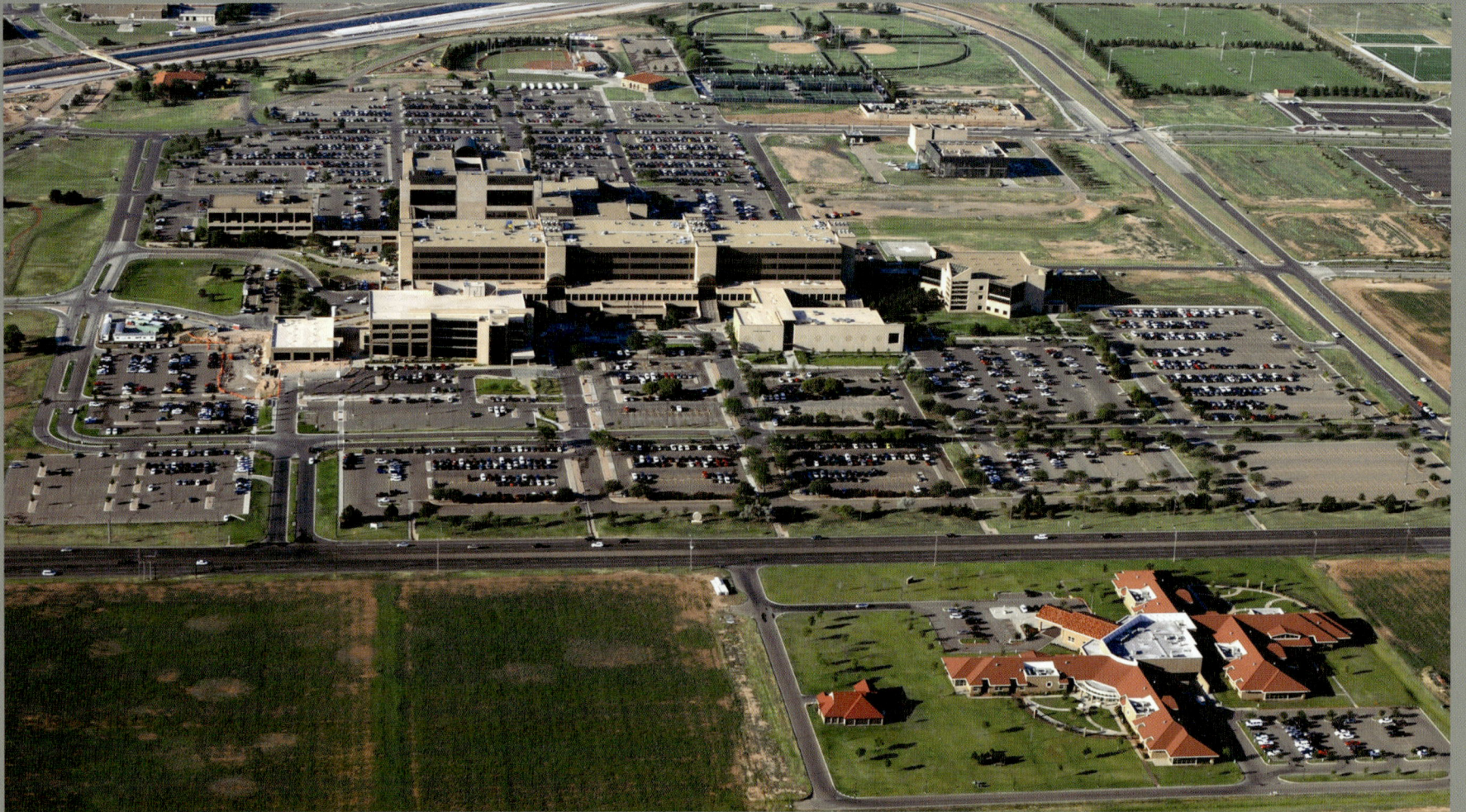
Aerial view of TTUHSC, 2008

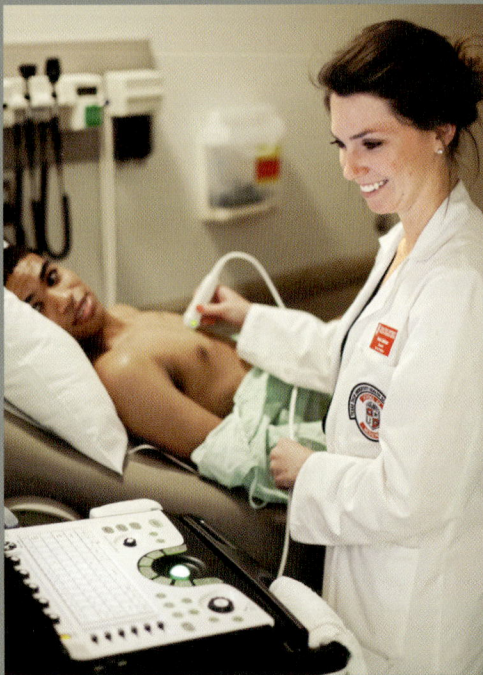
Student ultrasound

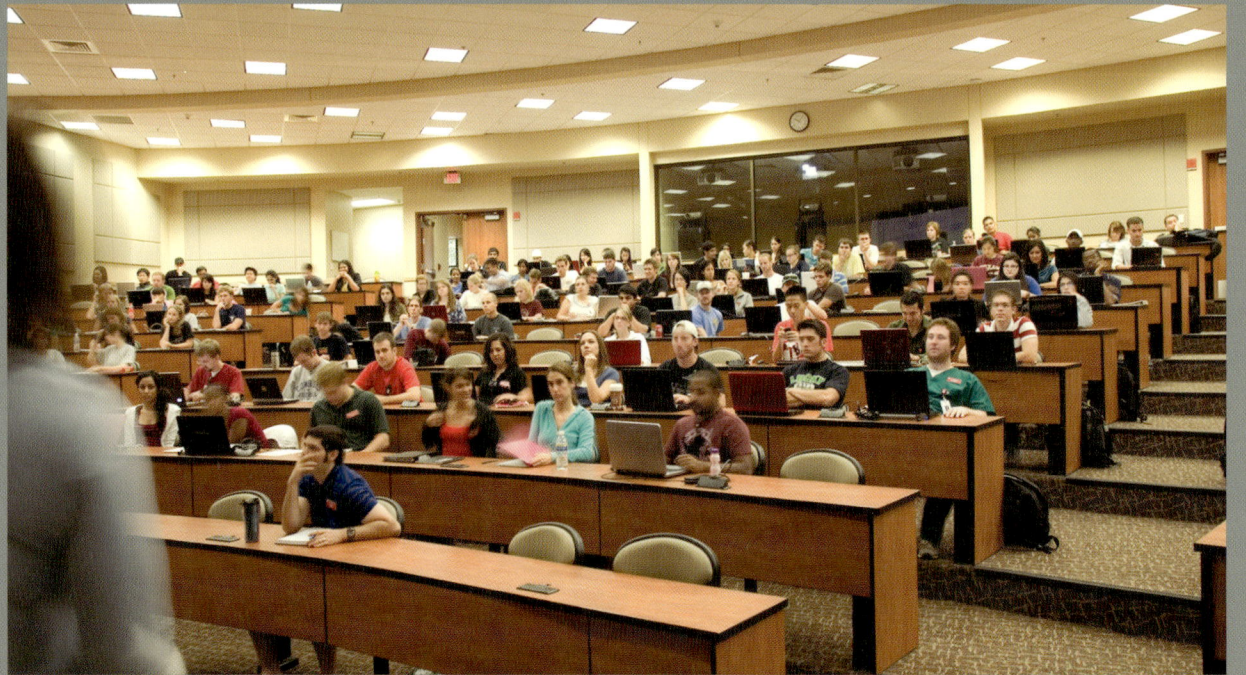
Academic Classroom Building with students

CHAPTER ONE

PIONEERS, INNOVATORS, AND VISIONARIES

The History behind the Texas Tech University Health Sciences Center

The Texas Tech University Health Sciences Center proudly celebrates 50 years of education and healthcare services for the people of West Texas and, through its basic and clinical research initiatives, the world beyond. From the beginning, the impetus for establishing a medical school affiliated with Texas Tech University was to produce more physicians to serve the rural population of West Texas, a service area comprised of 108 counties spread over 40 percent of the State of Texas. Access to health care has always been a challenge for this prairie region, an environment of vast ranchlands, cotton acreage, and oil fields, dotted by small towns and just a smattering of self-contained urban centers. When the Texas Tech School of Medicine was established in 1969, the physician to patient ratio was 1:1366. During the past 50 years, we have reduced that ratio by half and enhanced healthcare services for the populace through any number of innovative strategies.

While our flagship institution resides in Lubbock, the Texas Tech University Health Sciences Center also embraces campuses in the Permian Basin, Amarillo, Dallas, and Abilene to help bridge the distance for medical specialty needs and expand healthcare services throughout our area. Each TTUHSC campus offers education, research, and patient care through the School of Medicine, the School of Nursing, the School of Health Professions, the School of Pharmacy, and the Graduate School of Biomedical Sciences, with distinctive programs emerging from the particular needs of an area. The grassroots energy emanating from our campuses helps nourish the many programs that continue to grow at the Texas Tech University Health Sciences Center.

At the 50-year mark, the School of Medicine has graduated a total of 4,444 medical students, sending them out to their residency training with a rigorous and distinctive clinical background. A collegial and supportive educational and clinical model was operative at the medical school since its inception. Faculty and students often work shoulder-to-shoulder to provide diagnosis and treatment, and the seeds of this collaborative educational model were planted in the very beginning of the institution when this new medical school in West Texas was little more than a wild experiment.

Our Beginnings

In the 1960s, boosters for a medical school at Texas Tech University strongly argued that placing the school on the Texas Tech campus would add valuable academic resources to the new institution. To the deep chagrin of Lubbock leaders and West Texas politicians, especially Lieutenant Governor Preston E. Smith, in 1965, Governor John Connelly vetoed the first bill that had been exhaustingly nurtured through the Texas House and Senate to establish a

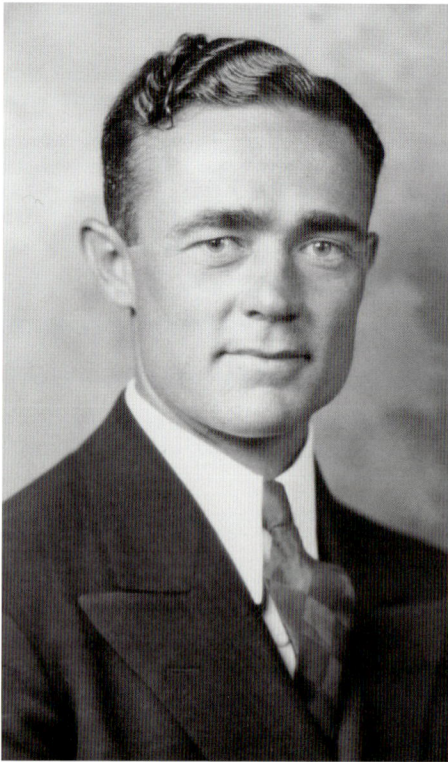

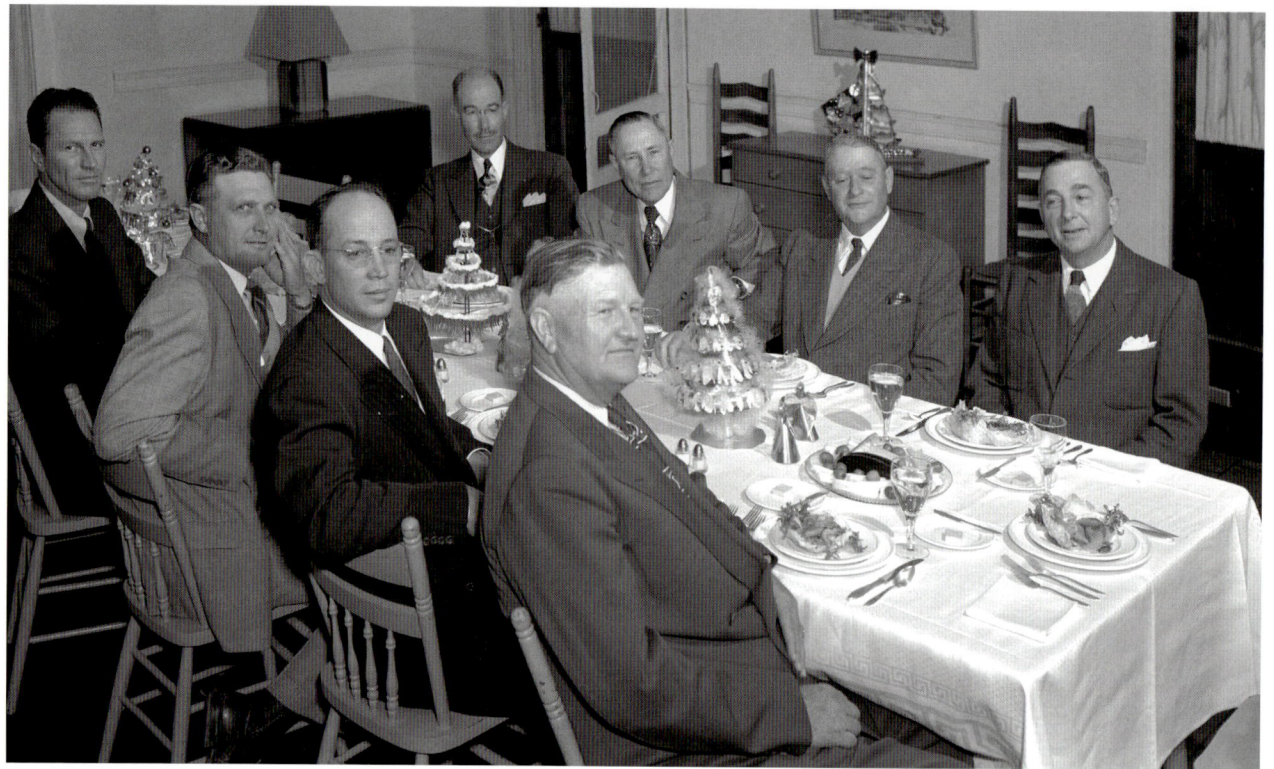

(ABOVE) Preston Smith (Brown Studio) 1931. Courtesy of the Southwest Collection/Special Collections Library

(RIGHT) Image of Texas Tech President E.N. Jones with members of the Board of Directors on March 24, 1953. Courtesy of the Southwest Collection/Special Collections Library

medical school at Texas Tech: House Bill No. 14. Connelly totally discounted the importance or significance of establishing a medical school on a contiguous campus with a university. However, besides the vital operations support from Texas Tech University in the early days of the medical school, interdisciplinary programs which resulted proved Connelly decidedly wrong in his assessment.

While the Texas Tech University Health Sciences Center and Texas Tech University have always been separate institutions, in the beginning, affiliation with the university played a crucial role in getting the medical school up and running within an unheard-of three years of its 1969 charter. To the local supporters of this new West Texas educational institution, time was of the essence. The Texas Tech Medical School had been established as part of a college that provided the credibility to apply for federal matching funds with rigorous deadlines. This was crucial to the development of the institution. Texas Tech president Grover E. Murray appointed John Buessler, MD, as founding vice president and dean of the nascent School of Medicine in 1970. Buessler had served as the founding chief of ophthalmology at the University of Missouri Medical Center and came to Lubbock directly from his position as executive director of Kansas

City General Hospital and Medical Center, University of Missouri–Kansas City School of Medicine. He was a dreamer, and his educational foresight in opening the Texas Tech School of Medicine is the stuff of legend.

In 1971, Buessler carved out a vision for the school in his famous "Red Book," which was a factor in securing interim accreditation from the National Institutes of Health (NIH). He hired a faculty—some from afar and many from local medical practices—and selected students for the 1972 entering class of 36 freshmen and 25 juniors. All of this happened with no designated facilities whatsoever. The Texas Tech administration came to the rescue by converting Drane Hall, a women's residence hall, to house the brand-new medical school. Cadavers were stored in the converted kitchen. Dissection and all things anatomical took place in the converted dining room. Thompson Hall, another traditional residence hall, was converted into clinical space. It was also turned into the student health center, providing medical and, some years later, nursing students the early hands-on experience that remains today a basic part of the Texas Tech University Health Sciences Center's educational model.

It was pretty much catch as catch can. William Seliger, DDS, PhD, founding chair of the Department of

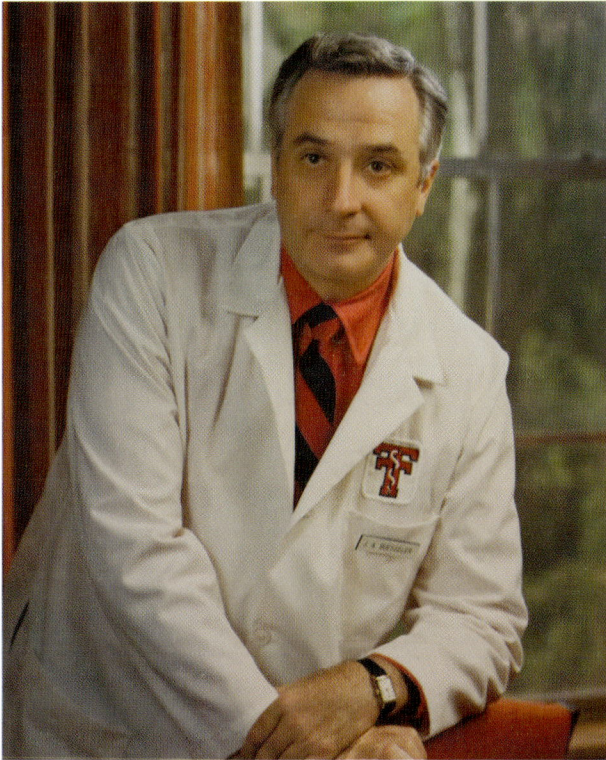

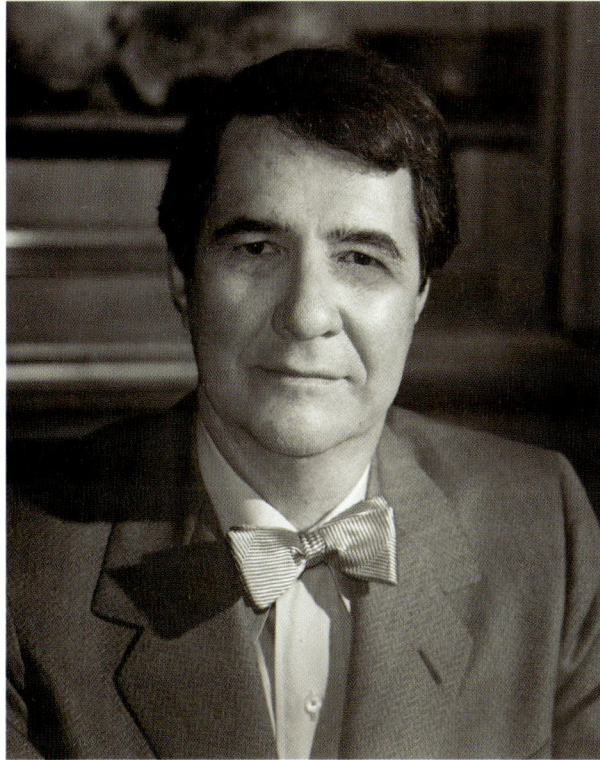

(LEFT) John A. Buesseler, MD, First President of the TTUHSC School of Medicine. Courtesy of the Southwest Collection/Special Collections Library

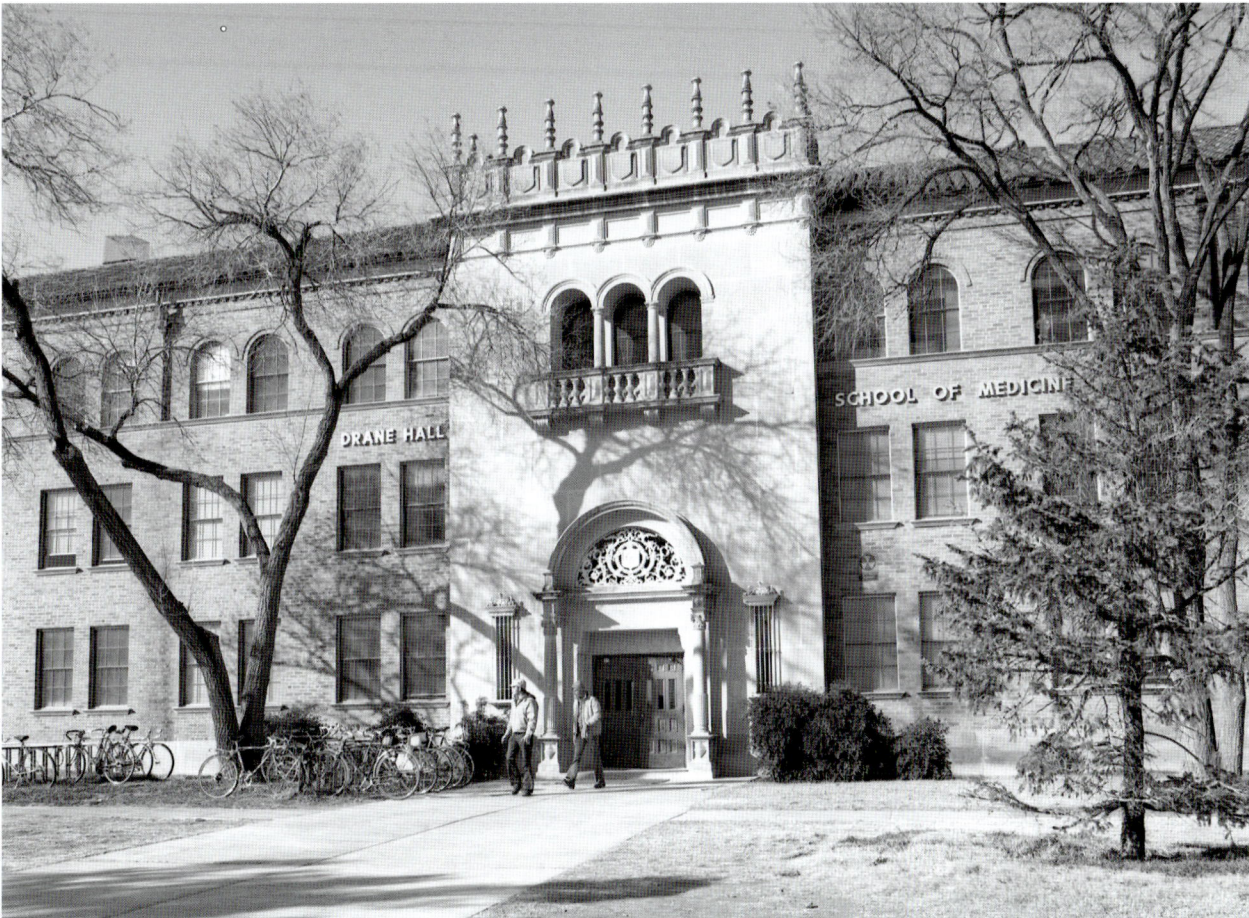

(RIGHT) Grover Elmer Murray, PhD, First President, Texas Tech University and School of Medicine. Courtesy of the Southwest Collection/Special Collections Library

Exterior view of the east entrance to the Drane Hall / School of Medicine Building on the Texas Tech University campus. Drane Hall served as the temporary building for the newly established School of Medicine while its new facility was being built west of campus. Courtesy of the Southwest Collection/Special Collections Library

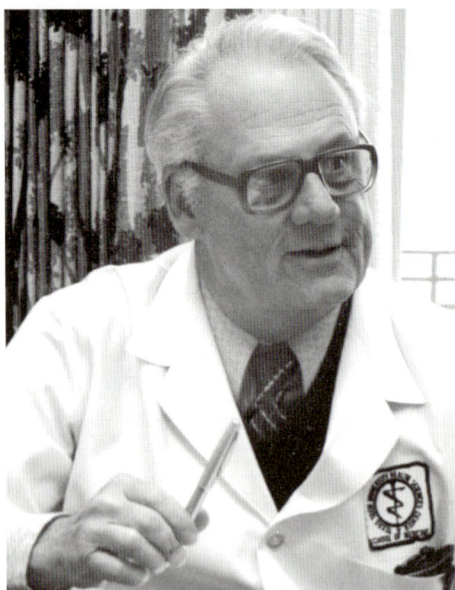

George Tyner, MD. Courtesy of the Southwest Collection/Special Collections Library

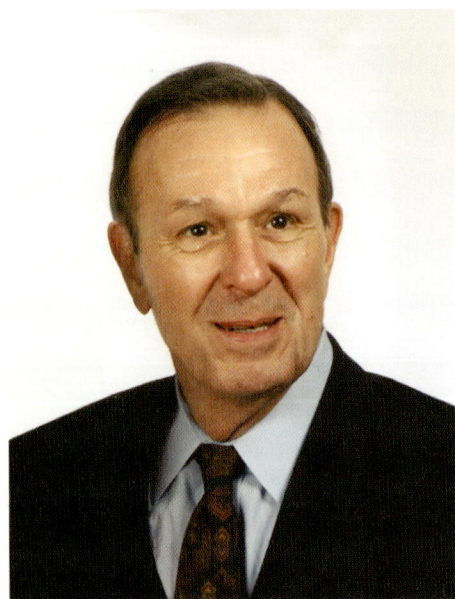

J. Ted Hartman, MD, Dean

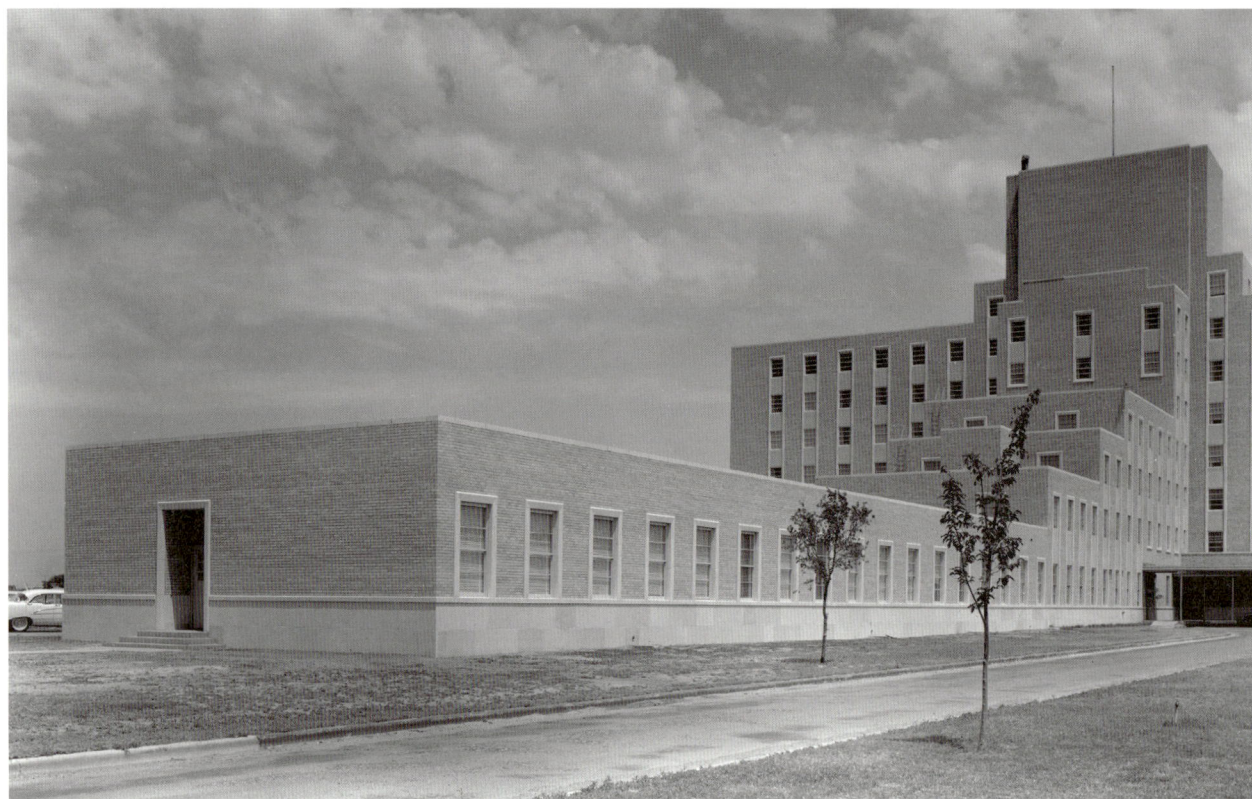

Image of the Methodist Hospital building on June 18, 1959. Courtesy of the Southwest Collection/Special Collections Library

Anatomy, had to scramble to find cadavers, finally driving all the way to Dallas to collect this crucial support for basic instruction (and unnerving Texas Tech campus security officers and their dog while the 12 cadavers Seliger procured were unloaded into the Drane Hall kitchen). Laboratory space was a constant challenge, leading to any number of territorial skirmishes between the new medical faculty and the departmental enclaves of biology and chemistry. Underused laboratory space was subject to quick claim with predicable uproar to follow.

George S. Tyner, MD, played a driving role in establishing the Texas Tech School of Medicine and was responsible for suggesting to President Grover E. Murray that he hire Buessler to plan the school. Tyner became chair of the Department of Ophthalmology, joining William G. Seliger, DDS, PhD, chair of anatomy; Francis Behal, PhD, chair of the Department of Biochemistry; and J. T. Hartman, MD, chair of the Department of Orthopedic Surgery, as a member of the original core faculty. Tyner and Hartman played crucial administrative roles in the development of the institution. Tyner became dean of the School of Medicine in 1974, and Hartman followed

him as interim dean in 1981 and dean in 1982. They both experienced the exciting and precarious rollercoaster ride involved in establishing the Texas Tech School of Medicine.

In 1986, Tyner joined historian Robert L. McCartor, PhD, in publishing the story of the founding of the Texas Tech School of Medicine, entitled *Eye of the Storm*. McCartor and Tyner explain the basic circumstances for the first class of incoming medical students:

> The students would be coming to a school without a building or hospital, one which spread throughout a different institution, a school which could not even present a reliable list of faculty (some students were actually selected . . . before their professors . . .) and they would be trusting their futures to an educational program which, at that time, did not exist. (*Eye of the Storm*, 173)

In spite of it all, the new school established temporary affiliations with Methodist Hospital and many of the smaller Lubbock hospitals, especially St. Mary of the Plains, for student rotations. The first students graduated feeling confident in their training, many praising the educational experience as exceptional. They were able to work closely with highly trained specialists in an unusually egalitarian atmosphere of frontier adventure. Dr. Andrew Hansen II, a member of the graduating class of 1975, assesses his experience:

> For me it was a great opportunity to go to medical school. The school was in Drane Hall on campus and it was like going to college all over again. The individual attention our class of 36 students enjoyed was fantastic. We became good friends with most of our professors and this certainly fostered the learning process. When we reached our clinical rotations, this continued as we were one-on-one with practicing physicians. I particularly enjoyed surgery as I was able to participate in care of patients without having to do all the "scut work" medical students have to do at a teaching hospital. In addition, the quality of the surgery was excellent. I saw top surgeons—Dr. Bob Salem, Dr. Jerry Stirman, and Dr. Jack Selby to name a few. It was a unique experience and one which cannot be reproduced today.

Lorenze Lutherer, who joined the faculty in 1972 as a PhD physiologist and received his medical degree from Texas Tech School of Medicine in the next few years, remained as a highly respected and productive faculty member until his retirement in 2014. He fondly remembers bowling with the students down the corridors of Drane Hall.

In 1974, the School of Medicine graduated 24 students in its first graduating class. In 2018, the School of Medicine graduated 171 students in its forty-fourth graduating class and, along the way, provided these students with state-of-the-art lecture, laboratory, and library facilities to support their endeavors. Today, the School of Medicine educates through a foundational blend of basic science, research, and interdisciplinary clinical practice, offering third- and fourth-year clerkships in Lubbock, Permian Basin, and Amarillo, with many residency positions to follow. The inclusive, collegial atmosphere of the school, however, still remains a point of great pride, pleasure, and honored history.

Today's Programs of Study

Since 2010, Dr. Steven Berk has been vice president and provost of the Texas Tech University Health Sciences Center. He began his affiliation with the Health Sciences Center as Amarillo dean and was appointed dean of the School of Medicine in 2006. Under his leadership, the school continues to grow in innovative ideas and educational resourcefulness. Responding to the ongoing need for family practitioners throughout the rural communities of West Texas, in 2010, Berk implemented the Family Medicine Accelerated Track, offering a way to finish medical school in three very concentrated years thereby saving students significant educational expenses and placing them in practice sooner. This new educational model is nationally recognized as a valued innovation by medical educators, inspiring other medical schools to adopt a similar program that encourages more students to choose family practice as their field and help overcome the national need for continuum of care services to families and communities.

At this 50-year milestone, sharing a contiguous flagship campus between the Texas Tech University Health Sciences Center and Texas Tech University is proving to add a dynamic educational synergy to both institutions. Faculty members in the basic sciences have established a number of collaborative research projects with Texas Tech University and both institutions are responsive to meaningful joint appointments. The School of Medicine has also established degree programs with the Texas Tech University School of Law where students can further their expertise in any number of areas of health law with an MD/JD dual degree. Through the Rawls College of Business, MD/MBA students can become specialists in the ongoing complications of medical financial and administrative business practices. Interestingly enough, in those very early days, it was part of John Buessler's dream for all of his faculty members to receive an MBA, whether surgeons, pediatricians, gynecologists, ophthalmologists, internists, and on and on. Some actually did. Many others, however, did not, thinking they had enough responsibilities already.

The School of Medicine also offers an MD/PhD degree, working in collaboration with the Graduate School of Biomedical Sciences, which was established in 1991 as the fourth school of the Texas Tech University Health Sciences Center. Students pursue a degree in medicine and a PhD through one of the basic science departments of Cell Biology and Biochemistry, Immunology and Molecular Microbiology, Cell Physiology and Molecular Biophysics, and Pharmacology and Neuroscience. This dual

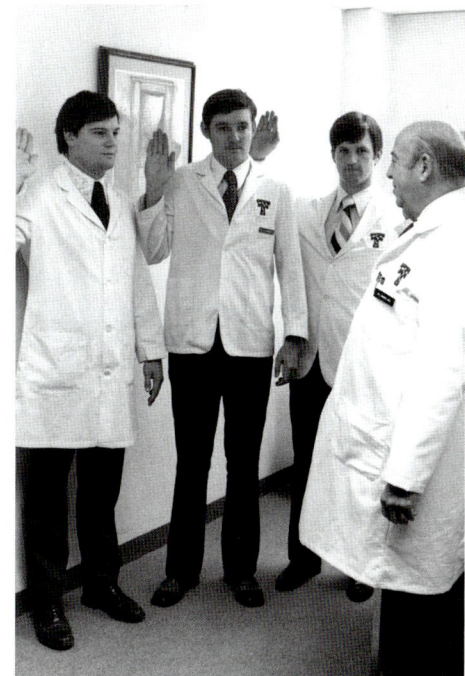

Taking the oath at the School of Medicine. Courtesy of the Southwest Collection/Special Collections Library

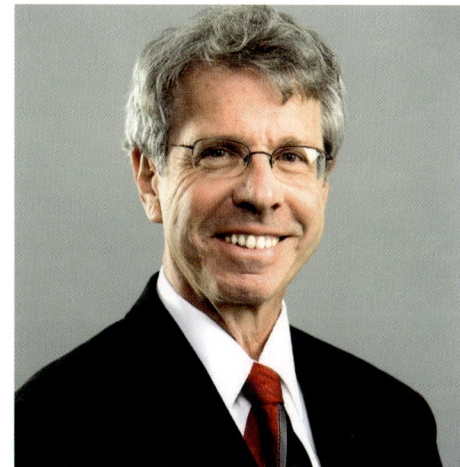

Steven L. Berk, MD. Dean TTUHSC SOM

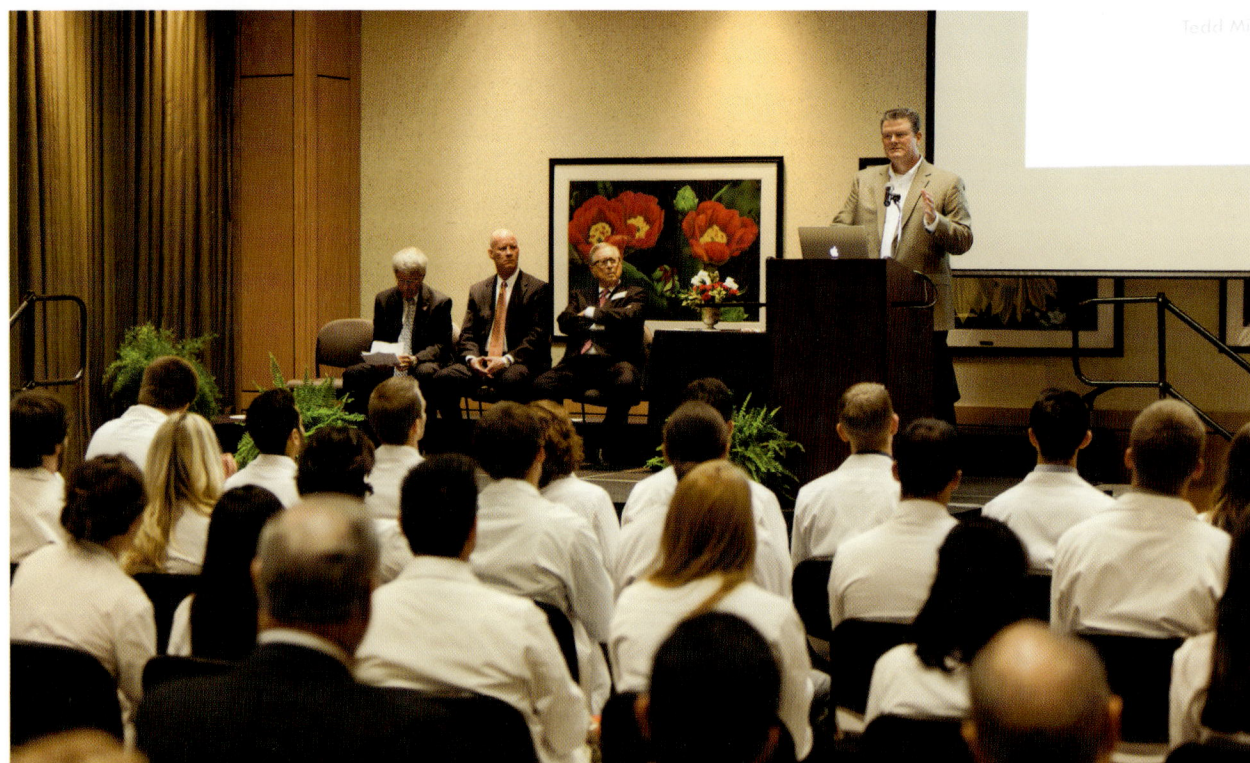

Tedd Mitchell, MD, President speaking to first Covenant Campus students with (seated) Steven L. Berk, MD, Richard Parks, CEO of Covenant Health System, and Robert Salem, MD, Regional Dean Covenant Campus

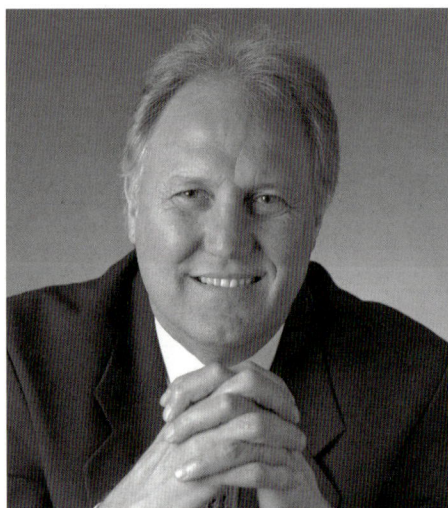

Douglas Stocco PhD. Douglas Stocco's groundbreaking research on Steroidogenic Acute Regulatory (StAR) (04–142) protein was published in 1994 *Journal of Biological Chemistry*. Cloning of StAR DNA helped to determine the cause of the potentially fatal disease Congenital Lipoid Adrenal Hyperplasia.

degree expands opportunities to become leading-edge scientists in the healthcare arena, engaged in breakthrough knowledge and scientific discoveries with the challenge to translate these discoveries into therapeutic strategies.

Innovative Research

In 1994, Douglas M. Stocco, PhD, professor in the Department of Cell Biology and Biochemistry, brought significant acclaim to the Health Sciences Center with his groundbreaking research on the Steroidogenic Acute Regulatory (StAR) protein. Cloning of StAR DNA helps determine the cause of the potentially fatal disease Congenital Lipoid Adrenal Hyperplasia. The results of his findings were published in the *Journal of Biological Chemistry* and earned Stocco a Merit Award from the National Institutes of Health in 1996. His rigorous research example was a catalyst for nationally significant research contributions from the Health Sciences Center faculty.

In 2007, John C. Baldwin, MD, became president of the Texas Tech University Health Sciences Center and during his tenure emphasized the importance of strengthening the research mission of the institution, characterizing the promise of a health science center as a center for basic

and translationional research. Baldwin named Stocco vice president of research, and during Stocco's tenure, the Texas Tech University Health Sciences Center has distinguished itself in the scientific arena with a number of important investigations with significant research findings and concomitant funding.

Working in the multidisciplinary School of Medicine Cancer Center, C. Patrick Reynolds, MD, PhD, and Min H. Kang, PharmD, were awarded grants from the Cancer Prevention and Research Institute of Texas in 2009 for their work on an oral formulation of a new anticancer drug called fenretinide, used to reverse multidrug resistance for pediatric cancer patients during chemotherapy. Dr. Afzal Siddiqui, PhD, MPhil, MS, director of the Center for Tropical Medicine and Infectious Diseases, received a Bill and Melinda Gates Foundation grant in 2014 of over $2.9 million to develop the vaccine that helps prevent blindness from schistosomiasis, a disease spread through parasites in contaminated water that affects many throughout the developing world. Faculty are also conducting ongoing research projects in fertility, Post-traumatic stress disorder (PTSD), and traumatic brain injury. Through multidisciplinary centers and institutes, the School of Medicine joins with the Graduate School of

Biomedical Sciences, the School of Pharmacy, the School of Health Professions, and the School of Nursing in a number of dynamic collaborations to further scientific discoveries and translational research resulting in improved patient care. Collaborative projects are ongoing at the Garrison Institute on Aging, the Center for Ethics, Humanities and Spirituality, and the Center of Excellence for Translational Neuroscience and Therapeutics.

Growing the Vision

The seeds of this interprofessional collaboration began in 1979 when the School of Nursing was established by the Texas Legislature, joining with the School of Medicine to become a part of the newly authorized Texas Tech University Health Sciences Center.

Politics being what it is, Texas governor Bill Clements made a campaign promise that he would not finance any new projects during the 1979 legislative session. He vetoed over 200 bills that year, and the School of Nursing was left in the wake with no financial support to open its doors until 1981. Founding Dean Teddy Langford Jones and Associate Dean Pat Yoder-Wise spent those two years carving out the most innovative and broad-based nursing degree program to be found. They knew their mandate. The region and the nation needed more nurses. The Texas Tech School of Nursing would embrace that challenge by developing many ways for talented and ambitious people to earn a rigorous yet flexible nursing degree through the newly designated Texas Tech University Health Sciences Center.

Today, the School of Nursing boasts over 12,000 alumni, many of whom are now providing health care throughout Texas and beyond. Always distinguished by a very high retention rate and high scores on the National Council Licensure Examination (NCLEX), the School of Nursing offers a traditional Bachelor of Science in Nursing (BSN) degree program, the RN to BSN degree program, an accelerated BSN program for second degree students and veteran to BSN program for military veterans with prior military healthcare experience.

In addition to a Master of Science in Nursing (MSN) with a focus in nursing administration, the School of Nursing also offers an MSN in nursing education, an MSN in nursing informatics, and the following specialties for the advanced practice registered nurse MSN degrees: Adult-Gerontology Acute Care NP, Pediatric Acute Care

NP, Family Nurse Practitioner (FNP), Pediatric Primary Care NP, Psychiatric-Mental Health NP, and the nurse midwifery MSN degree. The School of Nursing also offers a Doctor of Nursing Practice (DNP) degree. The DNP is a Post-Masters in Executive Leadership and in Advanced Nursing Practice. The school also offers the BSN to DNP option for FNP and Psychiatric-Mental Health NP.

Consistently in the vanguard of teaching and patient care innovations, the School of Nursing has paved the way to revolutionizing clinical education through simulation laboratories. Sharon Decker, RN, PhD, serves as the associate dean of simulation and executive director of the F. Marie Hall SimLife Center in the School of Nursing. Her groundbreaking work has led to the establishment of state-of-the-art simulation centers for multidisciplinary clinical education throughout the Health Sciences Center. Today, students in every clinical field on every campus have the resources to learn medical procedures through digital mannequins that breathe, perspire, bleed, and manifest every human murmur. The mannequins can present with pneumonia, congestive heart failure, kidney failure, diabetes, and other chronic ailments. To help refine diagnostic skills, they can be male or female, teenager or newborn. Now students can practice invasive procedures on

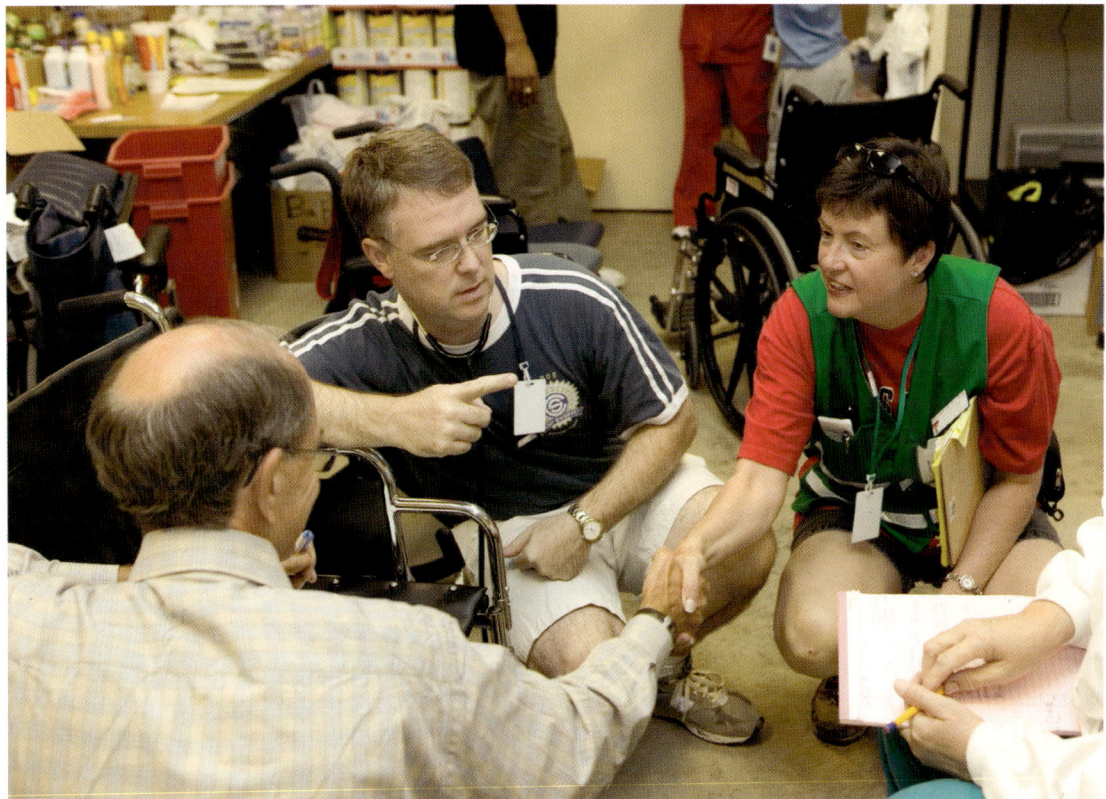

Interdisciplinary team: Mike Ragain, MD, Alexia Green, Dean SON, and Cloyce Stetson, MD, and other staff and students assisting in Hurricane Katrina Relief efforts

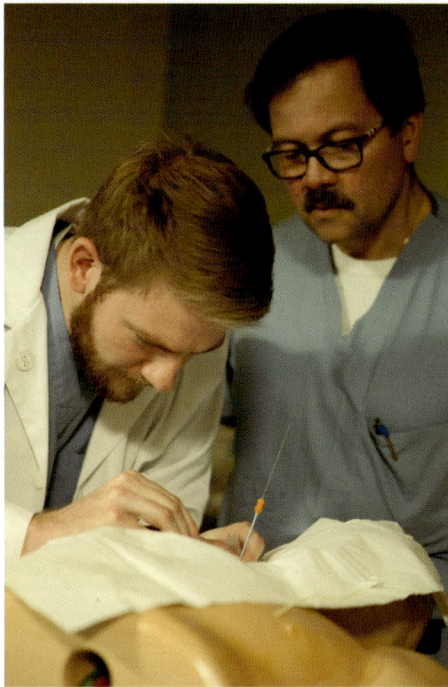
Student inserting a central line in the SimCenter

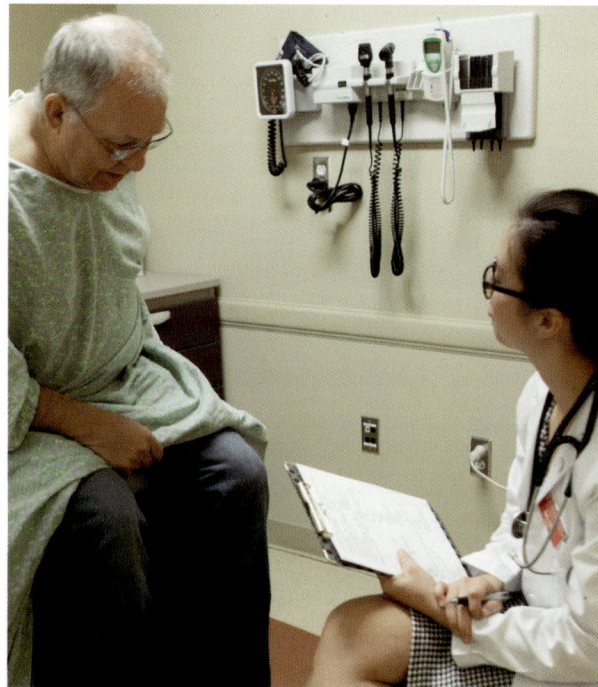
Demonstrating patient communication

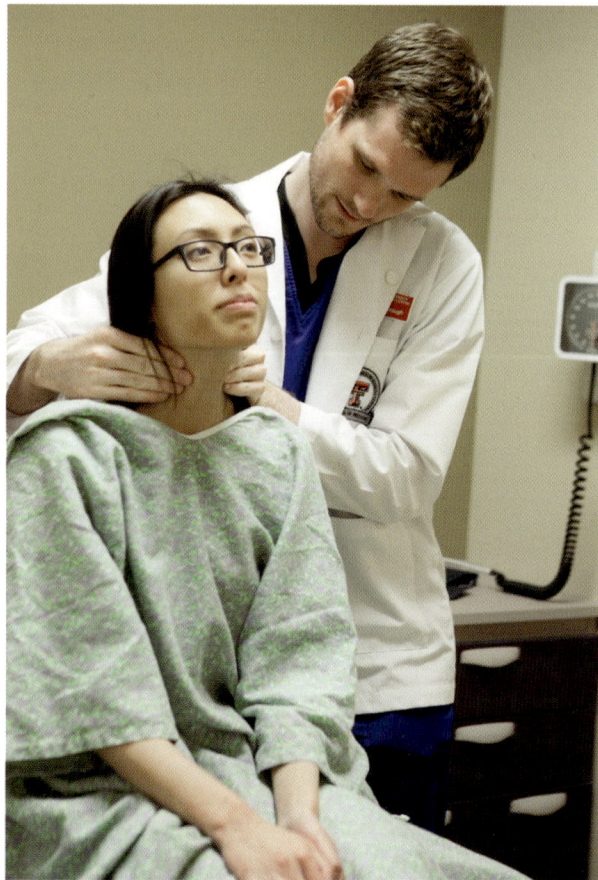
Performing a patient exam

mannequin patients without having to stick a human. They can also refine their communication skills and bedside manner through give-and-take with trained human simulated patients. The Health Sciences Center also employs mobile simulation units for continuing education and rural community outreach. Integrated ultrasound has become another significant teaching tool that was added to the curriculum in 2012.

The School of Nursing is as rooted in the community as in the classroom and is dedicated to reducing health disparities among high-risk populations. In 2007, under the leadership of Dean Alexia Green, the School of Nursing secured federal funding to establish the Larry Combest Community Health and Wellness Center, serving Lubbock and the surrounding area. The center is managed by the School of Nursing and integrates student clinical experiences and faculty practice into comprehensive healthcare delivery services for those in need. Currently, under the leadership of Dean Michael Evans, the School of Nursing has expanded its research mission, contributing valuable studies that address the challenges of effective healthcare delivery with evidence-based investigations into geriatric care and rural aging, breastfeeding outcomes, childhood sexual abuse, teen pregnancy in minority populations, childhood obesity, patient safety, and family caregivers.

Serving West Texas and Beyond

Responding to the vast geography of the West Texas service area, the School of Nursing and the School of Medicine have been on the leading edge of providing telehealth services to the rural hospitals and physicians of the region since 1990. They have led the way with internet outreach for medical consultations, second opinions, and direct patient care, offering medical support services to healthcare providers working in the isolated areas of the region. Today, our telehealth resources are available in 15 communities and are coordinated through the F. Marie Hall Institute for Rural and Community Health. Telehealth services include consultations for dermatology, cardiology, psychiatry, burn care, internal medicine, and screening for risk-based behavior in a school setting, in addition to providing psychiatric services over a telehealth link. Recently, the School of Nursing has added a psychiatric-mental health nurse practitioner program to this rural initiative, providing telehealth services to people in the region who cannot easily travel the distance for therapy sessions.

The challenges of primary care health delivery throughout our vast territory also inform the specialty areas offered through the School of Health Professions, known as the School of Allied Health until a name change in 2012. Established in 1983 under the leadership of Dean Shirley McManigal, PhD, MT, CLS Allied Health became the third school of the Texas Tech University Health Sciences Center and developed strong educational programs in clinical laboratory science, occupational therapy, and physical therapy. The School of Health Professions continues to respond to the growing need for professionals with the diagnostic and therapeutic expertise to improve and repair the physical and mental health of people with acute and chronic disabilities.

Paul P. Brooke, Jr., PhD followed McManigal as dean, and over his 14-year tenure, he tripled enrollment and expanded educational programs in laboratory science; physician assistants; rehabilitation science; healthcare management and leadership; clinical counseling and mental health; and speech, language, and hearing science. The Department of Speech, Language, and Hearing Science had been a part of Texas Tech University since 1928 and was transferred to the Texas Tech University Health Sciences, School of Health Professions (then School of Allied Health) in 1993 as a reflection of the growing technical and clinical applications of the science in the current healthcare environment. The School of Health Professions now offers a doctorate in audiology and, as another reflection of the growing body of knowledge in our digital age, established the first master of science degree in molecular pathology.

Today, under the leadership of Dean Lori Rice-Spearman, the School of Health Professions supports 20 programs through its five departments and offers interdisciplinary research opportunities through the Center for Brain Mapping and Cortical Studies and the Center for Clinical Rehabilitation Assessment. The school has received national recognition for the strength of its occupational therapy program and physical therapy program, providing state-of-the-art assistive technology and hands-on professional expertise to identify, correct, alleviate, or improve physical and mental dysfunction.

Since the beginning, distance learning has been a crucial dynamic in providing healthcare education to the region, with the first educational outreach programs

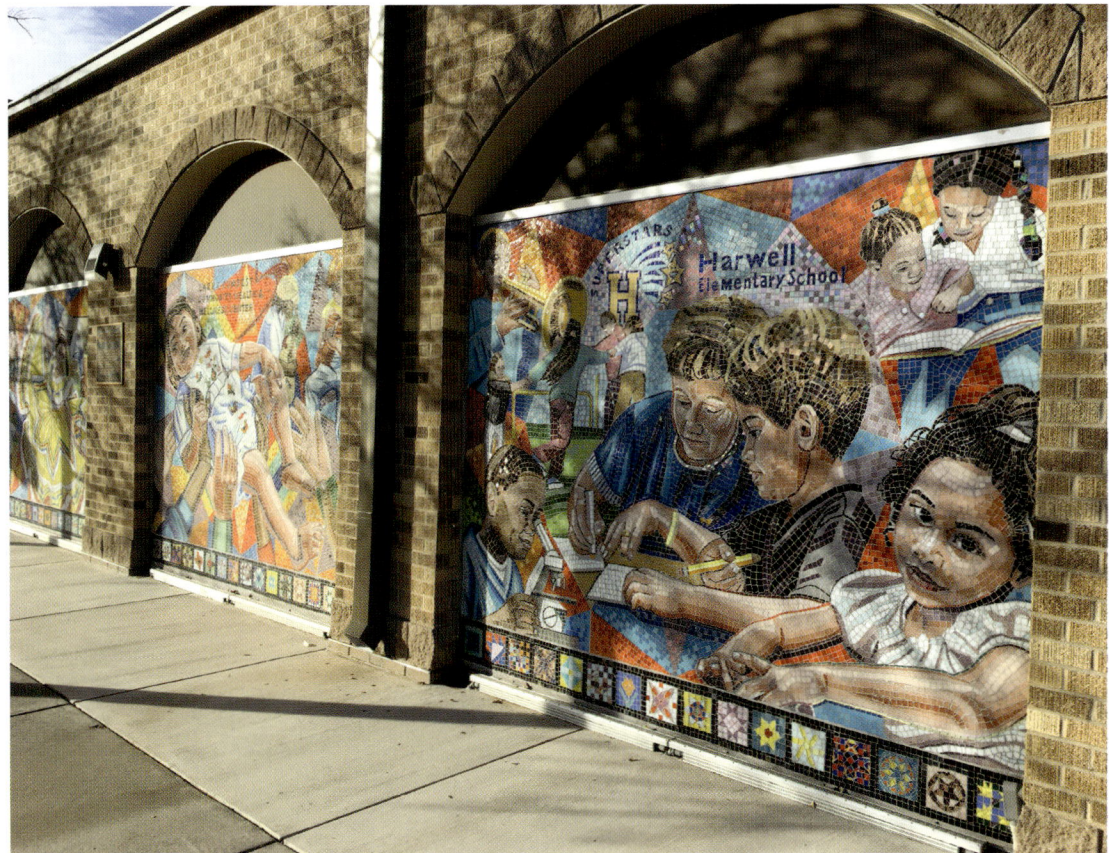

Mosaic at Combest Center

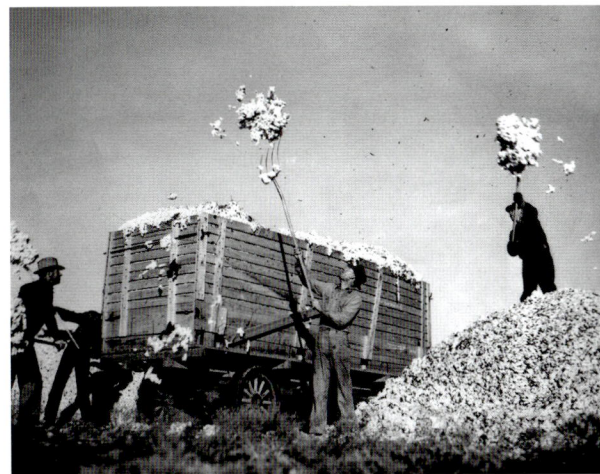

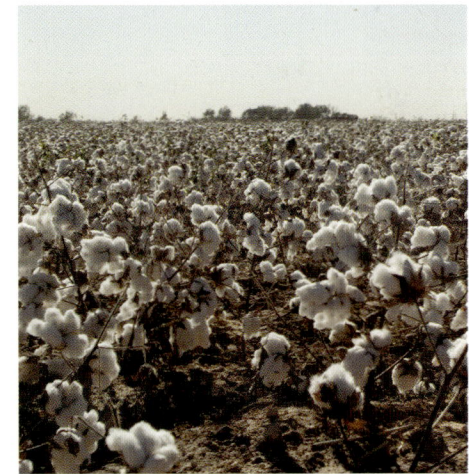

established by John Buessler and E. Jay Wheeler, MD, PhD, long before the internet was available to the institution and general public. Today, the Schools of Health Professions, Nursing, and the Department of Public Health all offer highly innovative opportunities for pursuing a degree through online program support and certification. While some degree programs require a strong

(LEFT) An original photograph by Winston Reeves of employees pitching cotton into a gin's wagons with pitchforks taken in 1938. Courtesy of the Southwest Collection/Special Collections Library

(RIGHT) Cotton fields. Margaret Vugrin, Photographer

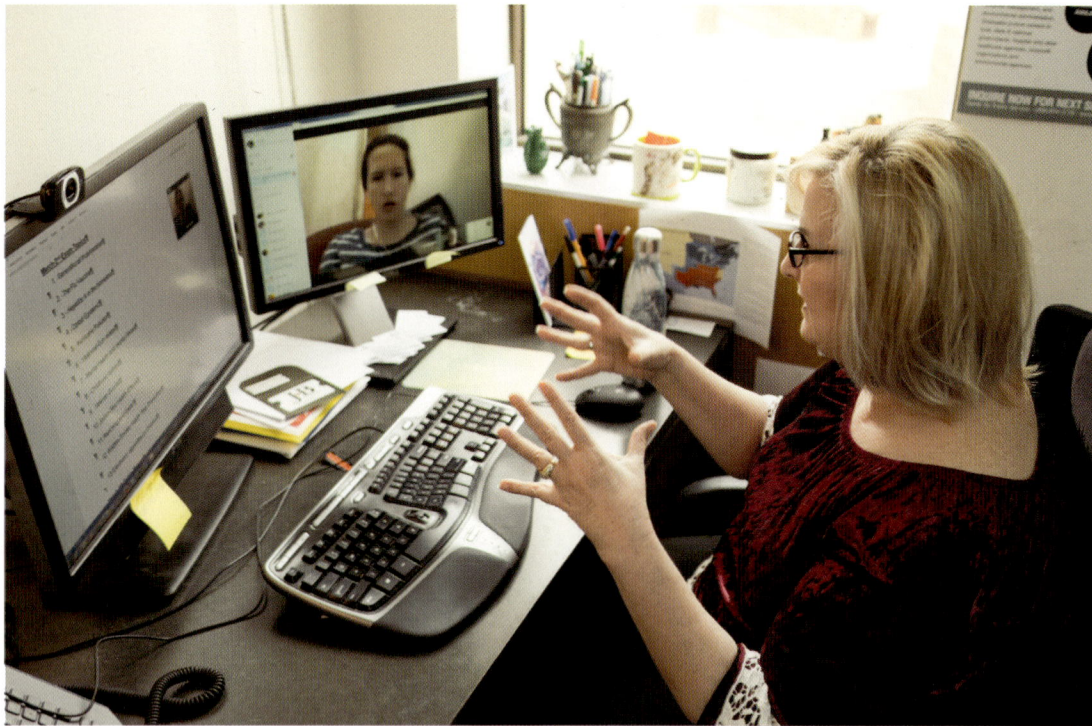

Lisaann Gittner, PhD, working with a distance student

pursue a MS degree in addiction counseling, clinical rehabilitation counseling, healthcare administration, and clinical mental health counseling supported by online courses. Students can also pursue a doctor of science in physical therapy with web-based course enhancement.

The campuses of the Health Sciences Center play a vital role in accommodating students pursuing degrees through distance learning, offering a way to complete their clinical requirements within a reasonable driving distance from home. The School of Nursing offers clinical instruction for web-based degree programs in Lubbock, Amarillo, Permian Basin, and Abilene and has spread its reach even beyond the Texas borders to include students around the world. The School of Health Professions degree programs also rely upon our campuses in Amarillo, Abilene, and Permian Basin. The Department of Public Health offers face-to-face or online course options, giving practicing professionals the opportunity to complete a Master's in Public Health degree anywhere they live and work. This support for distance learning degree programs has developed over the years as a vital supplement to the traditional mandates of the campuses as these centers continue to add their own distinctive dynamics to the mission of the Texas Tech University Health Sciences Center. Online educational methodologies are very important in the story of the creation of the Texas Tech School of Medicine and the success of this vast territorial experiment is worth noting as a cherished part of our fiftieth anniversary celebration.

Our Lubbock Roots

It is a fitting tribute that the library building at the Health Sciences Center campus in Lubbock is named the Preston Smith Library in honor of the governor of Texas who was a seminal force behind establishing the School of Medicine at Texas Tech 50 years ago. Smith was a true Lubbock loyalist and strong political champion for West Texas over his 30-year career. When the opportunity arose, he applied his seasoned political acumen to the goal of bringing a medical school to his alma mater in Lubbock.

Smith graduated from Lamesa High School in 1930 and enrolled in Texas Technological College that same year. The college was only five years old at the time, and Lubbock itself was only 21 years old, but with a population that had skyrocketed from 4,000 in 1920 to over 20,000 in 1930. Smith graduated from Tech in 1934 and set up shop in Lubbock, dabbling in real estate and investing in

clinical component, the didactic elements can be fulfilled at home. It is sometimes difficult to recruit healthcare professionals in the small towns of the region, especially in the 30 counties that do not have hospitals. However, there are great possibilities for talented and ambitious people who already live in those towns and love them to benefit their communities and themselves through rigorous healthcare degree programs and certification. The Texas Tech University Health Sciences Center has consistently cultivated the promises of distance learning to help accommodate the process of healthcare education throughout West Texas.

The School of Nursing offers distance learning opportunities for a BSN, accelerated second degree BSN, accelerated veterans to BSN, MSN degree, post-master's certificate, a BSN to DNP, a Rural Health Certificate, and a Global Health Certificate through web-based courses with preceptor-guided or campus clinical components included to complete the degrees. Many elements of the degree programs in the School of Health Professions are also available through distance learning, short campus stints, and weekend clinical clusters. Students can pursue a post-baccalaureate certificate in clinical laboratory science and a second BS in clinical laboratory science by completing the didactic elements of the degrees online. They can

a movie theater that, over the next decade, he expanded into a six-theater chain. In 1944, he was first elected to the Texas House of Representatives and served three terms, promoting farm-to-market roads, more small-town hospitals, better schools and teacher benefits, and the permanent building fund for state colleges. In 1956, he was elected to the Texas Senate, beating the father of actor Barry Corbin, incumbent Kilmer B. Corbin, in the primary. Again, he served three terms as state senator then ran successfully for lieutenant governor in 1962. Smith considered himself a conservative Democrat, combining a fiscal practicality with a passionate belief in state support for education. He was a very early champion for a medical school at Texas Tech.

As early as 1920, the Lubbock Chamber of Commerce was billing Lubbock as "The Hub City of the Plains," and it was already almost as much a medical center as an agribusiness center. By 1918, Lubbock had a School of Nursing with nursing students training at Lubbock Sanitarium, a hospital owned by Drs. J. T. Hutchinson, J. T. Krueger, and M. C. Overton. Lubbock Sanitarium ultimately became Methodist Hospital. Overton was the force behind the development of Lubbock as a medical center. He was a true pioneer physician, arriving in Lubbock by 1901 and traveling by horse and buggy to tend to his patients as far as 100 miles away on highways and byways that were barely more than ruts in the road. Soon he bought an automobile to help navigate the ruts and worked to establish hospitals in the city. Dr. Overton worked tirelessly as a family physician and a booster of the growing city of Lubbock. He bought land way out in the country, on the west side of what is now Avenue Q, right after Lubbock was incorporated in 1909. He was the only person to donate some of his land to build Texas Technological College. It was a noble overture and a very good investment. That donation paid off when he was able to sell lots to develop the first two neighborhoods adjacent to the new college, South Overton and North Overton.

By the time Smith arrived in town for college, Lubbock was already a vibrant medical hub, and Smith was aware of its future potential. In 1949, he tried to convince the Texas Tech administration into purchasing the failing Southwestern Medical College Foundation in Dallas. It was too early for the college to consider such things, but Smith always had big educational plans for Texas Tech, which were first made manifest in his political help establishing the 1965 Texas Tech University School of Law.

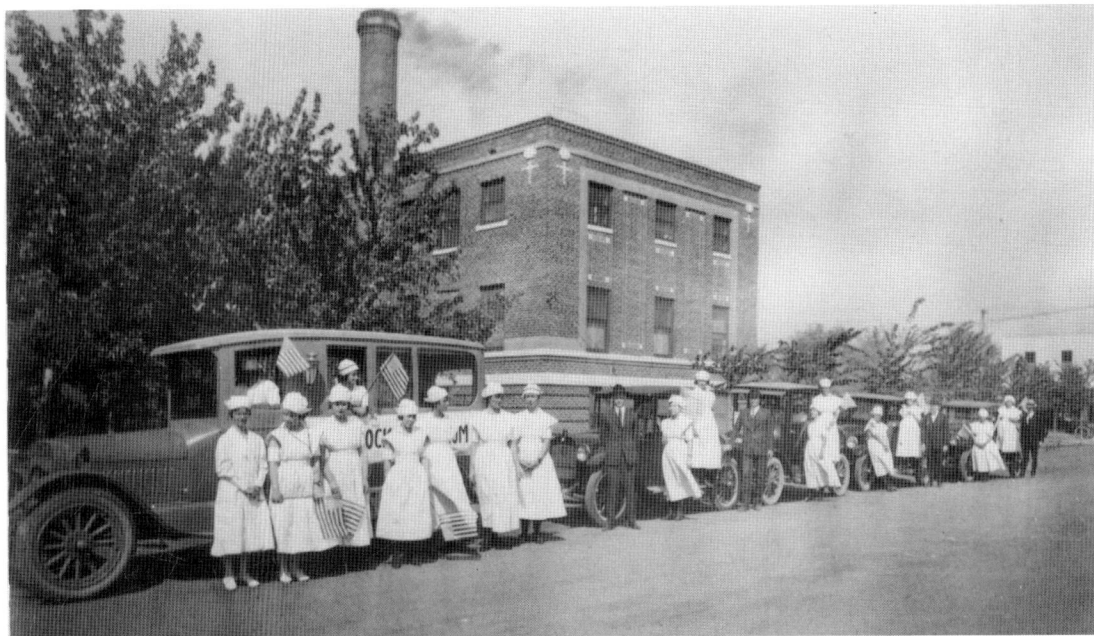

In front of the Lubbock Sanitarium, ca. 1920s. Courtesy of the Southwest Collection/Special Collections Library

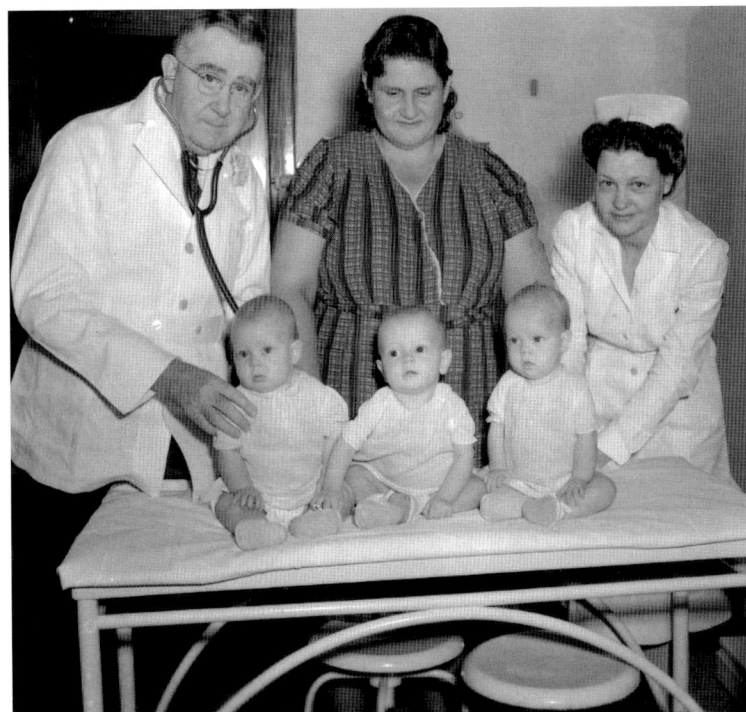

Dr. M.C. Overton in clinic. Courtesy of the Southwest Collection/Special Collections Library

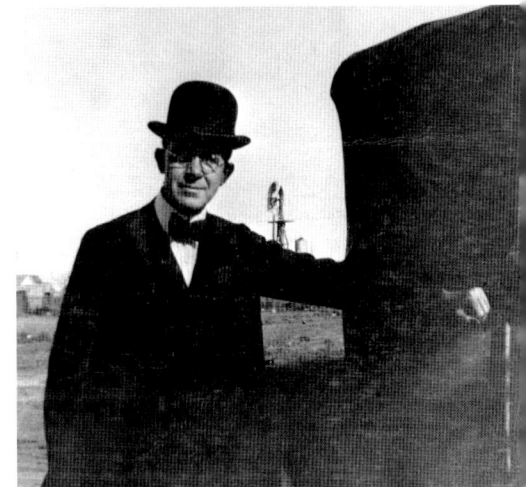

M.C. Overton, MD. Courtesy of the Southwest Collection/Special Collections Library

At the Texas Legislature

When Smith was elected lieutenant governor, he served with Governor John Connelly, who had dealt him a stunning personal and political blow with the previously mentioned 1965 veto of House Bill No. 14 to establish a medical school at Texas Tech. In 1968, Connelly decided not to run for reelection, and Smith stepped up, beating a long list of famous Texas Democrats to win the primary, including Ralph Yarborough, Dolph Briscoe, and Texas attorney general Waggoner Carr. Smith ran a folksy, grass-roots campaign, at one point sending letters to approximately 47,000 Texas families named "Smith" and asking, "Don't you think it is about time one of us was governor?"

Smith was elected to his first term as governor of Texas on January 16, 1969. Undeterred by the 1965 veto of HB14, Representative Delwin Jones sponsored a bill in the House and State Senator Doc Blanchard sponsored a bill in the Senate calling for appropriations to establish a medical school at Texas Technological College. Legislators from Houston also introduced a bill to establish a medical school as part of the University of Texas System. Both were quickly buried in what Governor Smith called "graveyard committees." Frank Erwin, chair of the University of Texas System Board of Regents and a powerful influence in the Texas conservative wing of the Democratic Party, approached the governor with consternation over the inaction on the Houston bill. Smith gave a very measured but meaningful response. He expressed frustration with the legislative inertia over medical school bills, then indicated that there was broad-based agreement that a new medical school should be established in West Texas and that he was banking on the

success of the Lubbock bill; however, he added that maybe the state should support two new medical schools. Erwin understood. Houston would get a medical school if Lubbock got a medical school. To Smith, a West Texas medical school in Lubbock took precedence. Erwin quickly went to work building vital bridges and lobbying forces to push both bills through to the governor's desk.

Houston had been an ongoing downstate battlefield for the Lubbock legislators. There were two more much closer to home. El Paso and Amarillo each felt a West Texas medical school should be established in their respective communities. El Paso had a very large population and Amarillo had solid affiliation agreements with teaching hospitals. Lubbock had Texas Technological College as a contiguous campus, a governor, and a forceful and enthusiastic local delegation of champions, constantly working the halls of the capitol. Hemphill-Wells, vice president B. E. Rushing, cardiologist Dr. O. Brandon Hull, Chamber of Commerce president John Logan, Texas Tech president Grover E. Murray, and Texas Tech vice president for academic affairs Dr. Sabe Kennedy all worked at collaring representatives and senators to generate support for the cause and were able to gather more and more legislators to their list of supporters. Bill Parsley, who had sponsored HB14, now worked for Texas Tech and had a wide network of contacts in Austin. The delegation missed no opportunity to corner them for support. Governor Smith's obvious commitment to Texas Tech convinced Erwin and the Houston delegation to throw their influence in favor of a Texas Tech School of Medicine; in return, Lubbock would reciprocate and support a University of Texas medical school in Houston.

The Lubbock momentum caused the Amarillo opposition to fade, with guarantees that Lubbock would use Amarillo's new medical resources as part of the school. Facing the inevitable, Senator Joe Christie of El Paso also dropped his bill for a medical school but supported two far-reaching amendments to the Lubbock bill. Christie wanted the bill to include a passage recommending that Tech establish some form of affiliation with Amarillo, El Paso, and Midland-Odessa. He also wanted the bill to contain a proviso that no state money could be used to support a teaching hospital for the school (McCartor and Tyner, *The Eye of the Storm*, 46).

Of the three West Texas cities, only Lubbock had no medical facility in place that could be used as a clinical resource for the school, and Christie believed spreading

IN AUSTIN HEARING

Lubbock Pushes Bid For Medical School

By SUE FLANAGAN
(Avalanche-Journal Austin Bureau)

AUSTIN — In an hour and 40-minute hearing Monday night, Lubbock put in its bid for Texas' fourth state supported medical school.

The bill to create a Texas Technological Medical School was referred to a sub-committee or representatives made up of Gene Hendryx of Alpine, Raleigh Brown, Abilene, and Randy Pendleton, Andrews.

Article: "Lubbock Pushes for Medical School." Courtesy of the Southwest Collection/Special Collections Library

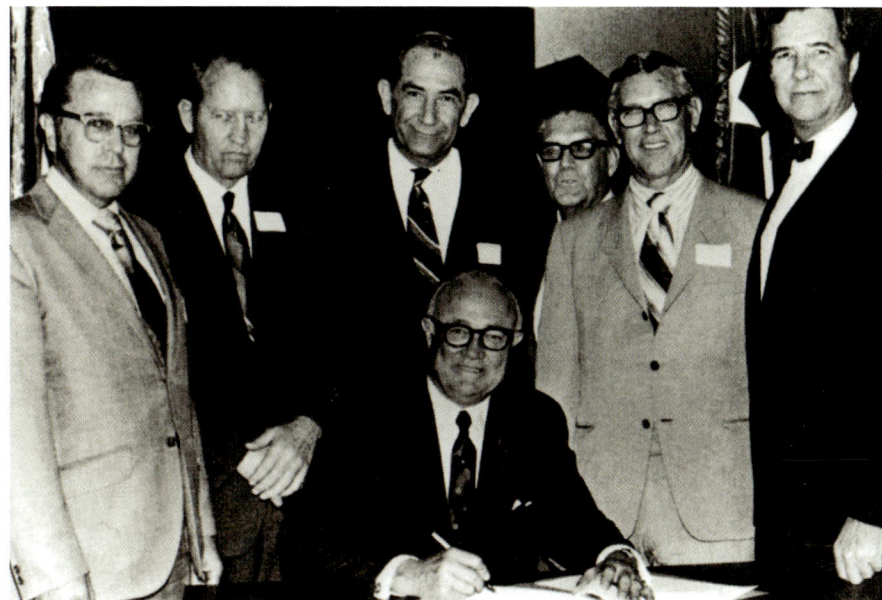

THE UNIVERSITY DAILY

Vol. 42   Texas Technological College, Lubbock, Texas, Thursday, February 9, 1967   No. 78

Tech med bill sees light again

By DAVID SNYDER
Editor

Sen. H. J. (Doc) Blanchard of Lubbock Wednesday introduced a bill in the Texas Senate which would authorize a medical school for Texas Tech, and said that he is "very optimistic" about its passage.

Blanchard's bill would also authorize a medical school at Houston and a dental school at Dallas, both of which would be under the University of Texas.

THE BILL provides no money, and requires that "adequate teaching facilities"—meaning public hospitals in both Houston and Lubbock, supported by local taxpayers—be available before appropriations are made for actual construction of a medical school in either city.

The bill, placed in the Senate hopper at 11:30 Wednesday morning, now goes to the Senate State Affairs Committee. Blanchard told the University Daily that a "crowded docket" would mean at least a month before the bill is heard in committee.

"IN THE MEANTIME, we (Blanchard and nine co-authors) intend to talk up the bill so we can kick it out as soon as it hits the floor," Blanchard said.

The 10 senators who co-authored the bill represent districts in and around Lubbock, Dallas and Houston, and form a substantial portion of the 31-member Senate. The large delegation prompted Blanchard to say he "feels optimistic" about passage of the bill in the Senate and the House of Representatives, since more than 35 members of the 150-member House are from one of the three cities.

BLANCHARD also said he had talked with Gov. John Connally about the bill, and that he was "optimistic" that the governor would sign it. Since he has no item veto on the bill, he would have to either sign all or none of it.

Gov. Connally vetoed a bill introduced by Blanchard two years ago which would have authorized a medical school at Tech because it was "inconsistent" with the then embryonic Coordinating Board's purpose of overseeing Texas higher education.

THE BILL Blanchard introduced Wednesday stipulated that the Coordinating Board would have to certify adequate teaching facilities and land before authorization of Tech's medical school would be complete.

"This is dependent on a first class public hospital," Blanchard said. "We won't put a brick into the medical school until such a hospital is completed."

BLANCHARD said this would avoid a situation such as recently happened with the South Texas Medical School of the University of Texas, located in San Antonio. Both a teaching hospital and medical school were under construction when a bond election necessary for completion and operation of the hospital failed, leaving the status of both in doubt.

Lack of any concrete action toward construction of a public hospital, which would double as a teaching hospital for medical students, has hampered Lubbock's and Tech's past efforts aimed at securing a medical school.

THE FIRST STEP toward construction of a public hospital would be creation of a hospital district by a vote of all property owners in the district, since a tax would be established.

The Lubbock County Commissioners Court, which would have to call such an election, has asked the legislature for permission to do so, as is required by the state constitution. The bill cannot be introduced into the legislature until 30 days after the Court authorizes publication of its intentions to seek an election, which it did Jan. 27.

THIS MEANS that a bill prepared by Rep. Delwin Jones of Lubbock which would grant permission for the election can be introduced in about two and a half weeks.

County Judge Rod Shaw, presiding officer of the Commissioners Court, said Wednesday afternoon that the Court would be "glad to cooperate in any way it can in doing what is possible for a medical school at Texas Tech."

"I ASSUME a vast majority of citizens are interested in Texas Tech and a medical school there," Shaw said.

He said the Commissioners Court would call an election as "soon as it is timely," as recommended by the Chamber of Commerce-Board of City Development Hospital and Medical School Committee.

"This will depend on how much time it will take to educate the people to cast an intelligent vote," Shaw said.
(See Page 5)

the school over separate campuses would cause an administrative nightmare. His amendments were meant to severely compromise the success of the medical school at Texas Tech and bring the issue back to Austin for reconsideration. The Lubbock delegation, however, saw value in this model, with Lubbock as the base, and had confidence in the Lubbock County Hospital District newly created by the citizens of Lubbock County to build a teaching hospital. The amendments were accepted, and after more negotiating and making modifications necessary to request federal funds, House Bill No. 498 passed the Senate on May 16, 1969, was accepted by the House of Representatives on May 19, 1969, and was signed into law on May 27, 1969. It was to go into effect on September 1, 1969. Through House Bill No. 923, which passed during the same session, Texas Technological College was reconstituted as Texas Tech University. The $10 million in appropriations necessary for Texas Tech to initiate a building program and solicit federal funds miraculously remained in the appropriations bill, and Governor Preston E. Smith signed it all into law.

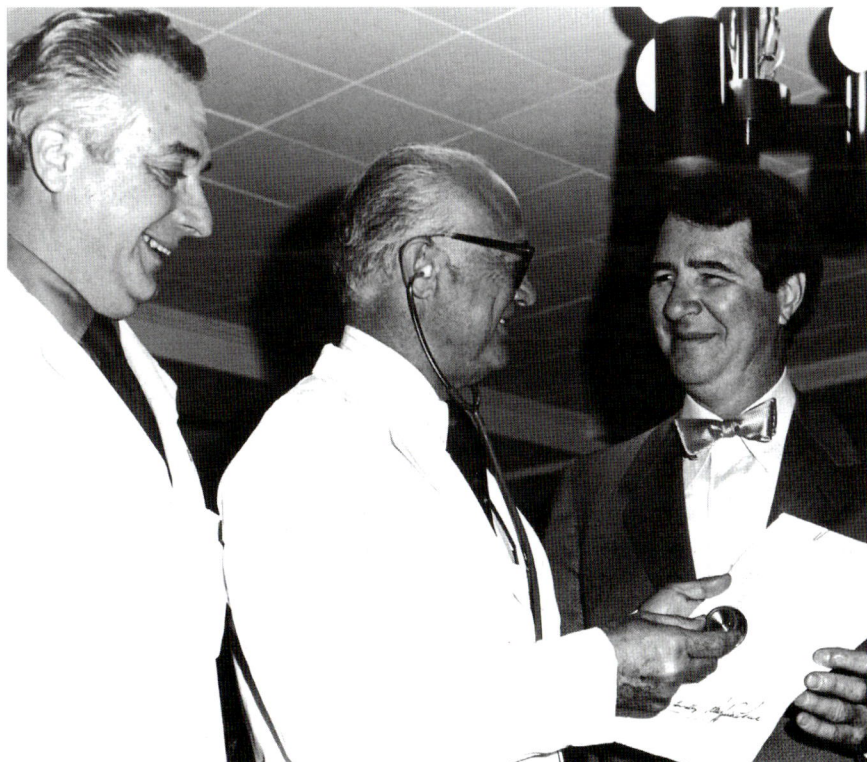

John A. Buesseler, MD; Governor Preston Smith; and Grover Murray, PhD, after signing of bill for creation of the medical school. Courtesy of the Southwest Collection/Special Collections Library

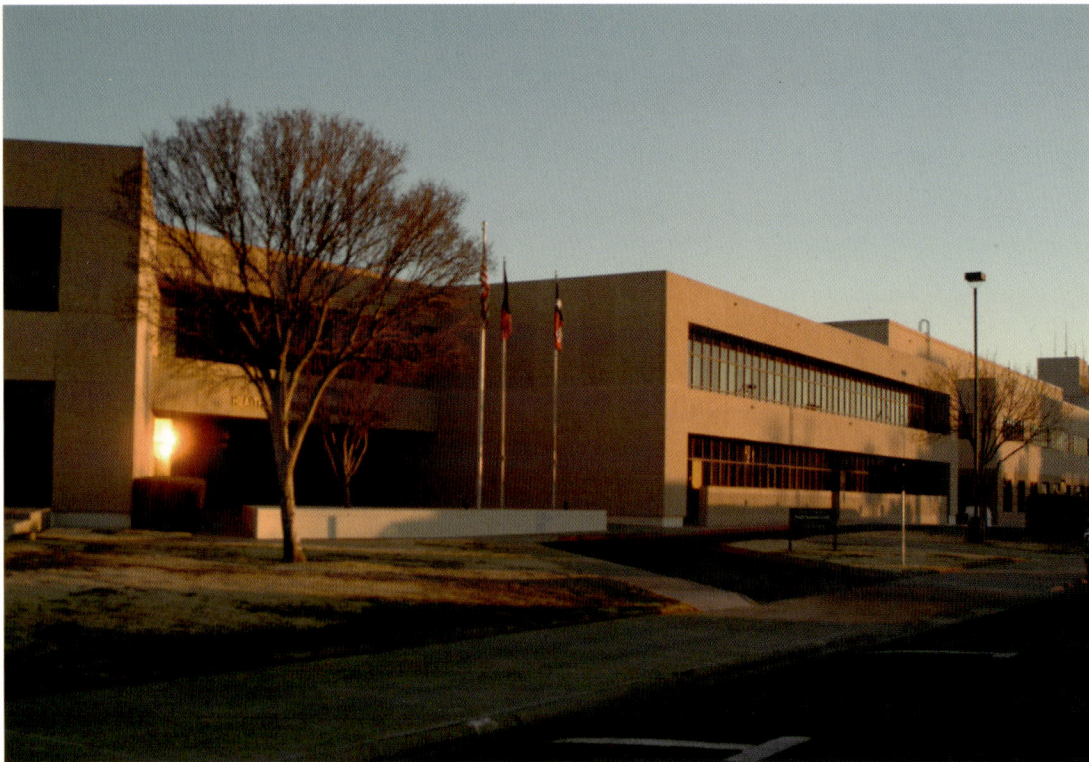

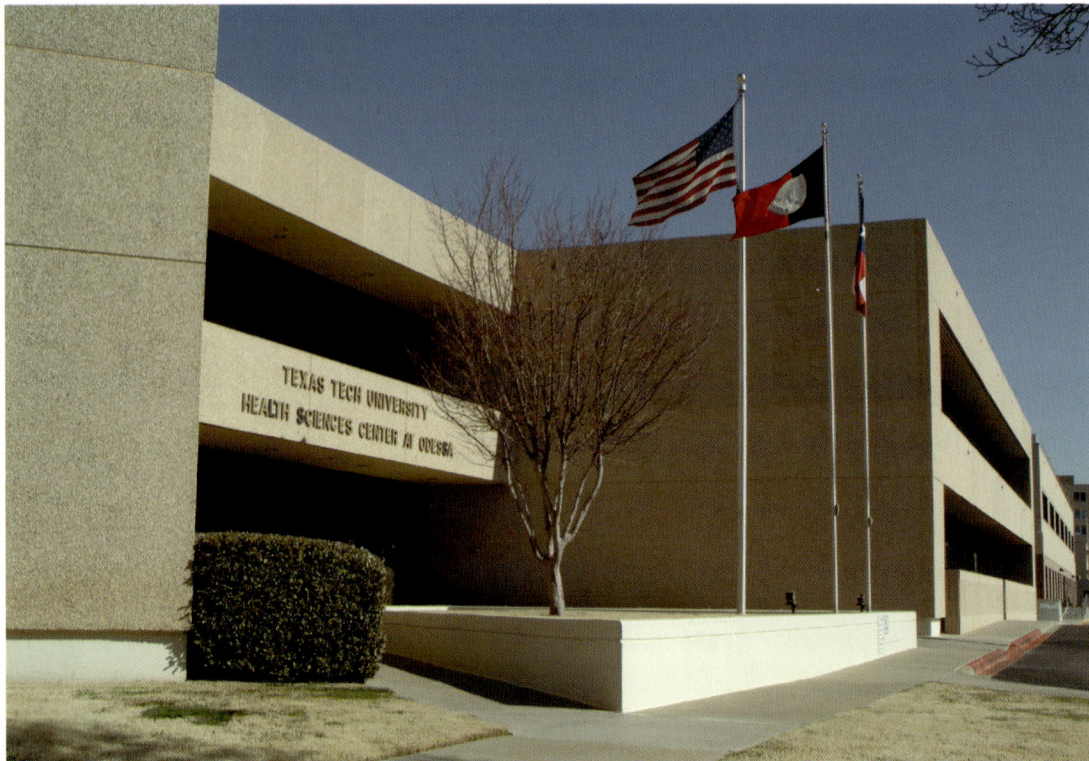

TTUHSC—Odessa Campus

Strong Connections

Over the past 50 years, the affiliations established with Amarillo, Permian Basin, and El Paso have turned out to be an invaluable part of the growth and promise of the Texas Tech University Health Sciences Center. Each Academic Health Center has contributed significantly and distinctively to the growth and promise of the institution.

The Permian Basin campus became an active part of the Health Sciences Center in 1985 when the School of Nursing established programs in Odessa with a faculty of three. Now, the School of Nursing, under the leadership of Sharon Cannon, RN, EdD, supports a faculty of 13, supported by three staff members, who provide innovative resources for highly trained and committed nurse professionals to the region in three prelicensure and four graduate programs. Carol Boswell PhD, RN, serves as the Co-Director of the Center of Excellence in Evidence-Based Practice. Dean Gary Ventolini, MD, directs the Permian Basin School of Medicine, located in Odessa, that offers patient care and medical education to third- and fourth-year students in all six core specialties. Permian Basin offers residencies in family medicine, internal medicine, obstetrics and gynecology, psychiatry and surgery (until 7/2019), as well as fellowships in Endocrinology, Geriatric Medicine, Child and Adolescent Psychiatry, Hospitalist Medicine, Emergency Medicine, Hospice and Palliative Medicine. With a long history of special emphasis on rural health care, Permian Basin also offers a rural medical residency through the Department of Family and Community Medicine, with residents completing their training in the small towns of Fort Stockton, Alpine, Andrews and Sweetwater. As a significant indication of the energy emanating from our campuses, Permian Basin serves as the headquarters for the TTUHSC Master of Physician Assistant Studies Program, administered through the School of Health Professions and located in Midland with clinical rotations in Abilene, Lubbock, Amarillo, El Paso, and Permian Basin. The Permian Basin campus is looking forward to expanding their physical presence with a new academic building that will open early in 2019.

The Amarillo campus of the Texas Tech University Health Sciences Center has been an integral part of the university since 1976, providing clerkships to third- and fourth-year medical students and residency training at three Amarillo hospitals. Currently over 70 medical students and over 75 residents receive training on the

Amarillo campus, noted for its bedside teaching and high faculty-to-student ratio. By reaching deep-down into the needs of the panhandle area, the Amarillo campus has developed into a powerful satellite of TTUHSC, serving as a dynamic testing field for a number of significant programs. Under the direction of Dean Richard Jordan, MD, Amarillo has recently joined with the VA Health Care System to establish a residency program in psychiatry to help address the mental health issues of our veterans in West Texas. The Laura W. Bush Institute for Women's Health began in Amarillo and now has a presence on all TTUHSC campuses. The institute conducts translational research on the distinctions of sex and gender in women's health issues and focuses on the accurate diagnosis and health needs of women throughout the continuum of life.

With strong and energetic support from the Amarillo community, in 1996, the TTUHSC School of Pharmacy was established on the Amarillo campus as the first school to be headquartered outside the Lubbock campus. The school offers a doctor of pharmacy, a dual-degree program in pharmacy and business, plus MS and PhD programs in pharmaceutical sciences and biotechnology, and a graduate pharmacy residency program. Under the leadership of founding dean Arthur A. Nelson, Jr., RPh, PhD, the school adopted a fresh approach to the challenges of the discipline, offering a faculty and student team structure with a case-based, practice component in all four years of the degree process. Today, the School of Pharmacy graduates the most and best-trained pharmacists in the State of Texas.

Inspired by the innovative spirit and impressive achievements of the School of Pharmacy, the people of Abilene mobilized to institute a Texas Tech School of Pharmacy in their town, establishing community partnerships with the Abilene Regional Medical Center, Hendrick Health System, and more than 50 community pharmacies in the Abilene area to provide opportunities for the Health Sciences Center to impact health care, education, and research in the region. The School of Pharmacy opened with 40 students in 2007 and has continued to grow each year. Today it resides on a campus with dedicated facilities for the School of Pharmacy, School of Nursing, and, a distinctive Abilene initiative, the establishment of the Julia Jones Matthews Department of Public Health. The idea of a public health program and eventually a school of public health started many years ago. Everyone involved in starting the program shared a vision of a public health

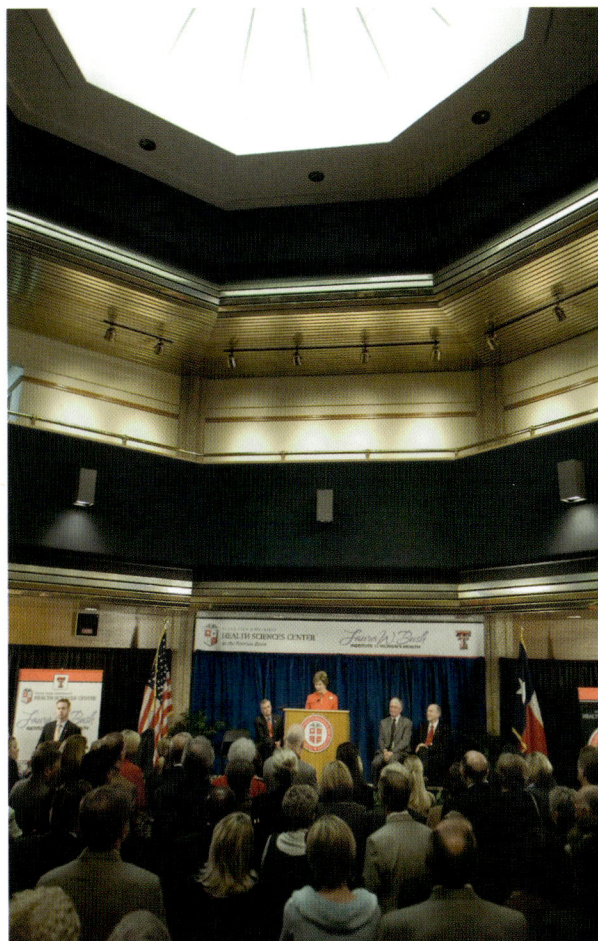

(LEFT) Laura Bush speaking at Laura W. Bush Institute for Women's Health event

(BELOW) Laura Bush

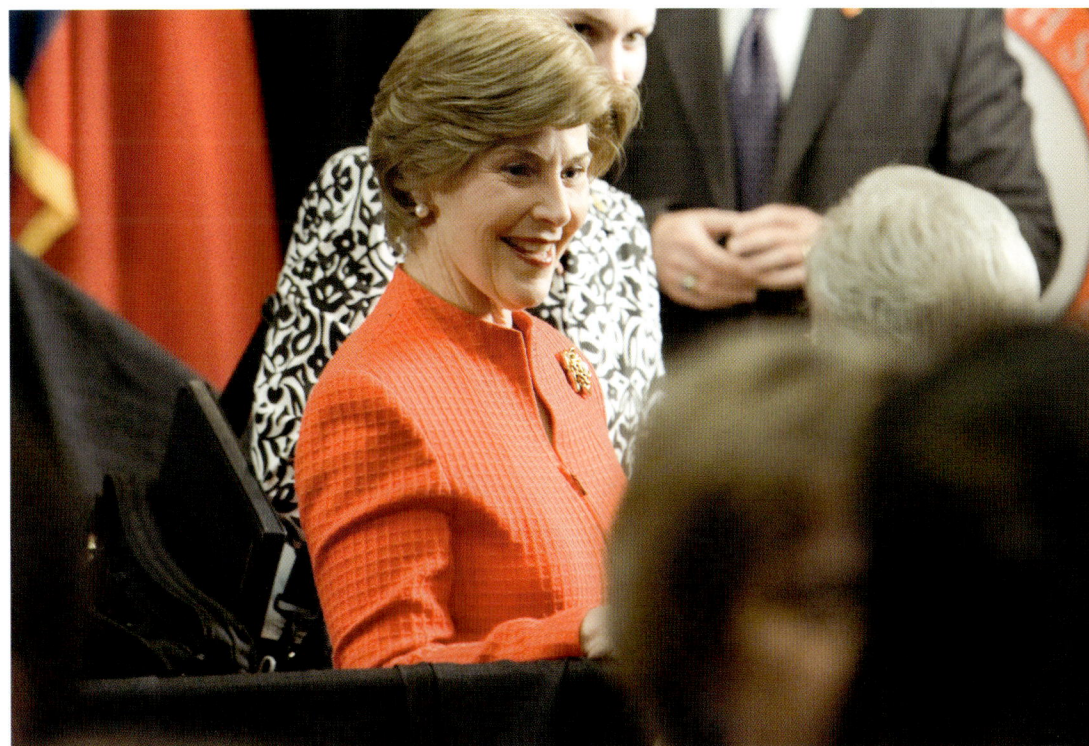

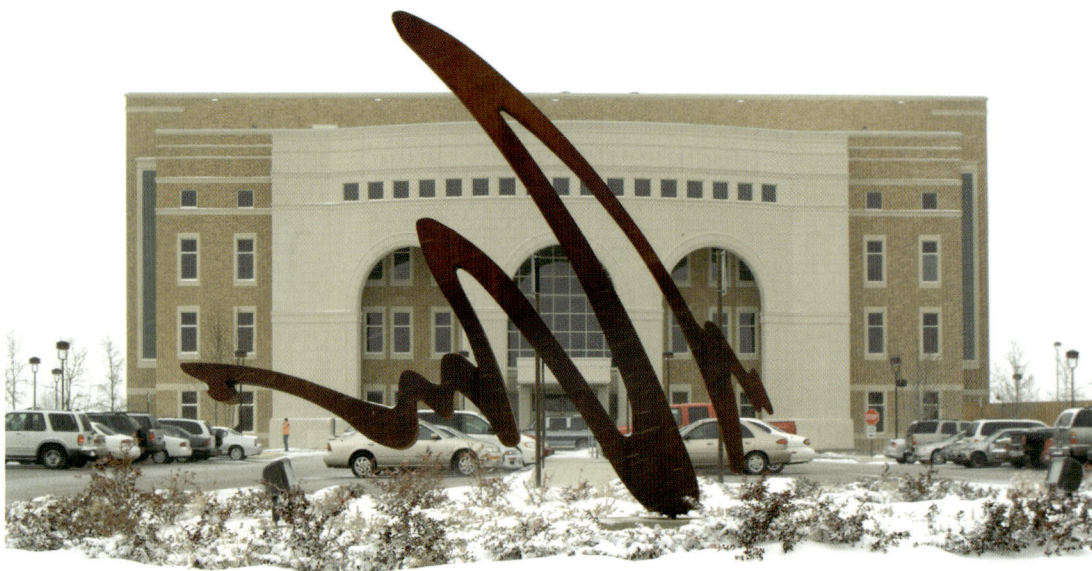

TTUHSC—Amarillo Campus

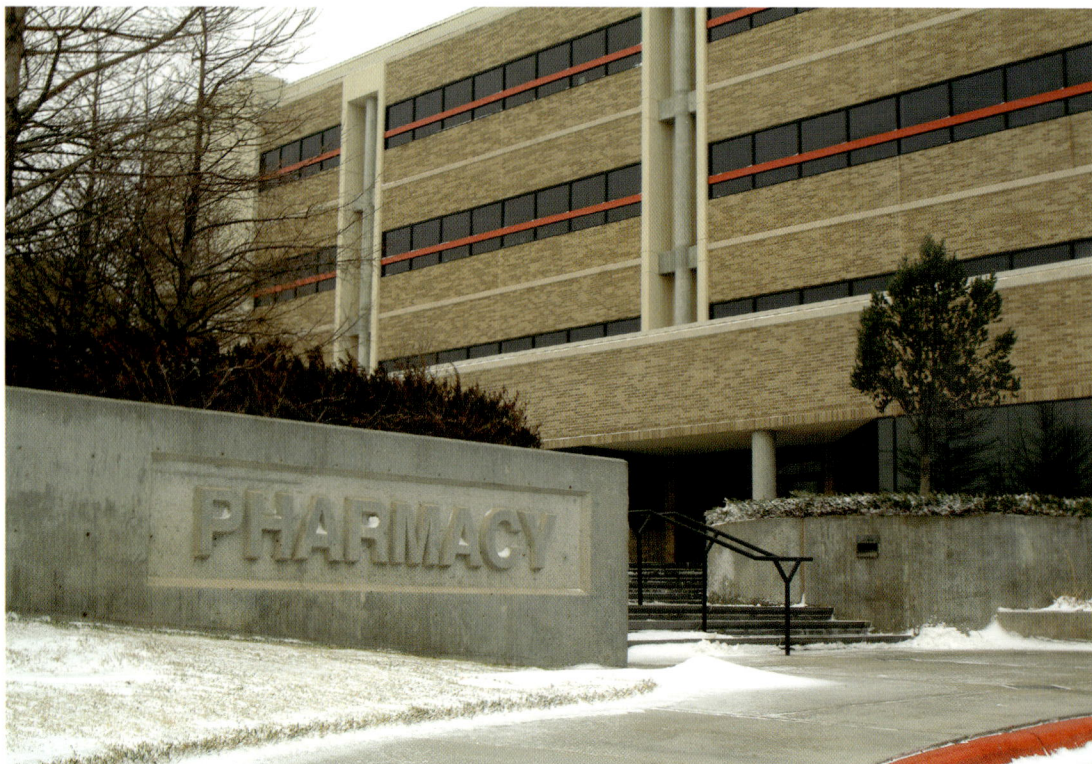

TTUHSC—Amarillo Campus—Pharmacy

program and set into motion the development of the program designed to serve the rural, West Texas population. West Texas has many medically underserved counties, and the health status in the rural areas is less favorable than many other parts of Texas and the United States. The Texas Coordinating Board approved the program in 2013 and the Department of Public Health program began in 2014. We have established campuses in Lubbock and Abilene and have graduated cohorts of students at both sites. With a focus on the health of our rural, West Texas region, TTUHSC Department of Public Health has clearly formulated a vision, a mission, and goals with measures for evaluation. The values support the mission by promoting student success and advancing the field of public health through the three main functions of programs of public health: education, research, and service. We prepare public health professionals who will be highly qualified practitioners and will serve communities in our rural region, as well as around the United States and internationally.

The School of Pharmacy has also expanded the Texas Tech University Health Sciences Center. In 1999, TTUHSC became the first pharmacy school with a Metroplex presence, placing some students there in their third and fourth years. Placements have grown over the years, and, in 2018, the TTUHSC School of Pharmacy now provides all four years of its doctor of pharmacy program at an established Dallas/Fort Worth campus. The Dallas School of Pharmacy residency program is one of the nation's strongest with 36 residents working in 16 post-doctoral programs.

Beginning in 1974, the Texas Tech Health Sciences Center supported a very dynamic campus in El Paso. Under the longtime leadership of Dean José Manuel De La Rosa, MD, the El Paso campus offered residents and third- and fourth-year medical students a distinctive medical experience in the socially and culturally diverse borderlands of Texas. In 2009, the Texas Tech Health Sciences Center in El Paso became the Paul L. Foster School of Medicine, an independent four-year medical school. Dr. De La Rosa played an integral part in helping establish this new Texas medical institution, and John T. Montford, then-chancellor of Texas Tech University, also played an important role in the process.

John Montford became the first chancellor of Texas Tech University in 1996. As a very effective Texas state senator, representing West Texas District 28 for over a decade, Montford had been actively engaged in issues affecting Texas Tech University and the Texas Tech University Health Sciences Center. As chancellor, he established the Texas Tech University System, and the Health Sciences Center became a completely autonomous university with David R. Smith, MD, as president. The Texas Tech University Health Sciences Center joined Texas Tech University and Angelo State University as the three universities comprising the Texas Tech University System.

Montford also used his political influence and position as chancellor to help establish a four-year medical school in El Paso. Through strong support from Texas Tech University and the El Paso community, the Texas Legislature moved to expand the Texas Tech Health Sciences Center El Paso into the independent, four-year Paul L. Foster School of Medicine. In 2013, the Paul L. Foster School of Medicine, the Gayle Greve Hunt School of Nursing, and the Graduate School of Biomedical Science became the Texas Tech University Health Sciences Center El Paso and the fourth freestanding university in the Texas Tech University System. Former El Paso senator Joe Christie

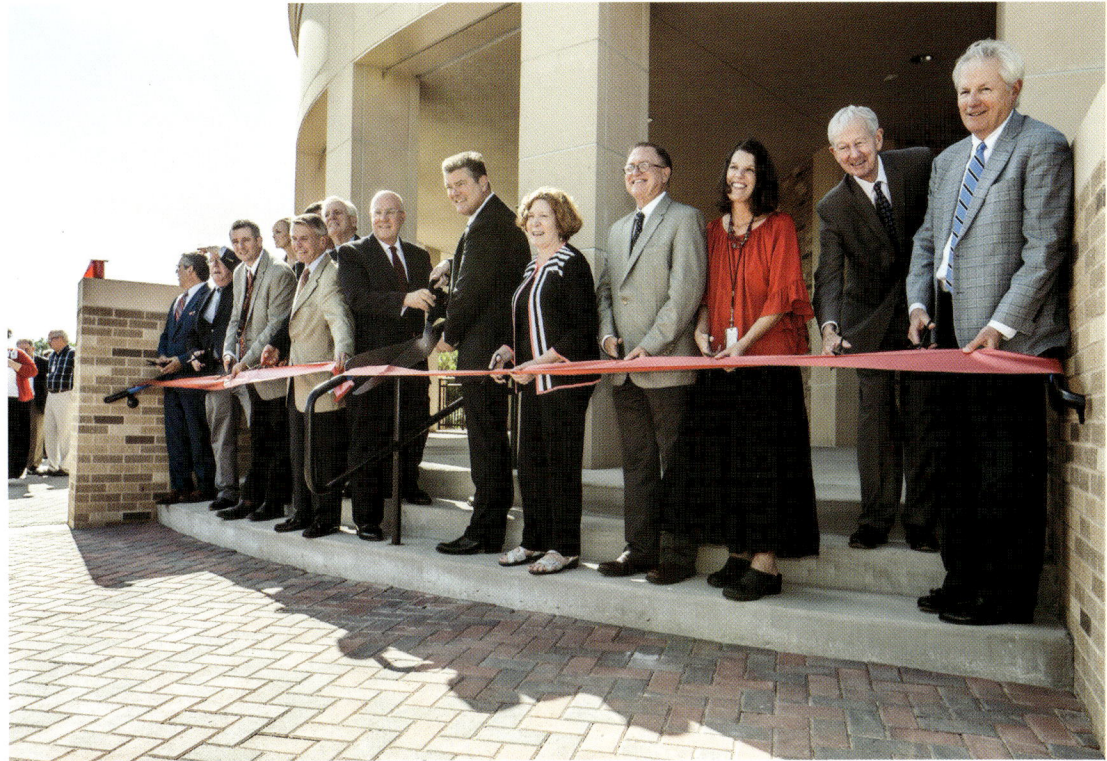

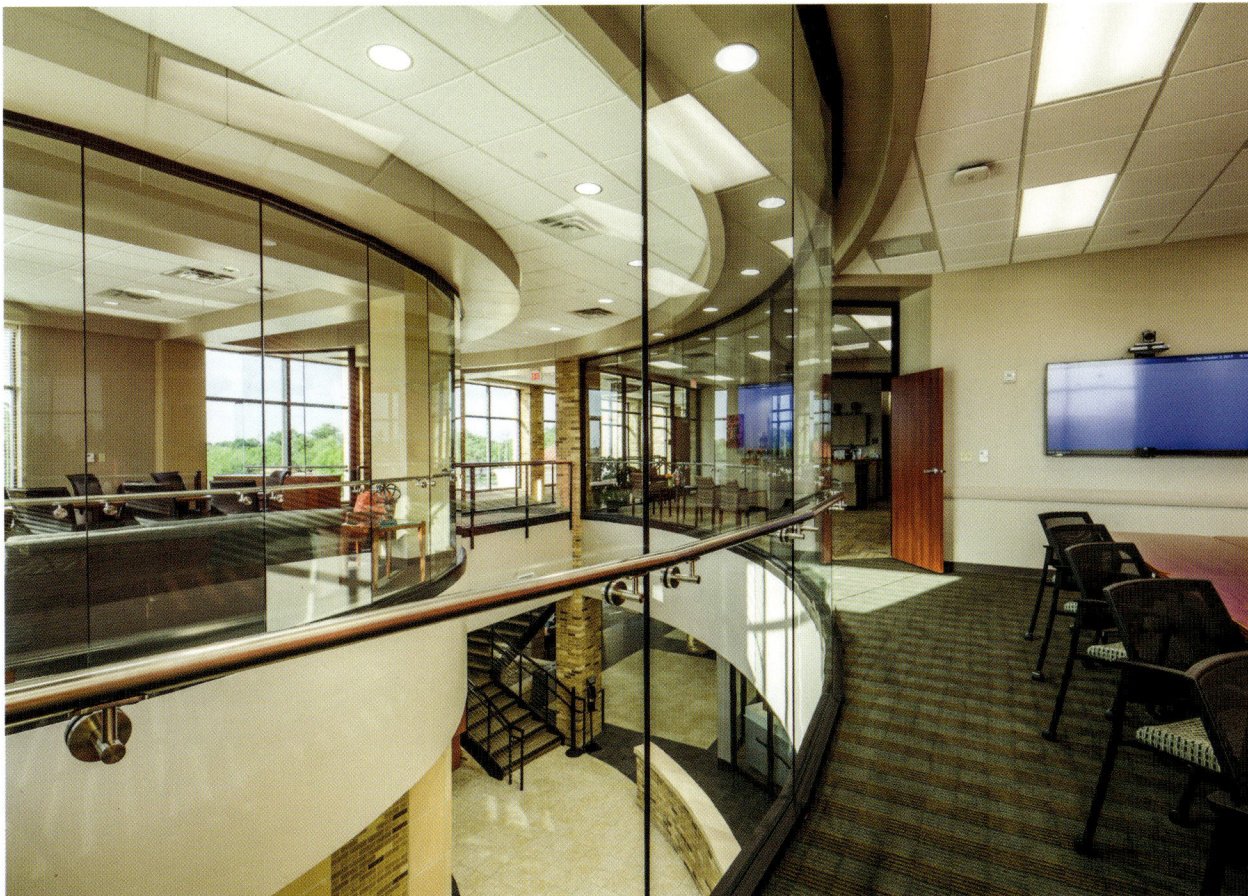

(ABOVE) Dedication of Abilene Campus
Photographer: Kevin Halliburton, AIA,
www.Ice-Imaging.com, Architect: TLP/PSC,
www.Team-PSC.com

(LEFT) TTUHSC—Abilene Campus—Interior
Photographer: Kevin Halliburton, AIA,
www.Ice-Imaging.com, Architect: TLP/PSC,
www.Team-PSC.com

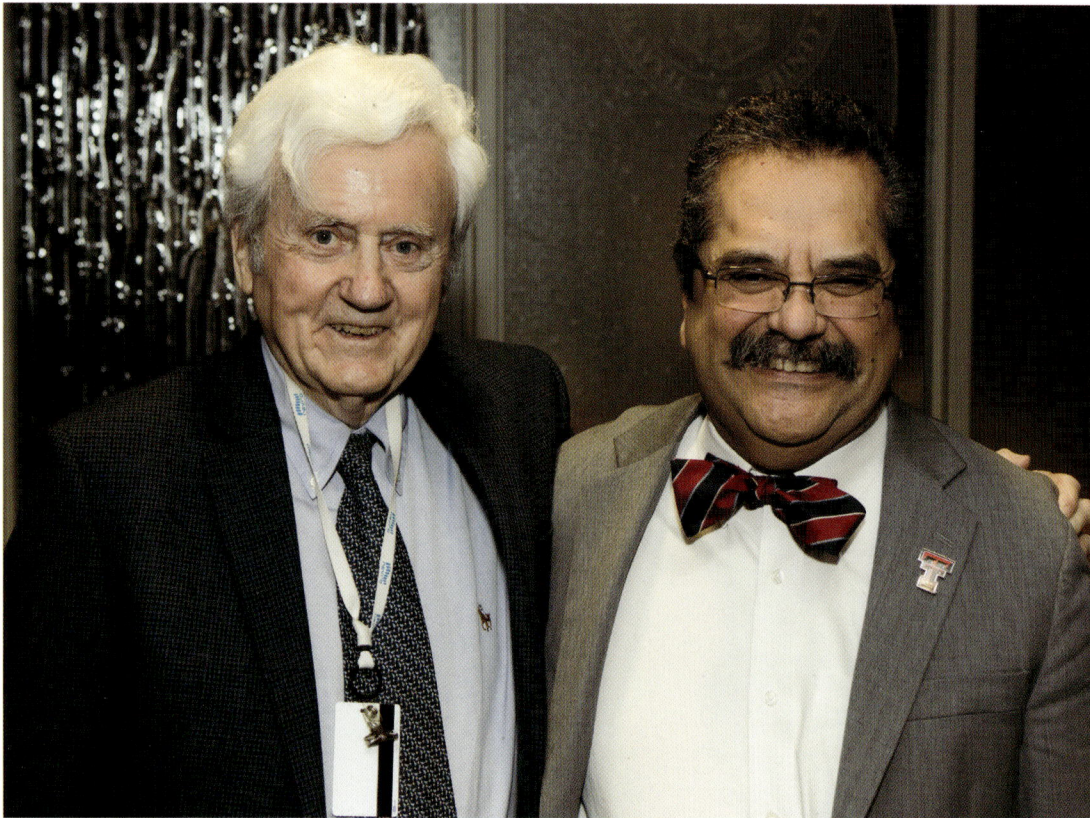

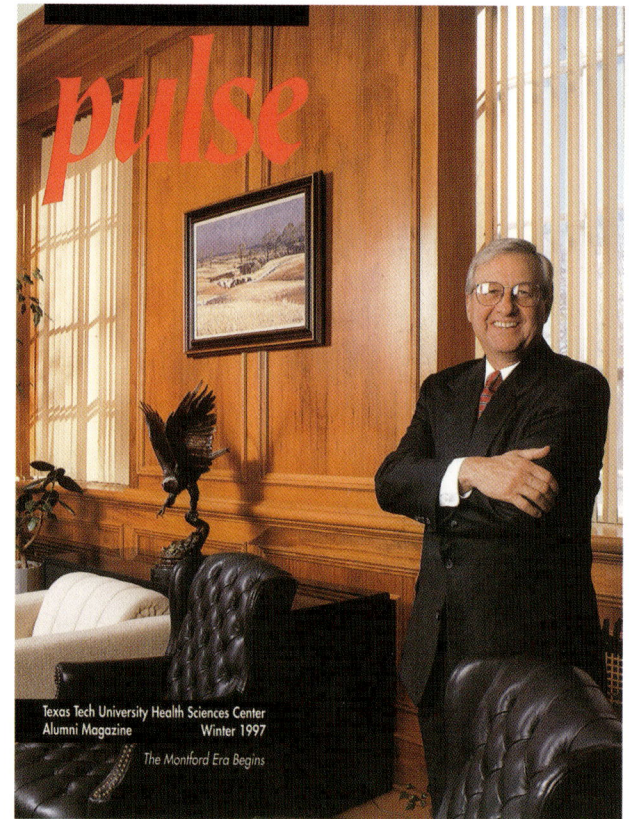

must be smiling wryly at this turn of events. In spite of his amendments, the Texas Tech University Health Sciences Center has succeeded stupendously with and through its vibrant satellite campuses, and 50 years later, El Paso has a full-fledged medical school under the aegis of the Texas Tech University System with strong support for the mission of this new educational institution.

El Paso thrives as a binational metroplex of 2 million people. Under the current leadership of President Richard Lange, MD, MBA, the Texas Tech University Health Sciences Center El Paso leads the nation in border health initiatives, serving as the largest multidisciplinary healthcare institution addressing the unique medical needs of the U.S.-Mexico border population. Through a curriculum steeped in clinical activities and its teaching affiliation with the Hospitals of Providence Transmountain, the TTUHSC El Paso remains in the vanguard of addressing the challenges of the medically underserved in Far West Texas. While the university offers a broad-based curriculum of healthcare education, the faculty is committed to addressing the unique healthcare challenges of the region, including a special border health track for pediatric residents, implementing strategies for preterm

birth prevention, and refining understanding and diagnosis of borderland infectious and chronic illnesses by enlisting traditionally underrepresented Hispanic subjects for clinical trials. The university anticipates the opening of the Woody L. Hunt School of Dental Medicine, the first dental school to open in Texas since 1970, with the promise of providing severely underserved far West Texans with dental practitioners to improve the dental and overall health care of the people of the region. The Texas Tech University Health Sciences Center proudly works in tandem with the Texas Tech University Health Sciences Center El Paso to serve the educational and medical needs of the vast rural lands of West Texas, supporting leading-edge educational and research initiatives that continue to reverberate throughout the world, especially in areas and nations that are medically underserved.

Establishing a Foundation

With the broad network of services, influences, and facilities representing the Texas Tech University Health Sciences Center today, it is difficult to remember just how precarious the existence of the Texas Tech School

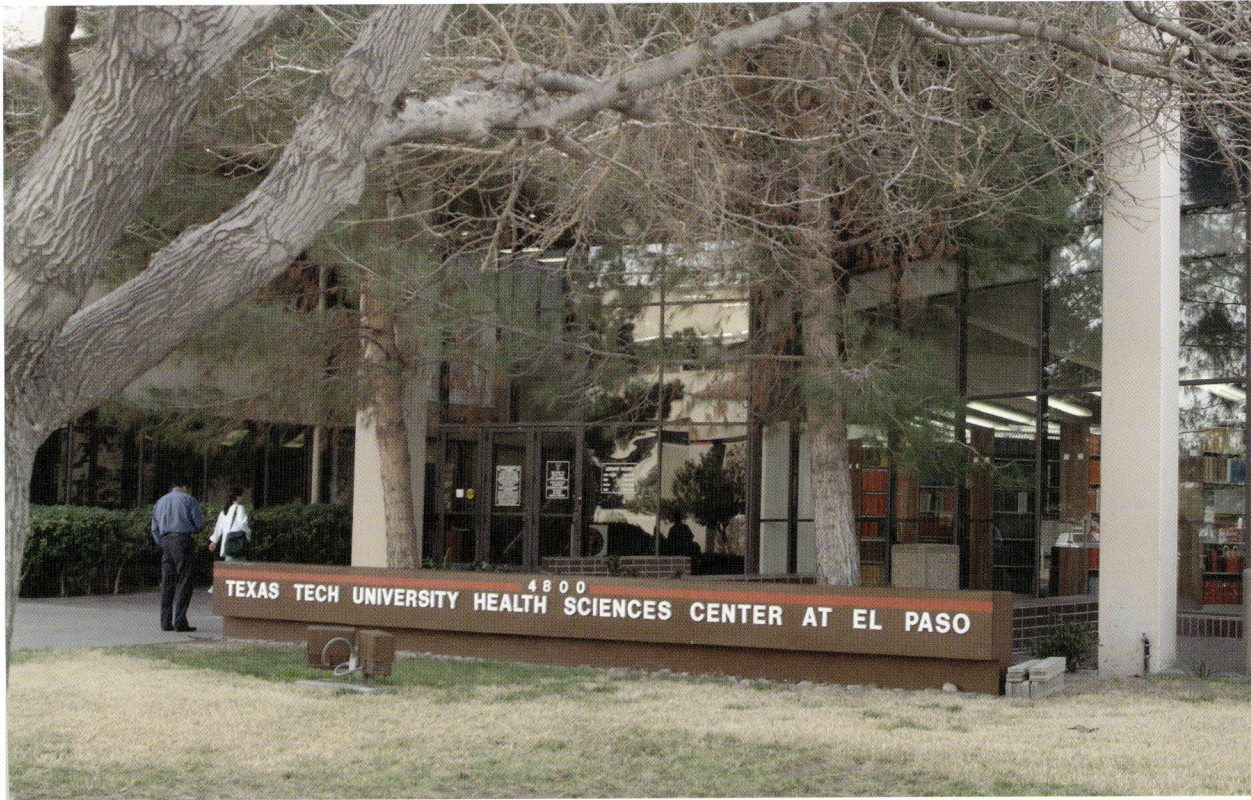

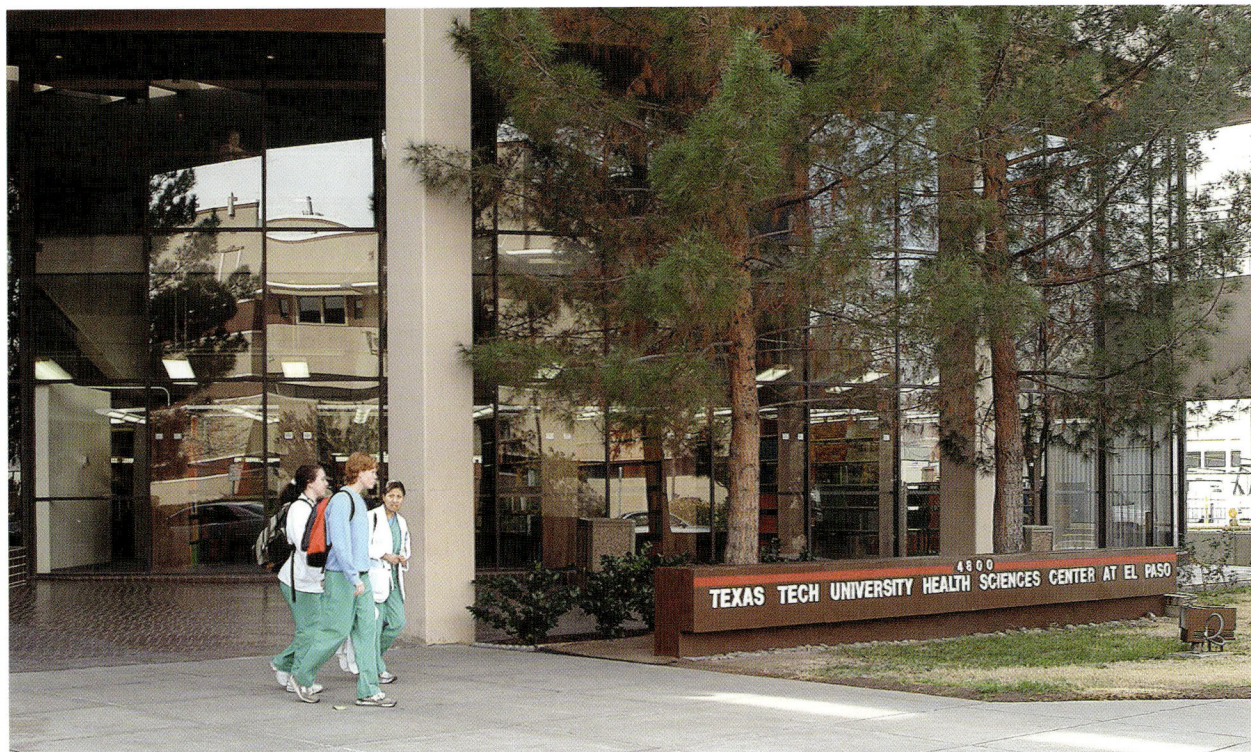

TTUHSC—El Paso Campus

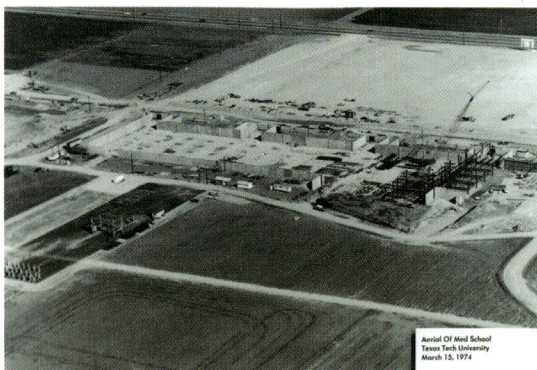
Aerial Of Med School
Texas Tech University
March 13, 1974

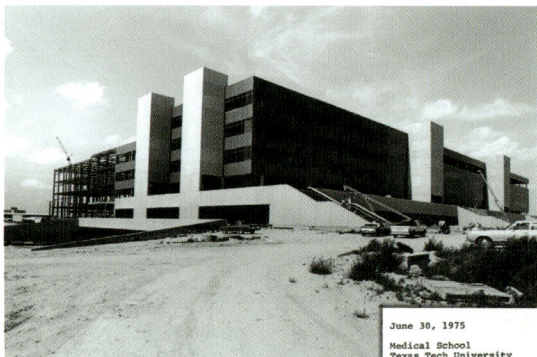
June 30, 1975
Medical School
Texas Tech University

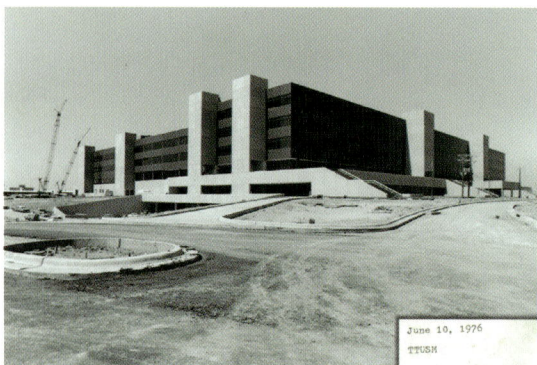
June 10, 1976
TTUSM

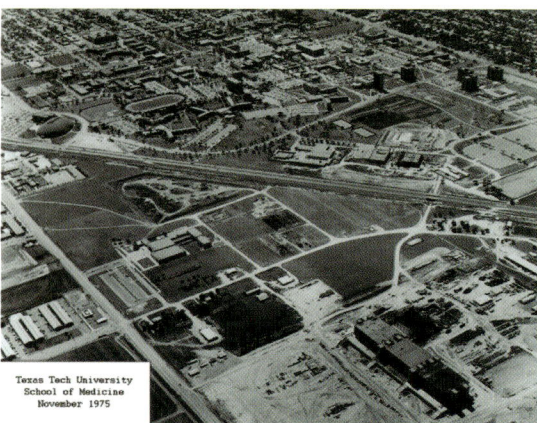
Texas Tech University
School of Medicine
November 1975

Construction

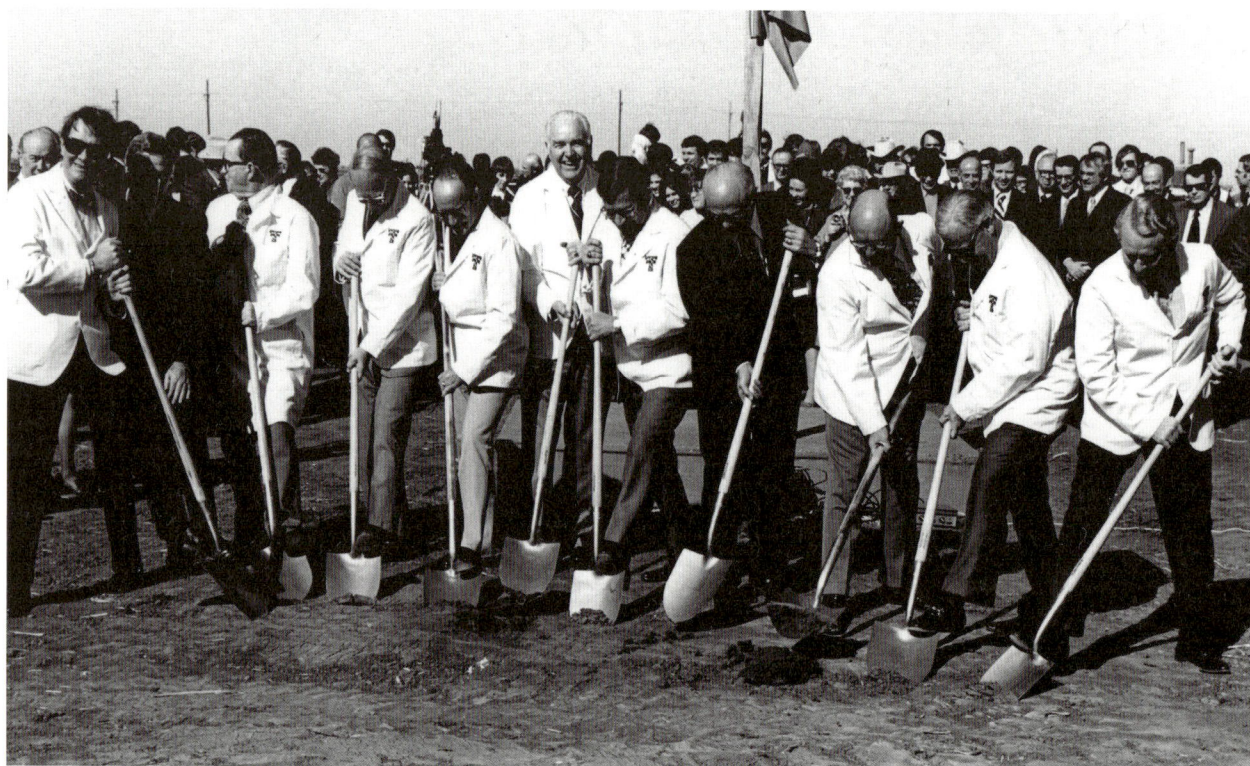
Photograph from the groundbreaking ceremony for the newly established Texas Tech School of Medicine. Pictured from left to right are: Dr. Grover Murray, Dr. S. M. Kennedy, Marshall Formby, Frank Junell, Dr. Judson Williams, Trent Campbell, Clint Formby, Preston Smith, Bill Collins, Field Scovell, and Waggoner Carr. Courtesy of the Southwest Collection/Special Collections Library

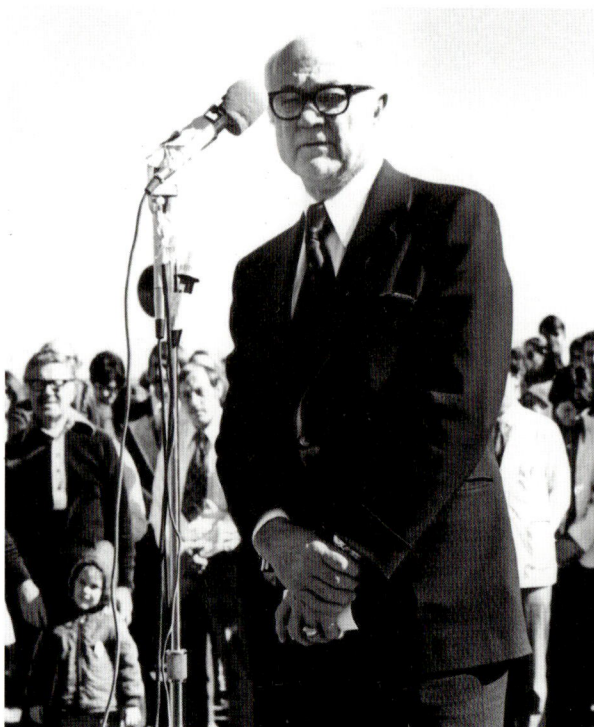
Preston Smith speaking at groundbreaking ceremony. Courtesy of the Southwest Collection/Special Collections Library

of Medicine was during its first decade. Educational pursuits continued at Drane and Thompson Halls in what McCartor and Tyner termed "the traveling medical school" for the first five years of teaching. In 1976, the medical school campus facility finally opened at 4th Street and Indiana as a massive, mile-long shell of a structure.

The Health Professions Educational Assistance Act of 1963 and the Comprehensive Health Manpower Training Act of 1971 provided federal funding for medical schools, increasing the national number from 86 in 1960 to over 125 by 1980. It was the recognition of a nationwide need for increased medical education, and the opportunity for federal financial support that had inspired an interest in expanding Texas medical education in the first place, and Texas Tech was a beneficiary. However, by the middle of the 1970s, this targeted federal funding was on the wane, and current circumstances required caution. President Murray understood that it was easier to secure financing for renovation than for new construction and advised that the money available be spent to build the largest structure possible, then finish out portions as the space was needed. The five-story medical school structure was divided into three areas, Pod A, Pod B, and Pod C. In 1976, Pod A was complete, and medical school faculty and students finally had a home of their own. Dr. De La Rosa remembers, as a student, playing handball off the walls and windows of Pod B in between medical school classes. By 1981, the finish-out of that cavernous Pod B had been thoroughly equipped for occupancy by the newly established School of Nursing and soon also housed the offices, laboratories, and classrooms of the School of Allied Health. However, when Pod A opened in 1976, the Texas Tech School of Medicine still did not have a permanent teaching hospital in Lubbock, a dilemma that had complicated clinical rotations, residency programs, and official accreditation from the very beginning of medical school enrollment.

When Governor Connelly vetoed that first 1965 bill to establish a medical school at Texas Tech, his primary point of contention was that Lubbock champions had not secured a hospital affiliation that would serve as the teaching hospital for the new medical school institution. As the largest hospital in Lubbock, Methodist was the obvious possibility, but President George Brewer had made it very clear from the beginning of medical school discussions that serving as a teaching hospital was not the mission of Methodist. It was a private hospital with paying patients and could not and would not consider fulfilling the responsibilities of a permanent teaching hospital.

After the 1965 veto, Lubbock medical school champions began immediately mobilizing the forces to campaign for a medical school in the next legislative session. The Lubbock Chamber of Commerce commissioned a study supporting the need for a medical school in West Texas located on the campus of Texas Tech. With Methodist out of the running, B. E. Rushing, Dr. Hull, John Logan, and Lubbock mayor Dub Rogers organized other local supporters to begin work on creating the financial means to build a county hospital. In a 1967 bill, they gained legislative approval to create a Lubbock County Hospital District, subject to voter approval. A Board of Managers reporting to the County Court of Commissioners would build a hospital to care for the citizens and the poor in Lubbock County. Voters were asked to approve three issues: (1) whether to create the district, (2) to provide tax funds for a teaching county hospital, and (3) to allow $4 million in construction bonds. On October 7, 1967, voters approved all three proposals and County Judge Rod Shaw celebrated by noting, "The people here are willing to provide funds for a teaching hospital and are willing to underwrite the

future growth of Lubbock and Lubbock County and the entire West Texas area." The downtown community, Texas Tech, the Lubbock-Crosby-Garza County Medical Society, and the Lubbock business community were all in support of establishing a medical school and teaching hospital. To emphasize backing from the financial community, in 1969, five banks teamed up to buy construction bonds well below the market rate, saving the hospital district more than $350,000 in costs for the hospital.

Murray Letter of Support, May 1971. Courtesy of the Southwest Collection/ Special Collections Library

Texas Tech University School of Medicine

P.O. Box 4349   Lubbock, Texas 79409   Phone (806) 742-2121

May 14, 1971

Mr. B. E. Rushing, Jr.
Chairman, Board of Managers
Lubbock County Hospital District
Room 108, Lubbock County Court House
Lubbock, Texas 79401

Dear Mr. Rushing:

This letter is in support of your application to the National Institutes of Health, Physician Manpower Division, for financial support in the construction of a 308 bed teaching hospital for Texas Tech University School of Medicine.

This joint venture of the Lubbock County Hospital District and the Texas Tech University School of Medicine shall have a very positive effect on the supply of physicians for this area and also should have a great impact on the delivery and cost of health care.

This joint program is an innovative one designed to produce two hundred physicians per year. It will place substantial emphasis on ambulatory care experience for students which should result in producing the type of physicians needed in this area.

The start-up and operating costs of this program are relatively minimal in comparison to the large number of physicians which it will provide. It is our hope that this innovative and exciting program will receive support from the National Institutes of Health. Texas Tech University School of Medicine enthusiastically endorses your application.

Sincerely,

Grover E. Murray
President

bc: Mr. Frank Junell
     Dr. John Hinchey
     Dr. John Buesseler ✓
     Dr. Judson Williams

With Texas Technological College newly authorized as Texas Tech University, passage of HR Bill 498 to create the Texas Tech School of Medicine, and the Lubbock County Hospital District in place to build a teaching hospital, Lubbock was poised for a dynamic new era of educational and medical growth. Unfortunately, it took almost a decade to work out all the kinks buried in this grand scheme, and the teaching hospital for the Texas Tech School of Medicine, so crucial to establishing that school in Lubbock, did not open its doors until 1978. In the meantime, Methodist, along with St. Mary's of the Plains, West Texas Hospital, Highland Hospital, and University Hospital, readily accommodated the need for student clinical rotations on a temporary basis, and St. Mary's was especially accommodating to the new medical school. Sister Maureen Van der Zee very willingly provided George Tyner and faculty from the Department of Psychiatry with a ten-bed area at the hospital for alcohol and addiction treatment, but St. Mary's was not equipped to be a permanent teaching facility.

For all intents and purposes, during those early years, each department in the medical school was left to its own devices in arranging affiliations for clinical teaching. The

TTUHSC—Lubbock

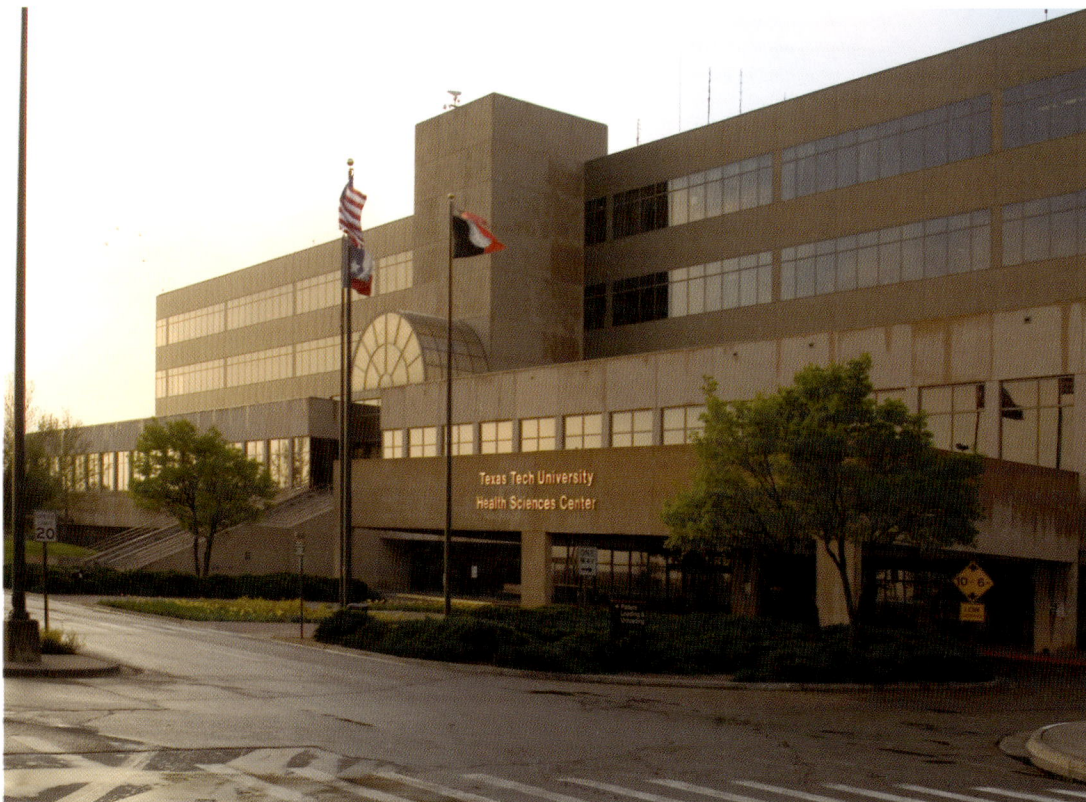

Department of Orthopedic Surgery established some clinical rotations with West Texas Hospital and from as far away as the Carrie Tingley Children's Hospital in Truth or Consequences, New Mexico. Necessity did, indeed, prove to be the proverbial mother of invention in the scramble for clinical teaching space. In 1974, when the Texas Tech School of Medicine established a teaching affiliation with R. E. Thomason General Hospital in El Paso, a selection of students were sent to the new El Paso Academic Health Center for their third-year clerkships, and a teaching model was born. To this day, a selection of third- and fourth-year medical students spend their clinical years either in Lubbock or on one of our campuses, Permian Basin, and Amarillo as well as at the new TTUHSC School of Medicine Covenant Campus established in July 2016.

Plain and simple, the complications surrounding the construction and opening of the county teaching hospital were hardwired into the structure of things. The Hospital District Board had to make sure the county could afford the new hospital, and the School of Medicine administration had to make sure the hospital accommodated its current and future teaching needs. The Hospital Board and the School of Medicine were two totally independent organizations with a vested interest in the number of beds, size of the facility, medical services, and administrative control of the hospital. Coming to a meeting of minds was a long and drawn out and many times contentious process. By 1978, however, they had resolved their major infrastructure differences, and the hospital finally opened as the Health Sciences Center Hospital. Constructed as an architecturally harmonious south-facing complement to the north-facing medical school building, the hospital provided care for the poor and offered medical school students a settled home for clinical clerkships. In 1980, the name was changed to Lubbock General Hospital and in 1990 to University Medical Center.

Today, University Medical Center serves as the largest and most successful tertiary care center in the region, extending its primary, specialty, and subspecialty services to West Texas, New Mexico, the Oklahoma panhandle, and western Kansas. University Medical Center and the Texas Tech University Health Sciences Center proceed in their teaching and patient care mission as a dynamic partnership, fostering medical innovations and gaining recognition for quality patient care. These two independent institutions work together in two-part harmony to serve the specialty care needs of the region through the UMC Children's Hospital, the Southwest Cancer Center, the Primary Stroke Center, the Timothy J. Harnar Burn Unit, and many other acute and chronic care centers unavailable anywhere else for hundreds and hundreds of miles. They have managed superbly to remove all of the major kinks from the system, combining UMC state-of-the-art medical facilities and staff with TTUHSC faculty physicians and students to provide the finest in-patient care and healthcare education. Currently, University Medical Center supports 13 residency programs and 11 fellowship programs with 212 graduate medical education positions. The hospital also supports 11 endowed chairs and one professorship at the Texas Tech University Health Sciences Center. Together, these institutions continue to make a profound impact on the quality of healthcare delivery and healthcare education in a multistate region.

Bernhard T. Mittemeyer, MD, had a great impact on the harmonizing and stabilizing of Health Sciences Center programs and services over a 24-year career with the institution. He joined the medical school faculty as a urologist after a 28-year career in the U.S. Army, serving as surgeon general from 1981 to 1985. During his years at the Health Sciences Center, he served as executive vice president and provost from 1986 to 1996, interim president in 2006, and more than once, interim dean of the School of Medicine. Few saw the evolution of the Texas Tech University Health Sciences Center from a greater vantage point than did Mittemeyer. He was in a position to navigate the institution through many challenges, and at his retirement, he opined in an article titled "Thanks for the Memories" for the summer 2011 issue of *Pulse*:

> These years at TTUHSC have given me opportunities that a 28-year career in military medicine could never have fulfilled. To witness and participate in what less than fifty years ago was but a governor's dream is hard to equal. To observe the amazing impact a much-maligned institution, at least in those early years, has had on the quality of life and health care of our citizens in a region larger than all of New England plus the state of New York combined, is hard to equal. Our growth and reputation has been phenomenal, and it gives me a sense of pride to see the success TTUHSC has made as an institution in the TTU System.

Building upon Excellence

As a strong emblem of that success and continued growth, the Texas Tech University Health Sciences Center ushered in the millennium with a flurry of new construction. The original Health Sciences Center's massive headquarters structure had been completely finished out and filled and was no longer adequate for the educational programs and student needs of the Texas Tech University Health Sciences Center.

New construction began in 1998 with the Preston Smith Library. This 50,000-square-foot library building was built on a slant to the original HSC complex with distinctive contemporary stone and glass embellishments. From the beginning, the library's collection has focused upon quality. In their history, McCartor and Tyner remark upon the library's distinction:

> Charles W. Sargent, Ph.D., assumed the duties of the director of the medical school library in 1972, replacing Helen Crawford. . . . The excellence of the library, especially one established in so brief a time, was noted in every accrediting review since the first visit in 1973. In addition to the expected printed material, the library provided audiovisual resources and computer services. The December 1973 LCME team prophesied that "This library should become an impressive resource for medical education in Western Texas," which it did. (*Eye of the Storm*, 171)

Guided by longtime executive director of libraries, Richard Wood, and current executive director Richard Nollan, the library has a presence in Lubbock, Permian Basin, and Amarillo and still coordinates resources with TTUHSC El Paso Library and ensures state-of-the-art healthcare resources for the expanding educational mission of the Texas Tech Health Sciences Center.

In 2003, the Lubbock campus opened the Academic Classroom Building, a sleek, contemporary structure complementing the original mile-long Health Sciences Center facility. The two-story, 60,000-square-foot addition contains two 200-seat tiered lecture halls, three medium classrooms, twelve smaller conference and seminar rooms, and a basic science teaching laboratory to ensure the finest in educational facilities for a growing student enrollment.

In 2007, the Texas Tech Physicians Medical Pavilion opened on the Lubbock campus, providing the medical

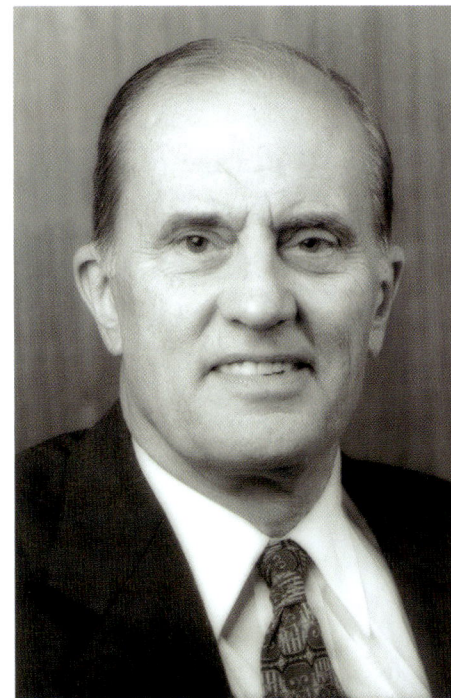

Bernhard Mittemeyer, MD, Vice President

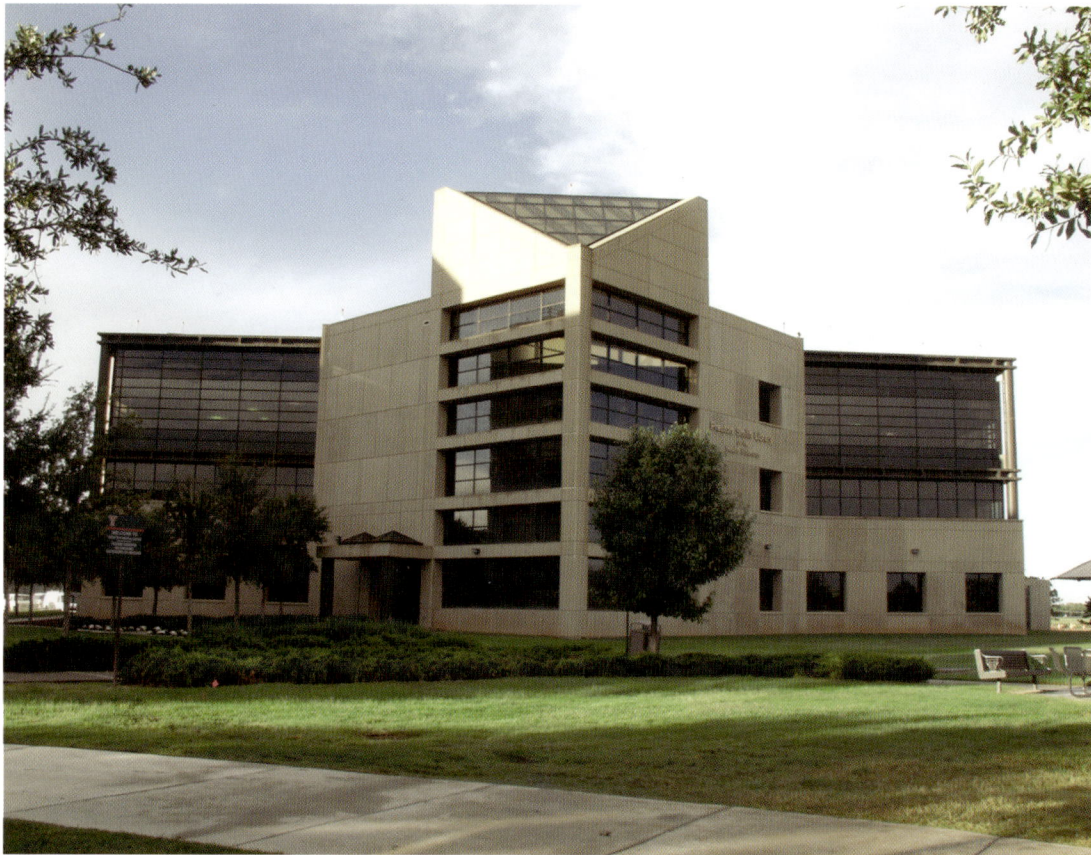
Preston Smith Library

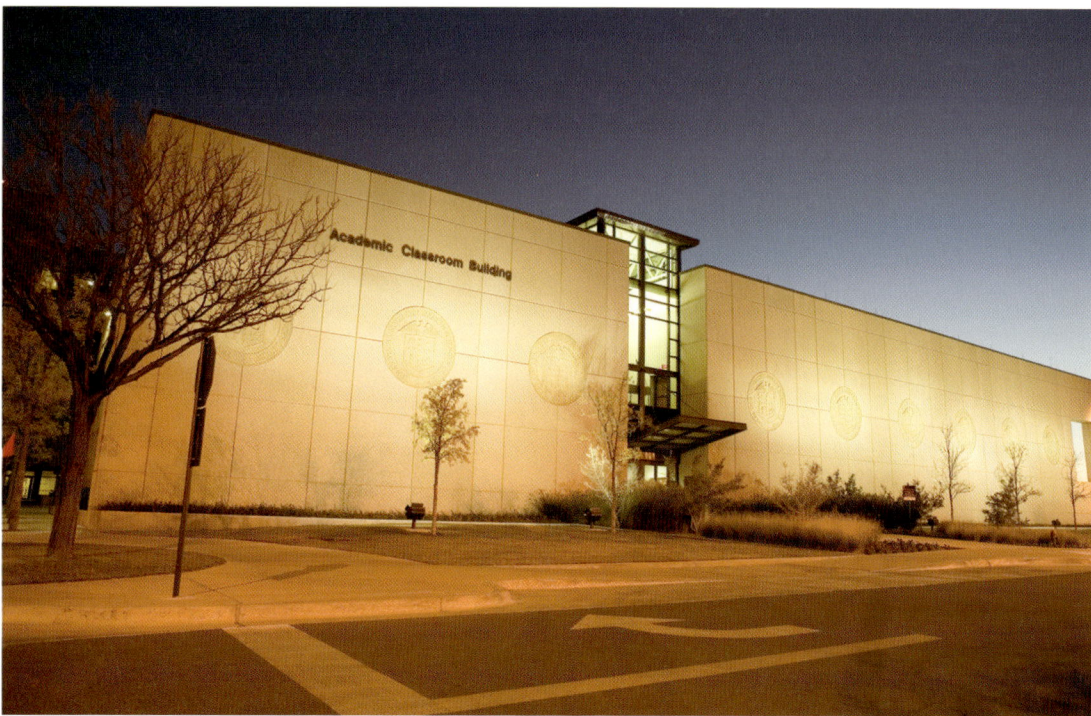
Academic Classroom Building at night

school faculty with increased space to conduct research and serve patients with primary and specialty medical care through hospital privileges with University Medical Center, celebrating the 40th anniversary of its foundation, the tertiary care center in West Texas and Covenant Health System, celebrating its 100th anniversary of foundation. The Physicians Medical Pavilion provides clinics for faculty physicians in the 14 clinical departments of the School of Medicine, comprised of Anesthesiology, Dermatology, Family and Community Medicine, Internal Medicine, Neurology, Obstetrics and Gynecology, Ophthalmology, Orthopedic Surgery, Otolaryngology, Pathology, Pediatrics, Psychiatry, Surgery, and Urology. Within these departments, residents and medical students receive training and patients receive treatment in over 40 specialty and subspecialty fields, including expertise in nephrology, endocrinology, infectious diseases, rheumatology, epilepsy, Alzheimer's disease, multiple sclerosis, Parkinson's disease, strokes, cleft palates, cochlear implants, thyroid surgery, cancer treatment and surgery, addictive diseases, burns, sports medicine, and many other specialty and subspecialty areas. Through these expansive clinical services, patients can receive the finest state-of-the-art specialty care within a reasonable distance from home.

In 2017, the Health Sciences Center conducted groundbreakings for three new buildings, which will complete the current master plan for the Lubbock campus and stand as an imposing visual statement on the strength and achievement of this multidimensional educational institution. The West Expansion represents Pod D of the original building and connects with the Preston Smith Library for a seamless campus experience, adding 125,000 square feet to the facility for a gross anatomy instructional laboratory, five classrooms, and administrative offices.

The University Center and the Academic Event Center are both freestanding facilities on the north side of the campus designed to greet patients and the public to the Health Sciences Center. As of the writing of this volume, the Academic Event Center is just at the groundbreaking stage. The University Center, however, is close to completion and will serve as the official welcoming center to the campus. It will contain admission offices, a bookstore, the clinical simulation center, and administrative offices with a true campus entrance off 4th Street to frame the whole Health Sciences Center campus complex. The architecture of the University Center and the Academic Event

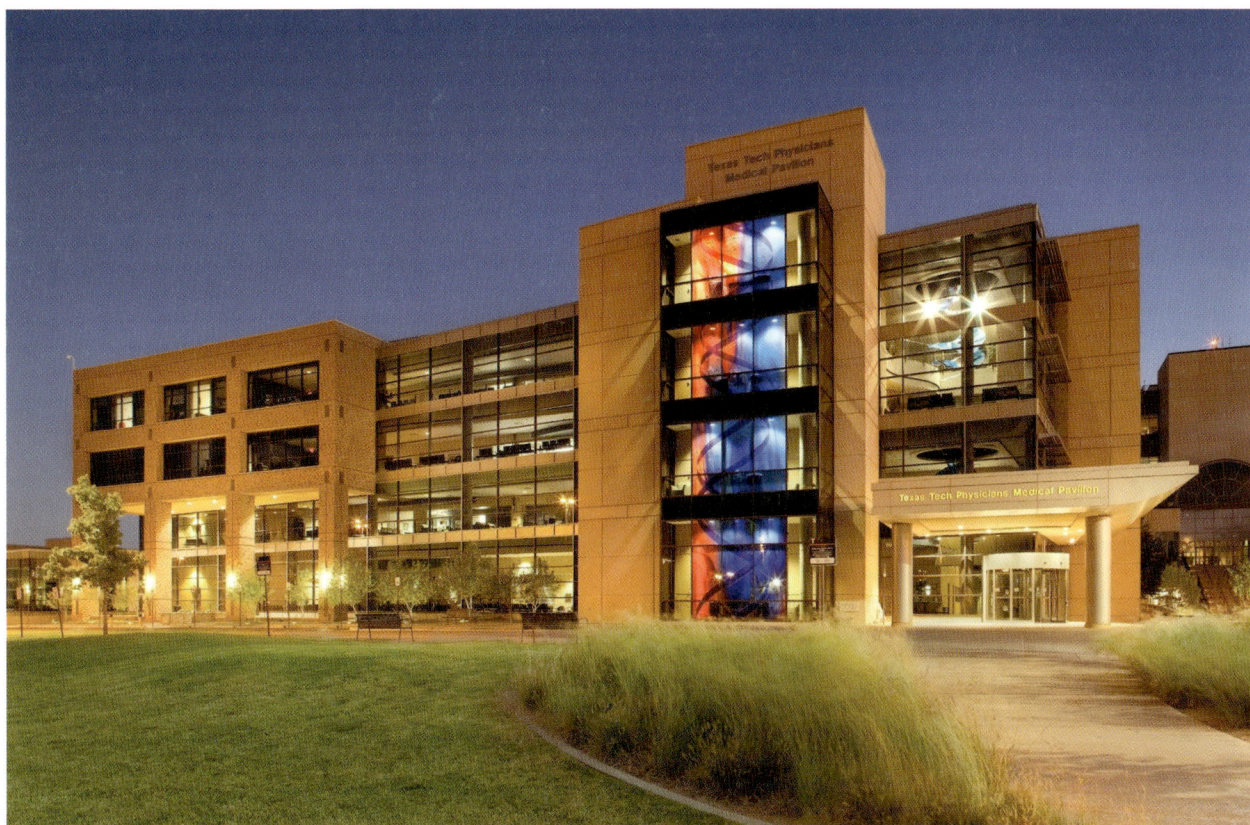

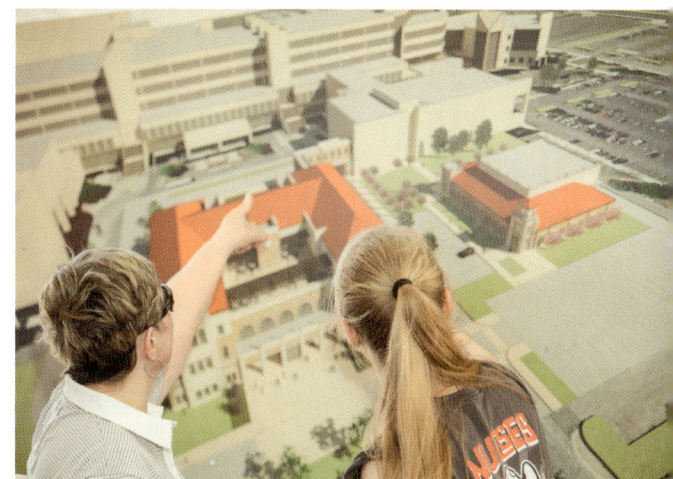

Center stand in significant contrast to the contemporary glass and stone style of the rest of the campus structures. It reflects the distinctive Spanish Renaissance architectural style of Texas Tech University, confirming the meaningful ties that proudly bind these two institutions through a shared campus, history, and promise of dynamic collaborations to come.

Since 2010, Dr. Tedd L. Mitchell has served as president of the Texas Tech University Health Sciences Center, leading the institution into this new era of strength and achievement. As its longest serving president, Mitchell has successfully led a period of record growth in enrollment, academic excellence, and physical expansion on all campuses. Texas Tech University Health Sciences Center now graduates more healthcare professionals than any other health-related institution in Texas. Mitchell has promoted interprofessional concentrations and novel research initiatives in the School of Medicine, School of Nursing, School of Pharmacy, and the School of Health Professions. The opening of the Julia Jones Matthews Department of Public Health in the Graduate School of Biomedical Sciences, headquartered on the Abilene campus, will add important new avenues for exploration.

In 2014, Mitchell supported School of Medicine dean Berk's effort to expand enrollment by an additional 30 medical students who will complete third- and fourth-year clerkships at Covenant Health Systems. University Medical Center is at educational capacity, serving the Health Sciences Center with exceptional support. An affiliation with Covenant Health Systems adds a second teaching hospital to the institution to provide expanded clinical opportunities for medical students and residents as the Health Sciences Center continues to grow. In 1998, St. Mary's of the Plains, as part of the Sisters of Saint Joseph, incorporated Lubbock's Methodist Hospital into its organization, creating Covenant Health System. Clearly, Methodist Hospital has finally become an important teaching hospital for the Texas Tech University Health Sciences Center, especially for the new Covenant Branch Campus students and residents. We think George Brewer would approve this time.

In 2018, Dr. Tedd L. Mitchell was appointed chancellor of the Texas Tech University System while continuing as president of the Texas Tech University Health Sciences Center. As chancellor, Mitchell brings his listening and negotiation skills to the table to work collaboratively with

(LEFT) Texas Tech Physicians Medical Pavilion

(ABOVE) Viewing the University Center and West Expansion Plan

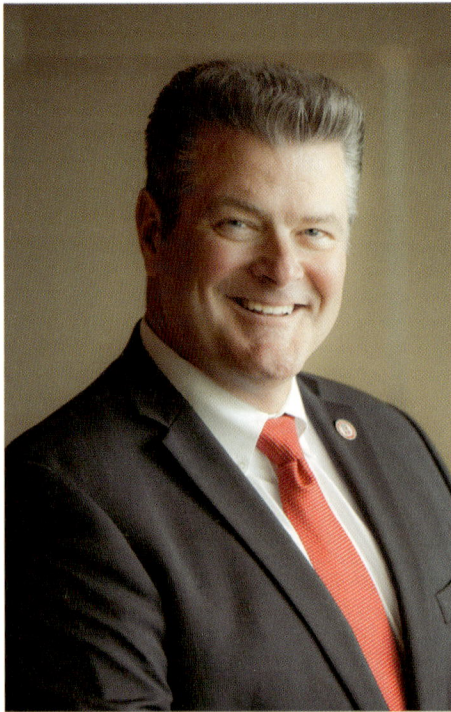

Tedd Mitchell, MD

(RIGHT) Tedd Mitchell, MD, and Staff

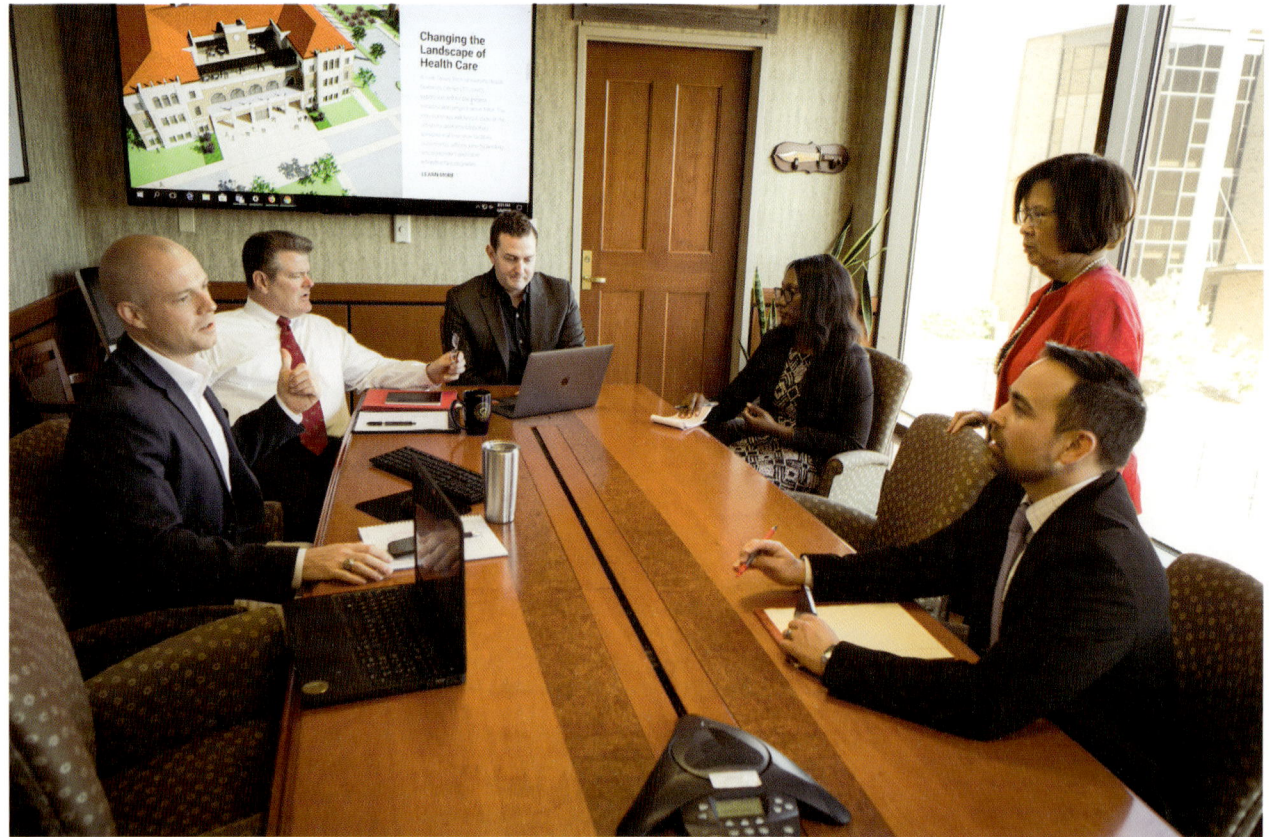

university presidents to establish a vision of meaningful initiatives, innovation, and purposeful growth to the system of institutions that operate on 17 campuses statewide and internationally. He also brings to this dual administrative role a strong dedication to advancing higher education, health care, research, and outreach and will add his energy and enthusiasm to advancing the influence of the Texas Tech University System as he continues to build programs at the Texas Tech University Health Sciences Center.

Fifty years ago, John Buessler put forth a wide-ranging concept of what this new medical school at Texas Tech could become. He wasn't what we might call "a detail person," and all indications suggest he could have used some help with interpersonal skills, but when it came to vision, literally as well as figuratively, few could best him.

Shortly after he had assumed his new position as founding vice president and dean of the Texas Tech School of Medicine, Buessler decided that he needed to make a brief military tour of Vietnam in the thick of the war. President Murray prevailed upon Lubbock's very influential congressman George Mahon to intervene, and

Buessler, who was a colonel in the Army Reserves, left Lubbock to visit Vietnam for two months of active duty in June 1970. He was interested in learning the details of helicopter medical rescue protocols that had evolved over the many years of this combat-heavy jungle conflict. Buessler thought emergency flights would have meaningful applications for serving crisis care patients in the many isolated parts of West Texas. At that time, domestic medical helicopters were virtually unheard of, and his brief Vietnam War tour served as little more than a very dramatic academic exercise. Today, however, University Medical Center relies upon Aerocare helicopters and small jets to transport over 400 critical care patients annually to the state-of-the-art Emergency Care facilities in Lubbock. University Medical Center is the first hospital in Texas to received TraumaI designation and often flies in and treats emergency care patients from the multistate area of New Mexico, the Oklahoma panhandle, western Kansas, and West Texas. Many patients, injured in oil fields in this area, are brought to UMC's Timothy J. Harnar Regional Burn Center, which is one of only four American Burn Association (ABA) accredited burn centers in Texas and is

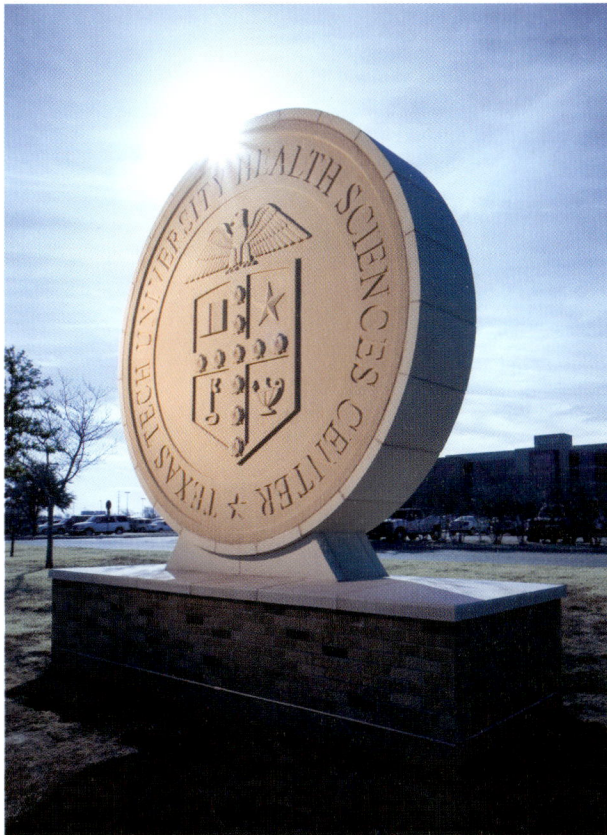

Seal of the Texas Tech University Health Sciences Center

carrels and 35 new classmates. The prospect of gaining our MD degree in three years was great, but little did we know then of the toll it would take and the high price we would pay for that in less than one year." For the health and well-being of the exhausted students and faculty, the School of Medicine adopted a traditional four-year curriculum in 1976. However, today, thanks to Dean Steven Berk, a very talented "detail person," the concept has been revived and significantly refined to create the Family Medicine Accelerated Track, now serving as an educational model nationwide.

Buessler envisioned a medical school with "porous walls" where students could learn in a seminar environment, eschewing the academic, scientific, and clinical silos of traditional medical education. The plan remained too ephemeral for meaningful application back then. Today, however, through rigorous restructuring and evaluation, the Health Sciences Center has implemented Curricular Theme Teams to focus on the teaching of body systems and disease processes rather than individual basic science disciplines. The old intellectual walls are, indeed, tumbling down as more and more programs emphasize translational goals for the basic and clinical sciences.

Buessler's dreams were as big as the West Texas sky and often as amorphous as the clouds floating by. It took some doing to bring things down to earth, but in spite of all the reconnoitering back then, his experimental ways infused the Texas Tech University Health Sciences Center with a sense of educational adventure that still characterizes the institution today. At this fiftieth anniversary milestone, we continue to embrace the fearless spirit of problem solving that has placed the Texas Tech University Health Sciences Center in the vanguard of new and better ways to improve healthcare education and medical practices throughout our history. As president and chancellor Tedd L. Mitchell proclaims, "We are not standing still. We are ever growing and looking forward to changing the landscape of health care for future generations."

one of only 47 regional burn centers in the United States. Director John Griswold, MD, and his staff of physicians, nurses, and other healthcare personnel provide specialized care to these badly burned patients.

To help resolve the physician crisis in significantly underserved West Texas, Buessler implemented an expedited three-year degree program for the new medical school that was put into place without the guidance of existing three year programs. William H. Gorman, MD, class of 1975, recalls his experience within what proved to be a challenging program, stating, "The first day at 'Drane Hall' School of Medicine was typical—exciting with new, short white coats; newly remodeled lecture rooms; nice study

CHAPTER TWO

SCHOOL OF MEDICINE

Steven L. Berk, MD, Dean

In 1969, there was one physician for every 1,366 residents in the West Texas region, and today this ratio has improved to one doctor for every 719 residents. The original emphasis on primary care medicine shows up today in the three-year Family Medicine Accelerated Track. As the first program of its kind in the country, it allows students to complete requirements for the medical doctorate in three years, reducing the time and expense of medical school. Graduates enter TTUHSC Family Medicine residency programs and upon completion are prepared to practice—oftentimes in rural areas of the state.

Over the past five years, an average of 53 percent of all TTUHSC medical school graduates have elected to enter the primary care specialties of family medicine, internal medicine, obstetrics and gynecology, and pediatrics. In 2017, 52 percent of graduates elected primary care specialties.

The introduction of electronic teaching aids proposed 50 years ago led to distance learning and the integration of technology and state-of-the art simulation centers to train students on all TTUHSC campuses. Jay Wheeler, MD, PhD, was an early proponent of telemedicine at TTUHSC.

The patient care programs of the School of Medicine have served as the base for clinical education of medical students and residents, introducing the students to clinical settings early in their training, drawing on community physicians and healthcare settings as it was envisioned

50 years ago. Affiliation agreements were signed with the St. Mary of the Plains Hospital and Methodist Hospital (now Covenant Health Systems), and the Lubbock County Hospital District (now University Medical Center) for training and clinical care.

In 2016, the school again expanded clinical training in Lubbock through a collaborative partnership with Covenant Health Systems. With the support of volunteer faculty, 30 students are assigned to complete third- and fourth-year clerkships at Covenant Medical Center. The patient care programs of the School of Medicine also serve as the base for clinical research and as a major source of patient care for West Texans. In fiscal year 2017, the School of Medicine provided more than half a million clinical visits of care.

The School of Medicine opened for classes in 1972 with 36 first-year students and 25 third-year transfer students. John Buessler, MD, had been appointed founding dean of the Texas Tech School of Medicine. A faculty-student directory from the winter of 1973 listed 75 faculty members, including several technicians and librarians, 61 full-time students, and 3 part-time students. The first class of 24 students graduated from the Texas Tech School of Medicine in March 1974.

A decade later, the Texas Tech School of Medicine graduated 90 students in its tenth class, and the multi campus design was in full swing. Students completed their first two years of basic sciences coursework in Lubbock, before

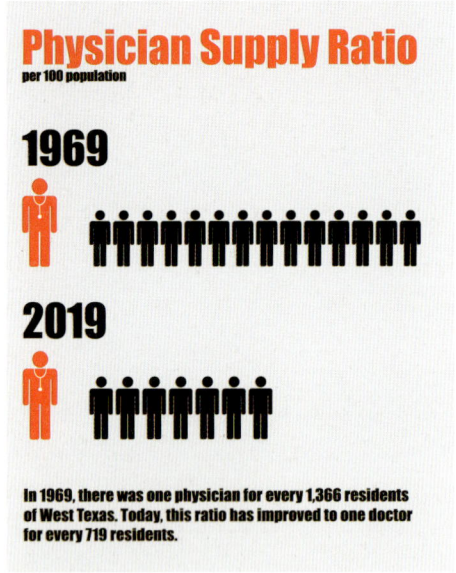

Physician Supply Ratio
per 100 population

1969

2019

In 1969, there was one physician for every 1,366 residents of West Texas. Today, this ratio has improved to one doctor for every 719 residents.

Infographic: Comparing physician numbers between 1969 and 2018

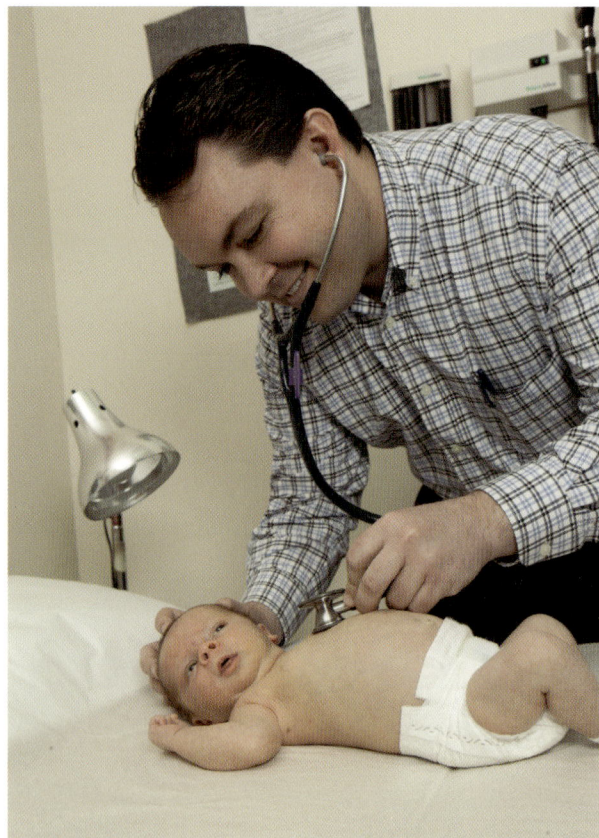

Family Medicine Clinic—infant check up

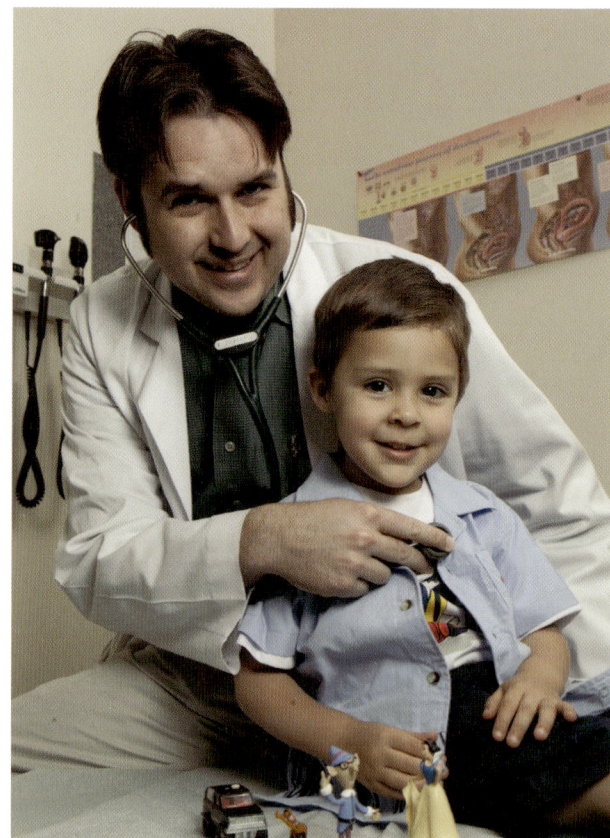

Family Medicine Clinic—well child check up

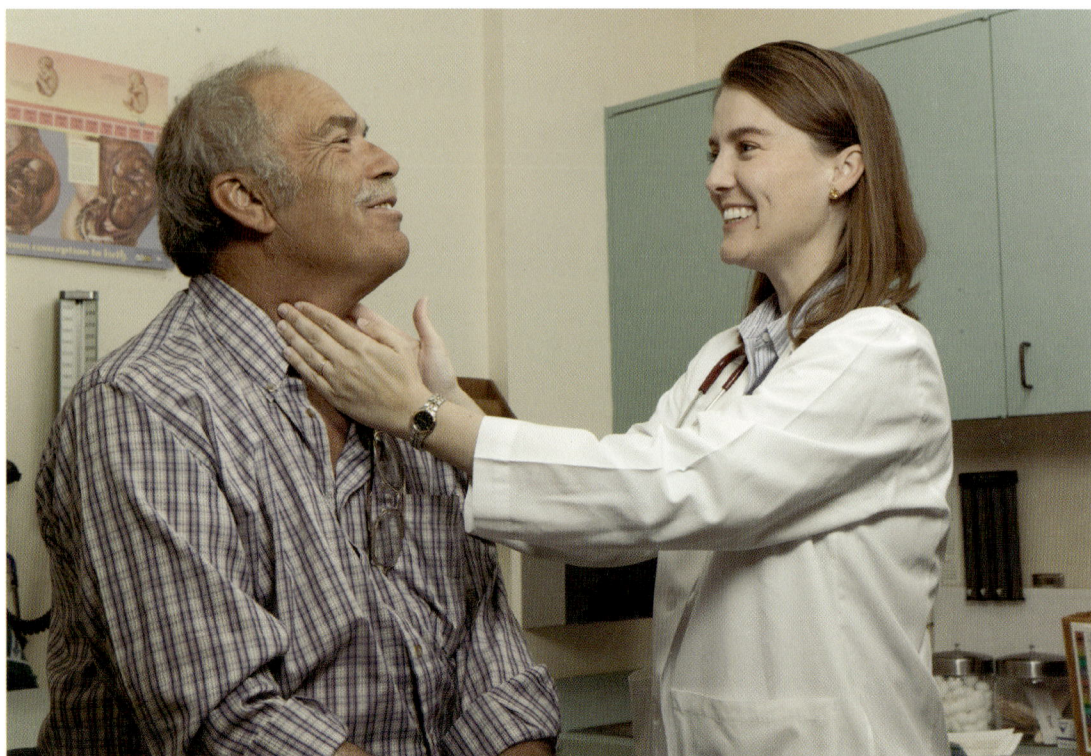

Family Medicine Clinic—geriatric check up

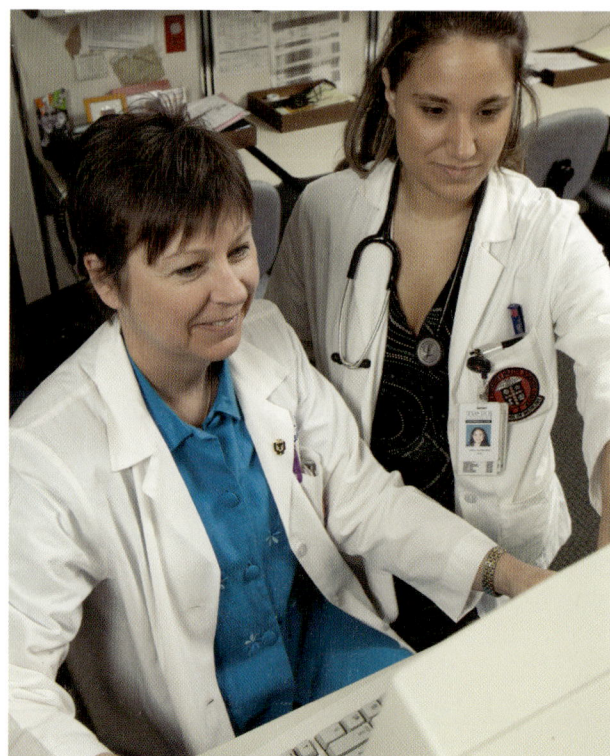

Family Medicine Clinic—Laura Baker, MD

distributing among the campuses in Amarillo, El Paso, and Lubbock. The 2017–2018 entering class was the first year that more female students were accepted than males (51%) and the following year, 2018–2019, 107 of the 180 students are females (58%). Residency education was introduced in 1973, with the February provisional approval of programs in family medicine at both the Lubbock and Amarillo campuses. Family medicine residency programs were later approved in El Paso in 1976 and in Odessa in 1984, all as the first such programs on their respective campuses. The campuses of the School of Medicine operate 20 individually accredited residency programs and 15 fellowship programs in West Texas. As of October 2017, these programs had 487 total residents in training, which includes 46 fellows, of which 309 (63.5%) were in primary care fields. Of the 309 total primary care residents in training, 103 are specifically in family medicine, thus fulfilling the initial idea of producing more health professionals for West Texas. The 35 residency and fellowship programs have 147 first-year trainees and will graduate approximately 139 residents and fellows in 2018.

The education of medical students and residents has been traditionally provided within departments encompassed by the Basic Sciences and Clinical Medicine. The following section will recount the activities of both areas starting with the Departments of Basic Sciences.

Cell Physiology and Molecular Biophysics— Guillermo Altenberg, M.D., Ph.D., Professor and Chair

The Department of Cell Physiology and Molecular Biophysics grew out of the Department of Physiology, where the faculty's first charge was to teach medical students. As TTUHSC expanded, biomedical research in the basic science departments has become more important over the last 10–15 years. The department became a modern teaching/research unit. Its faculty, whose primary job was teaching, became a modern teaching/research unit and has received more than $20 million in research funding. The department's research focus is membrane proteins and it has created the Center for Membrane Protein Research. These proteins are the targets for most drugs used in medicine today and have pivotal roles in genetic and acquired disorders such as cystic fibrosis, stroke, and resistance of cancers to chemotherapy. The center currently has 17 faculty members from seven TTUHSC departments,

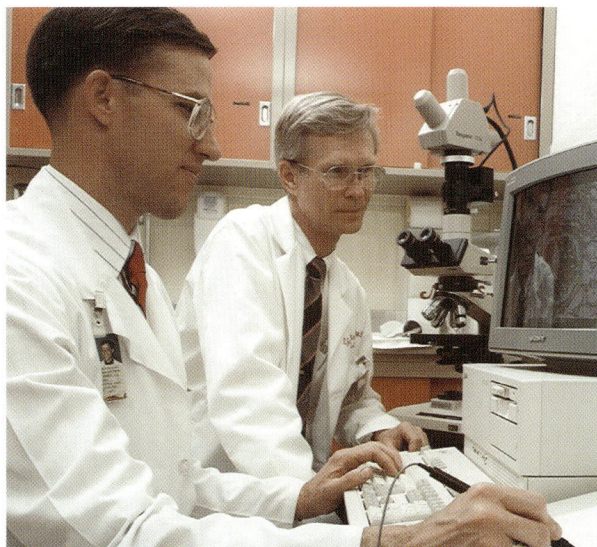

E. Jay Wheeler, MD, PhD, Associate Dean for Developing and Special Programs

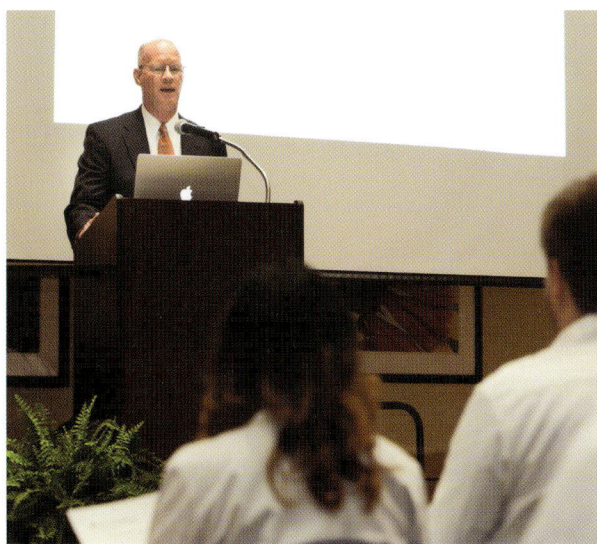

Richard Parks, President/CEO of Covenant Health addressing first class of Covenant Campus MSI students

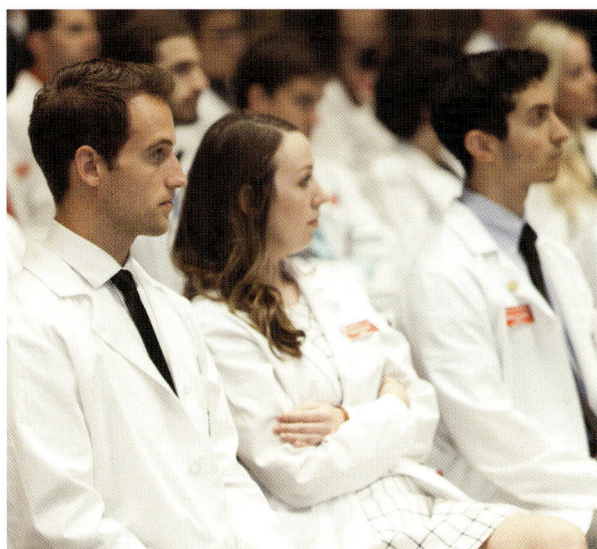

First cohort of Covenant Campus students

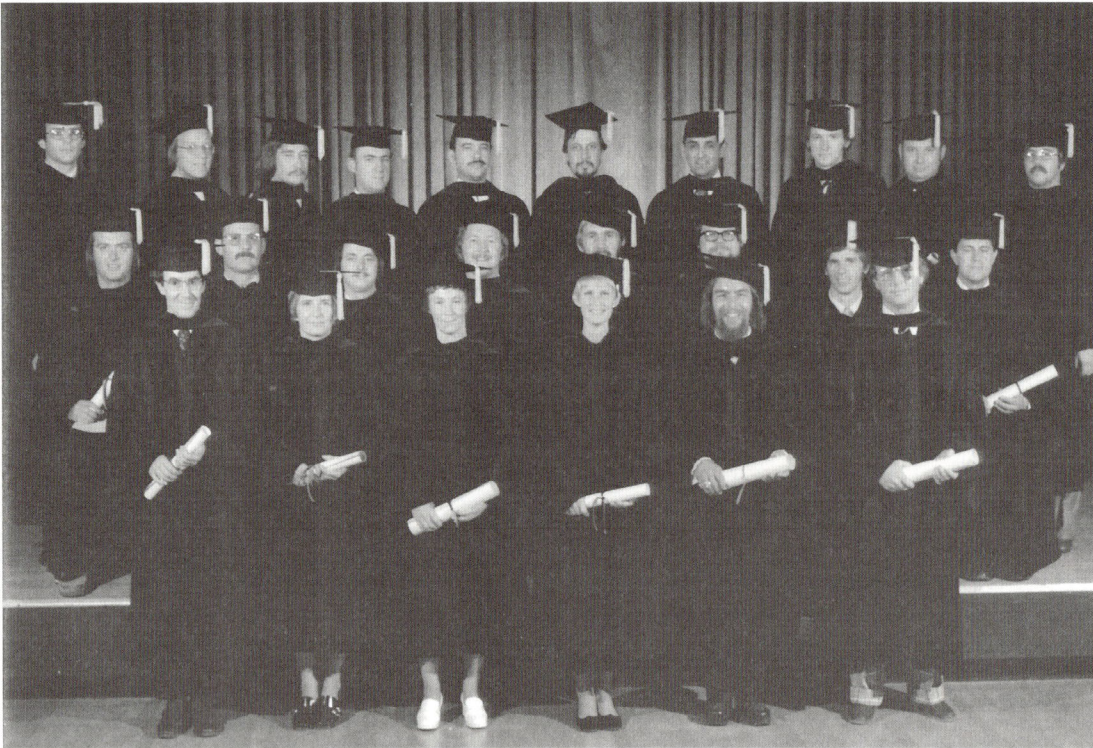
First SOM graduating class 1974

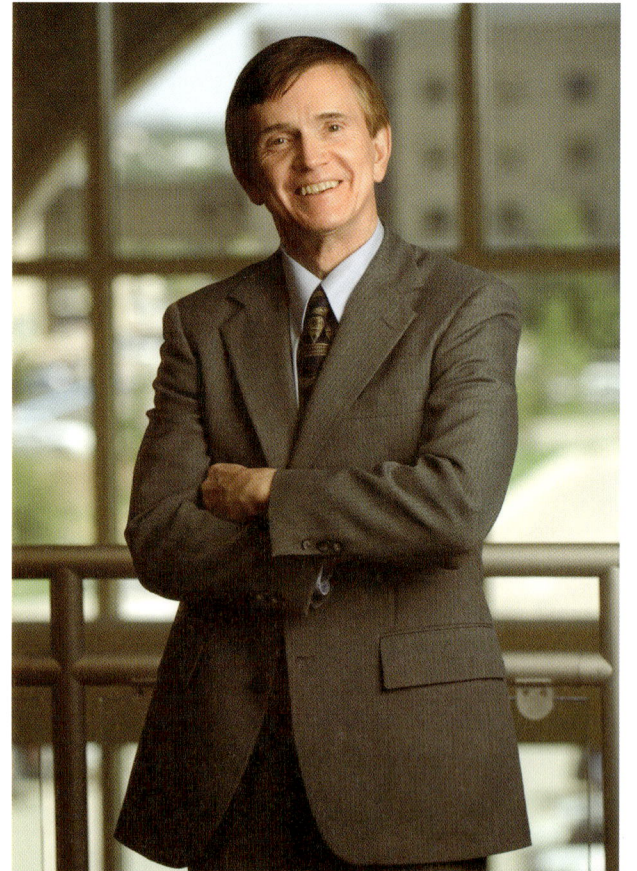
Richard M. Jordan, MD, Dean, Amarillo

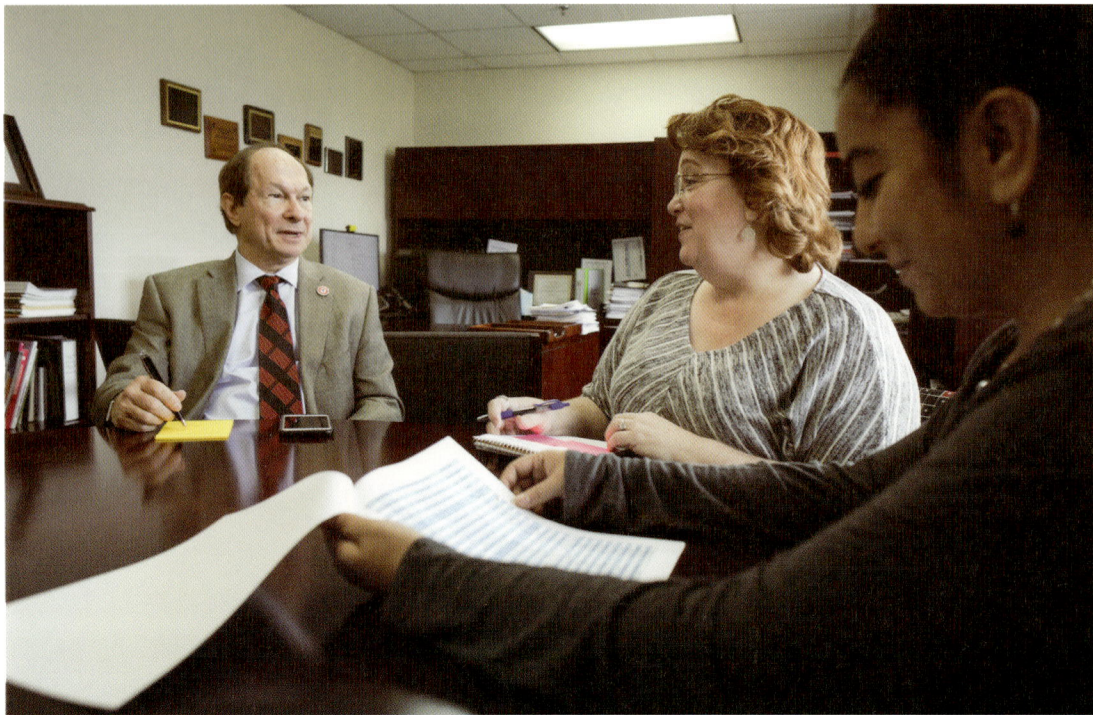
Gary Ventolini, MD, Dean for Permian Basin and staff

(RIGHT) Manny de la Rosa, MD, Founding Dean for the Paul L. Foster School of Medicine and current Vice President for Outreach and Community Engagement

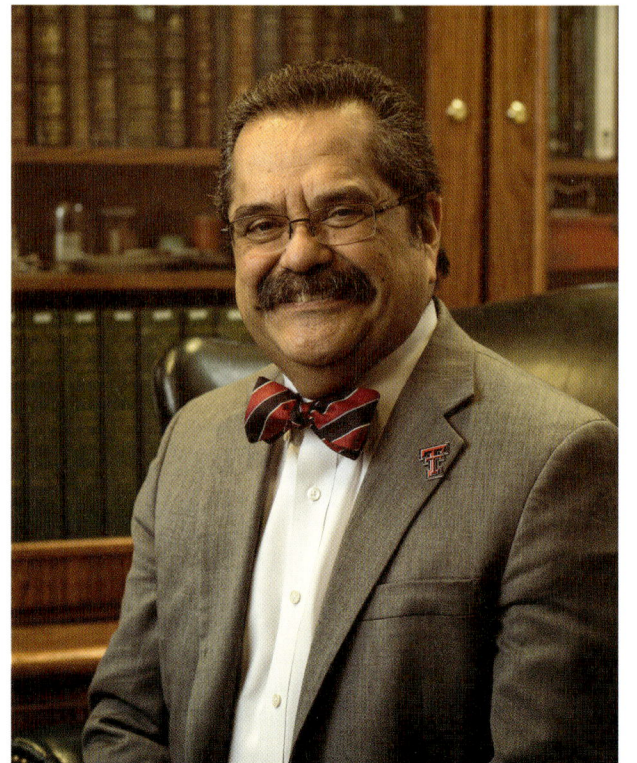

and, with the support of leadership, it has been able to recruit exceptional investigators from across the nation.

Immunology and Molecular Microbiology— Matthew B. Grisham, PhD, Professor and Chair

The department's faculty along with faculty from seven other departments are part of the Graduate School of Biomedical Science's concentration in immunology and infectious diseases (IID), a PhD and MS program, or a second PhD in medical microbiology. Research programs focus on mucosal and tumor immunology, cancer biology, microbial pathogenesis, and infectious diseases and vaccine development. A major theme is translating cutting-edge scientific discoveries into new therapeutic strategies that may be used to treat immunological and infectious diseases. Since 1990, the IID faculty has graduated more than 55 PhD and MS students, the large majority of whom took positions in universities, health sciences centers, biotech and pharmaceutical companies, clinical laboratories, and government research facilities.

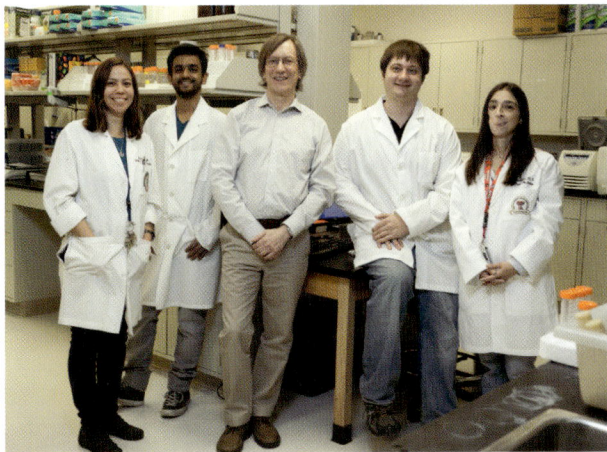

Guillermo Altenberg, MD, PhD, Chair Cell Physiology & Molecular Biophysics

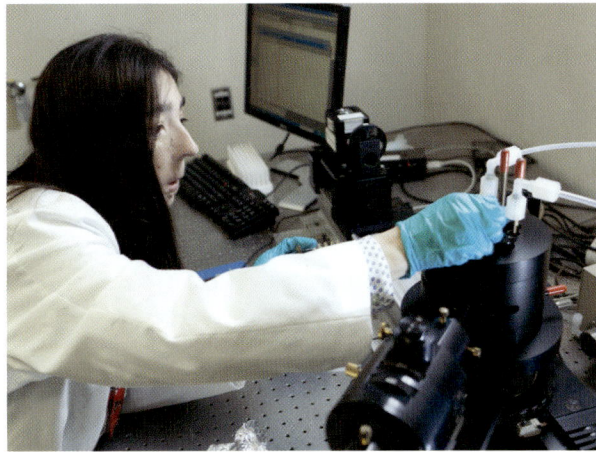

Grad student working in Altenberg lab

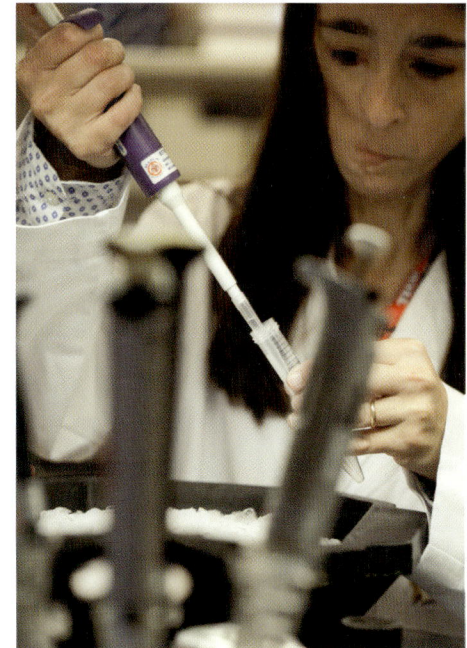

Grad student working in Altenberg lab

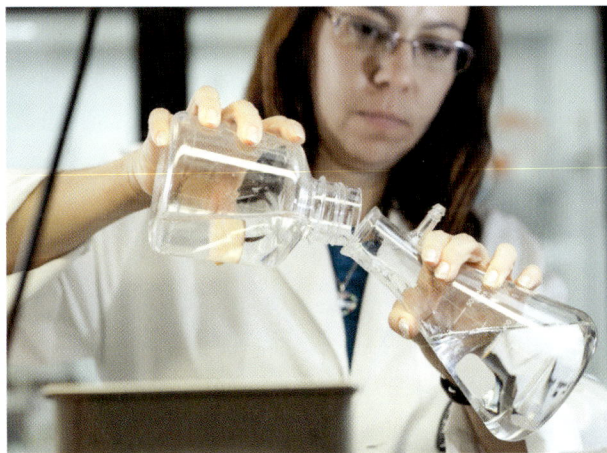

Grad student working in Altenberg lab

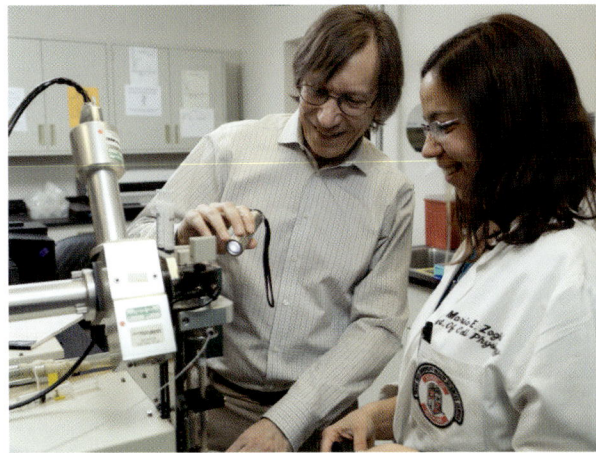

Grad student working in lab with Dr. Altenberg

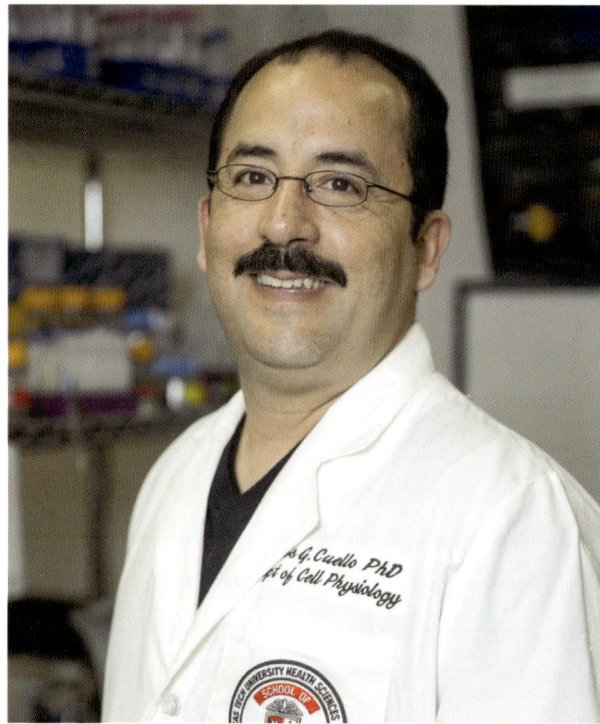
Luis Cuello, PhD

Cell Biology and Biochemistry—
Vadivel Ganapathy, PhD, Professor and Chair

The Department of Cell Biology and Biochemistry was created in 1995 by combining the Department of Anatomy and the Department of Biochemistry with Harry Weitlauf, MD, as the chair of this new department. Under Dr. Weitlauf's leadership, the departmental faculty pursued research in biochemistry, reproductive biology, and cancer. After Dr. Weitlauf's passing, Douglas Stocco, PhD, stepped up to chair the department and presided over its transition to new leadership: Vadivel Ganapathy, PhD, was appointed as chair in 2014. He is the Grover E. Murray Professor and Welch Endowed Chair in Biochemistry. Since then, the department has been expanded with the hiring of six new faculty members; this thanks to the support of Steven L. Berk, MD, the dean of the School of Medicine, and Quentin Smith, PhD, Senior Vice President for Research. The research focus has also shifted more towards cancer, but other areas of strength including reproductive biology, diabetes, obesity, neurological diseases, and renal biology remain vibrant. In addition to research, the department is actively engaged in medical student and graduate student teaching. Also of importance to the department are stronger ties to the clinical departments to intensify the bench-to-bedside translational aspects of research.

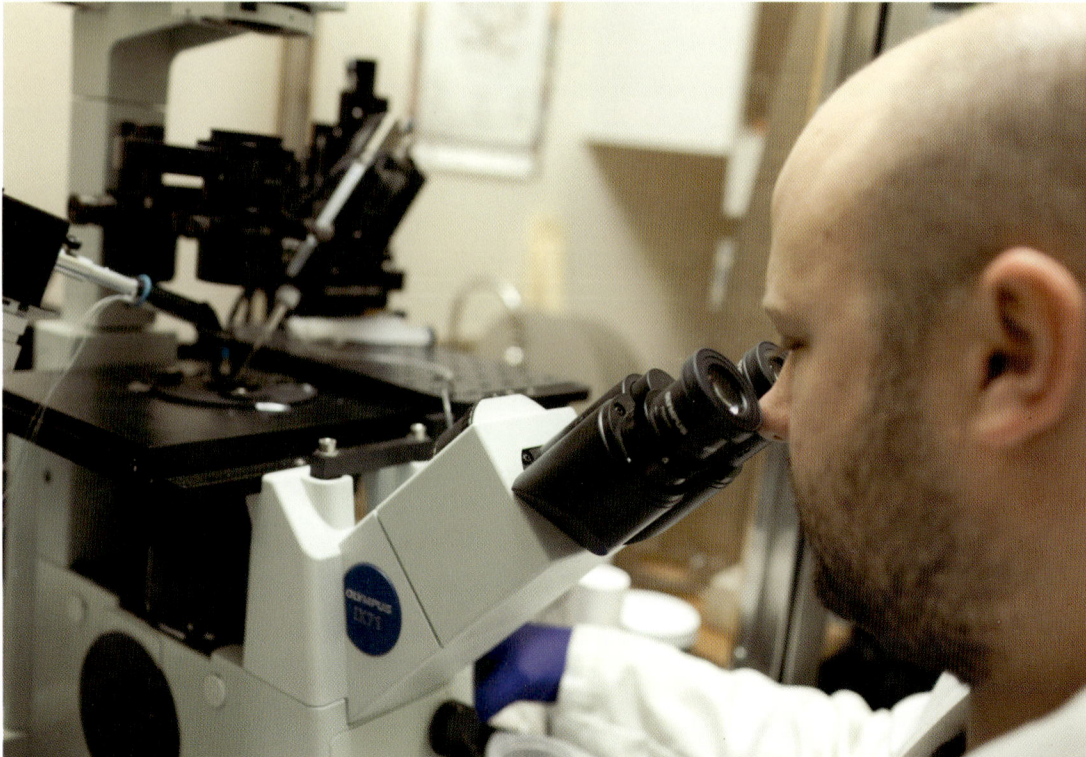

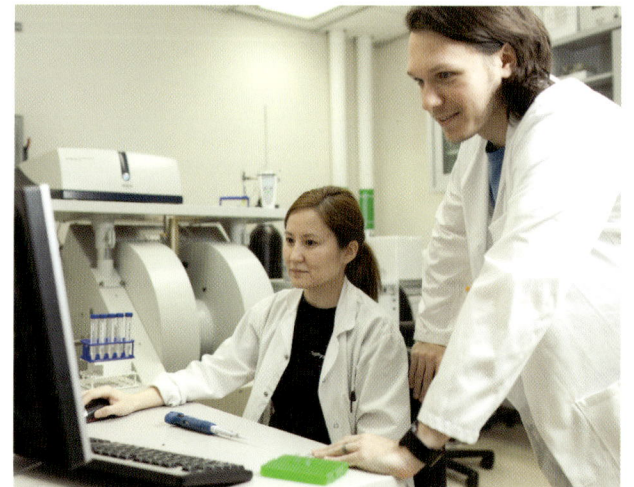
Grad students working in Luis Cuello lab

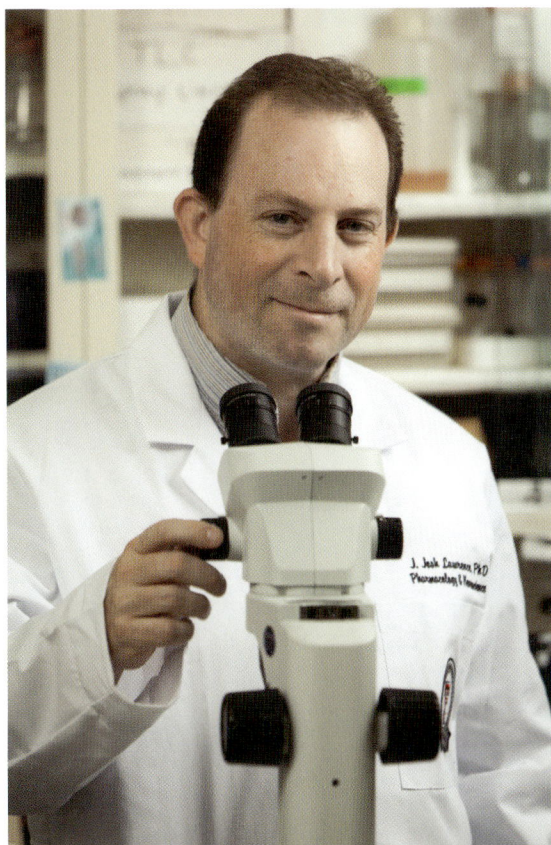
J. Josh Lawrence, PhD

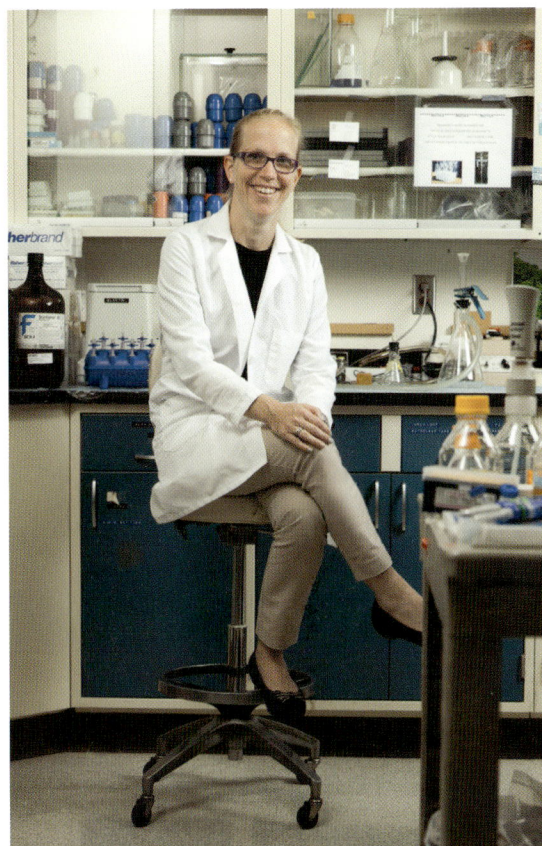
Josee Guindon, PhD

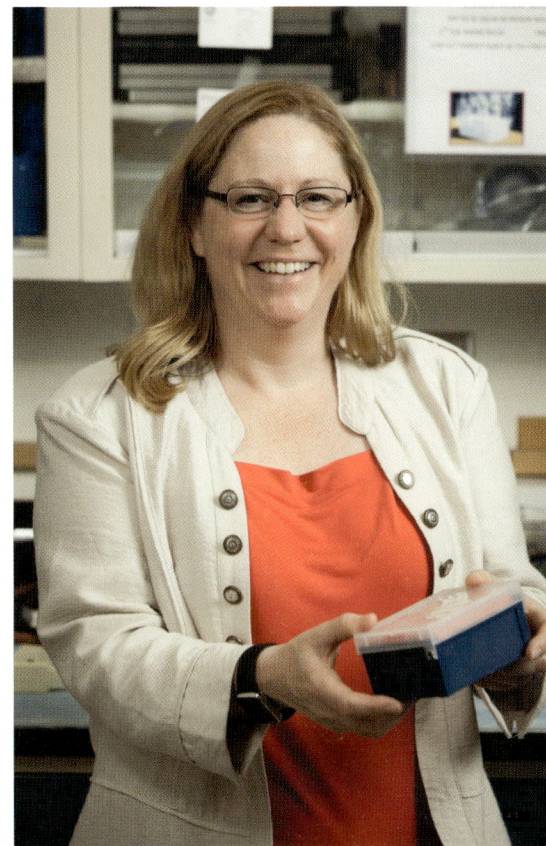
Jannette Dufour, PhD

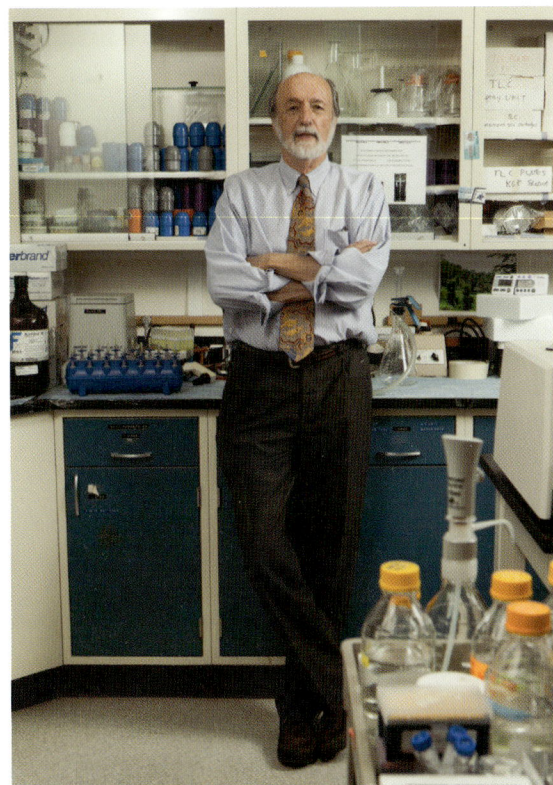
Ted Reid, PhD

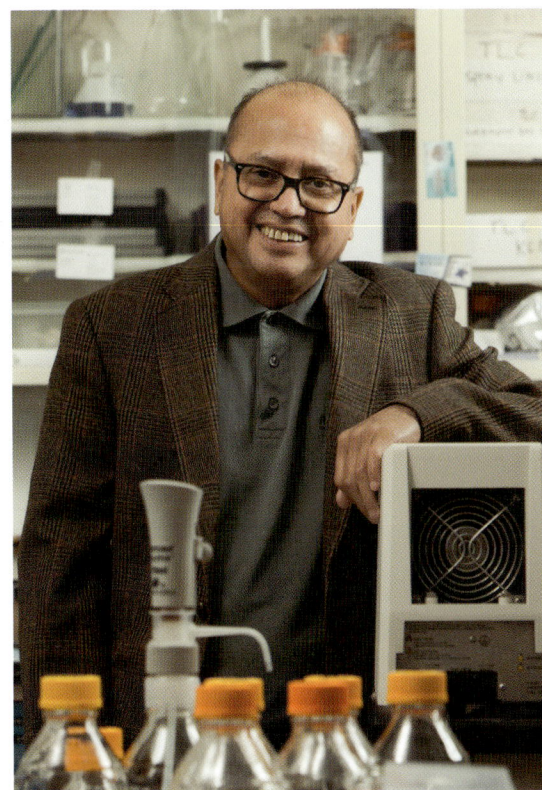
Raul Martinez-Zaguilan, PhD

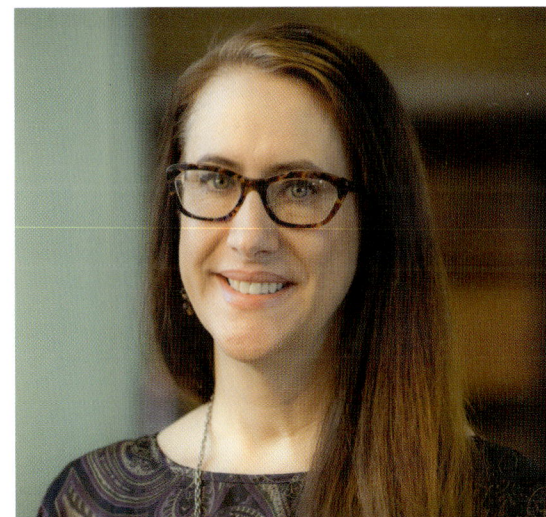
Kendra Rambaugh, PhD
Artie Limmer, Photographer, Associate
Director, Institutional Advancement

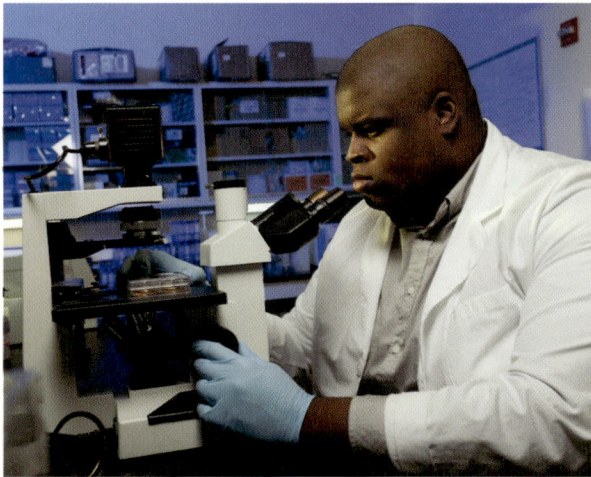

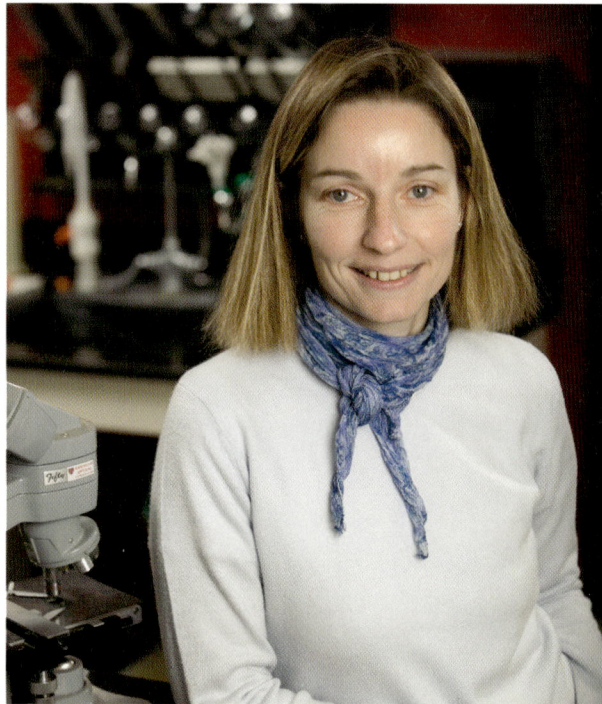

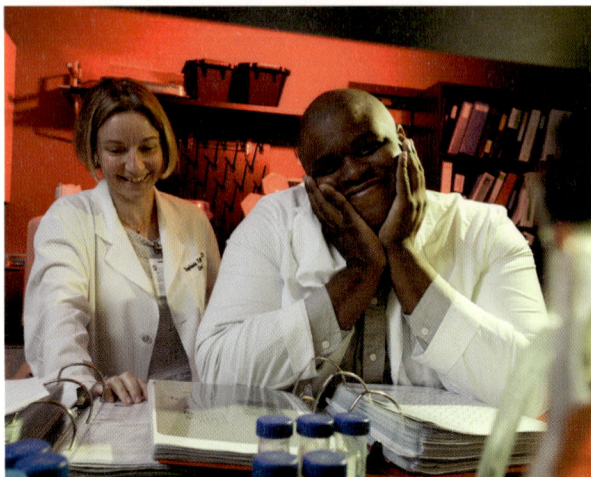

Grad students working in Filleur lab

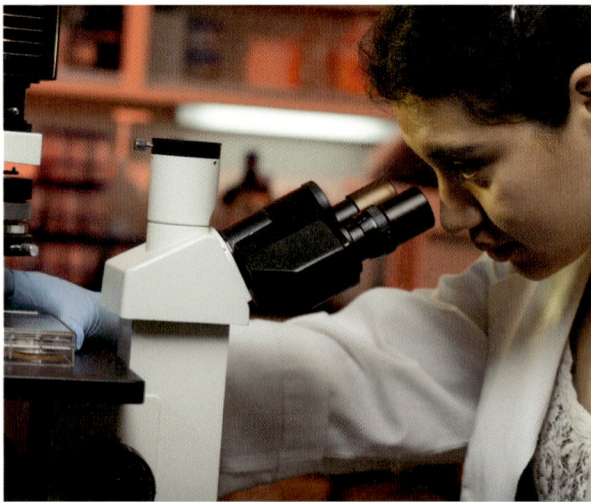

Stephanie Filleur, PhD

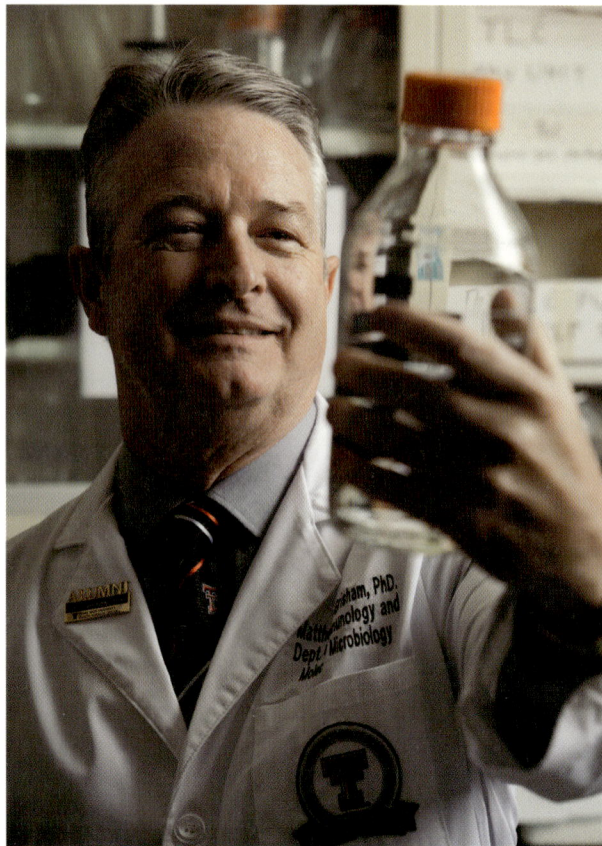

Matthew B. Grisham, PhD, Professor and Chair of the Department of Immunology and Molecular Microbiology

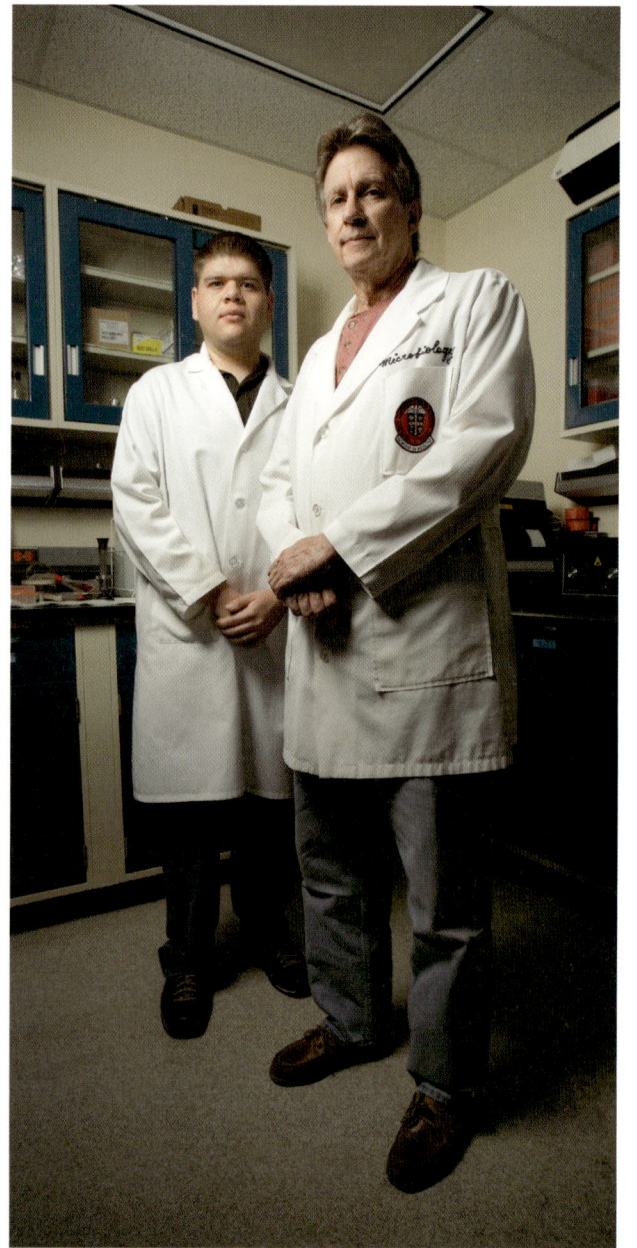

David Strauss, PhD, and associate

Pharmacology and Neuroscience—Volker Neugebauer, M.D., Ph.D., Professor and Chair

The Department of Pharmacology was among the small number of basic science departments when the School of Medicine began, but it has grown steadily as its mission expanded to include the field of neuroscience and the number of faculty in the department doubled by 1993. Under the leadership of Reid Norman, PhD, from 2000–2014, the department became the home of the South Plains Alcohol and Addiction Center. Now, chaired by Volker Neugebauer, MD, PhD, the department is moving from its traditionally strong expertise in the area of alcohol and addiction to pain and related neuropsychiatric disorders. At the same time, it is building bridges to translate this new knowledge to clinical staff with its Center of Excellence for Translational Neuroscience and Therapeutics. The center is well-equipped for collaborative research and training in clinically relevant conditions such as chronic pain, opioid addiction, alcohol abuse disorder, epileptogenesis, and autism.

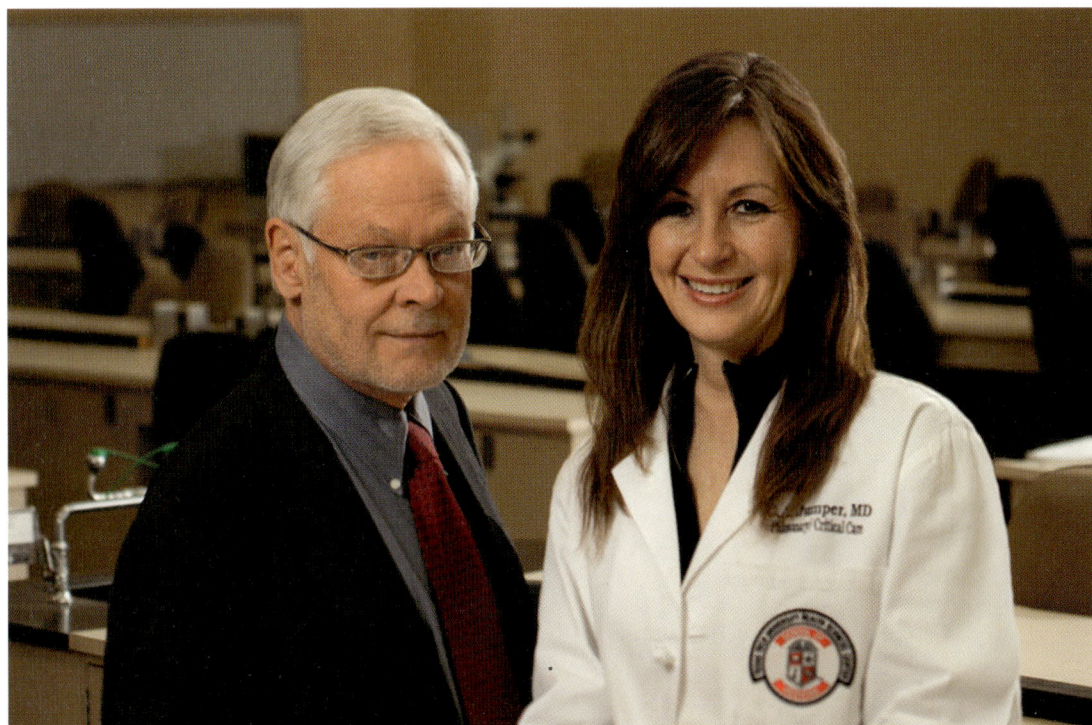

Reid Norman, PhD, and Cynthia Jumper, MD

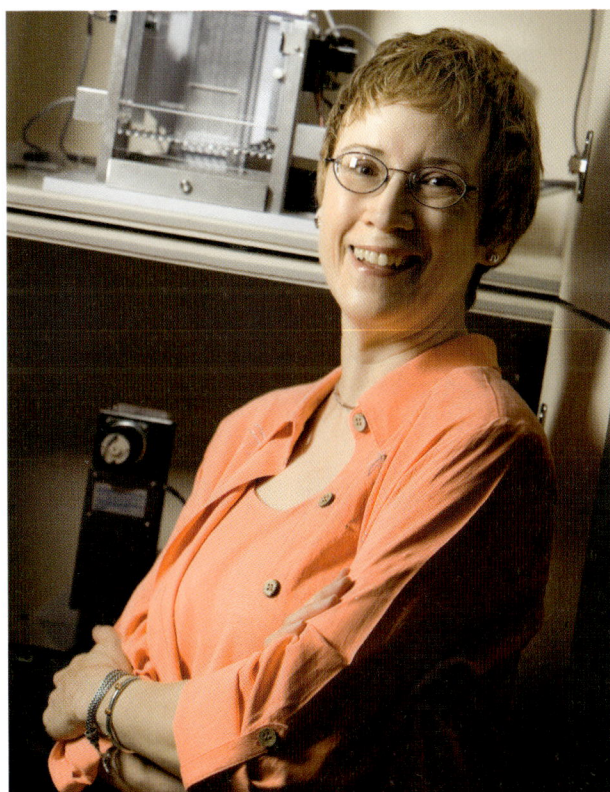

Alice Young, PhD

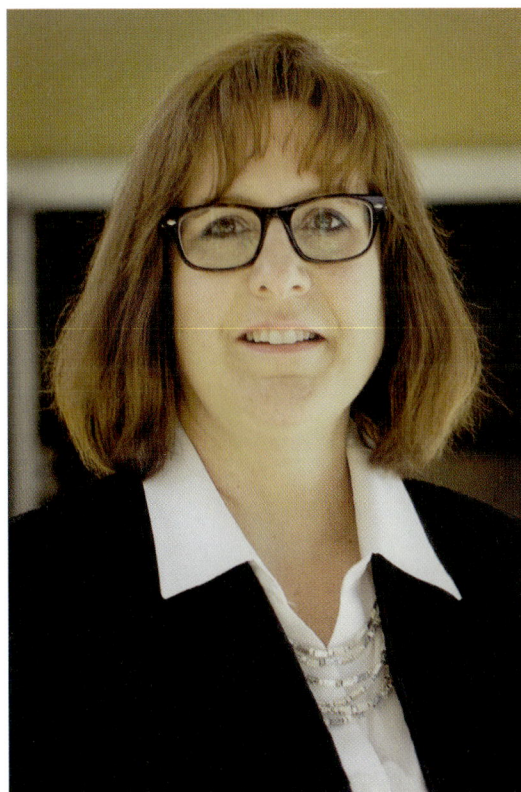

Susan Bergeson, PhD

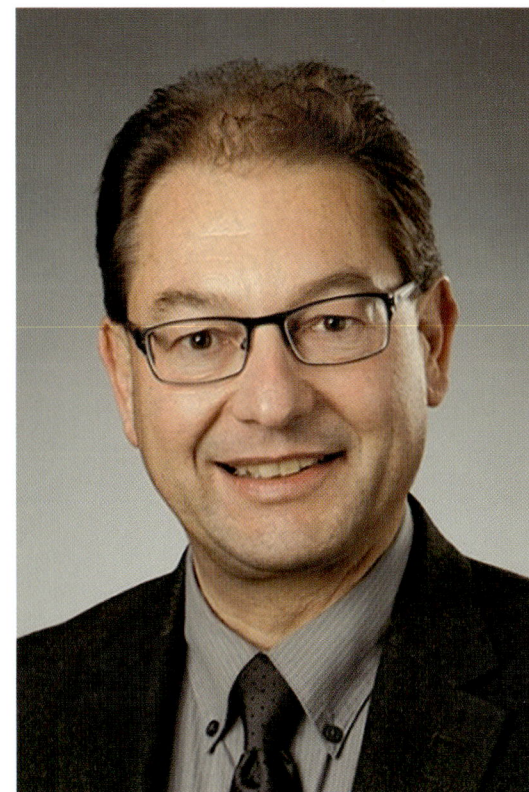

Volker Neugebauer, MD, PhD, Chair

Internal Medicine

The Department of Internal Medicine has provided a strong backbone for the School of Medicine since its inception. This department currently has 29 fellows, 42 residents and 48 full-time faculty, and 139 community faculty. It trains approximately 100 physicians and ancillary healthcare students on a daily basis. Internal Medicine leads the school in publications, size, and budget. The core values of this department are unity and diversity, excellence through innovation, celebration of ownership, and integrity with grace. These values inspire the department's involvement in telemedicine, community outreach, staffing the free clinic, global health electives, interprofessional training, care of veterans, and care of one another. A collaborative spirit has characterized the department in its growth over the years, with faculty, residents, students and staff co-operating in its healing mission. Santhosh Koshy, MD, MBA, was appointed the new chair of internal medicine at TTUHSC in August 2018, following in the tradition of outstanding leadership established by William Holmes, MD, Neil Kurtzman, MD, Don Wesson, MD and Cynthia Jumper, MD, MPH.

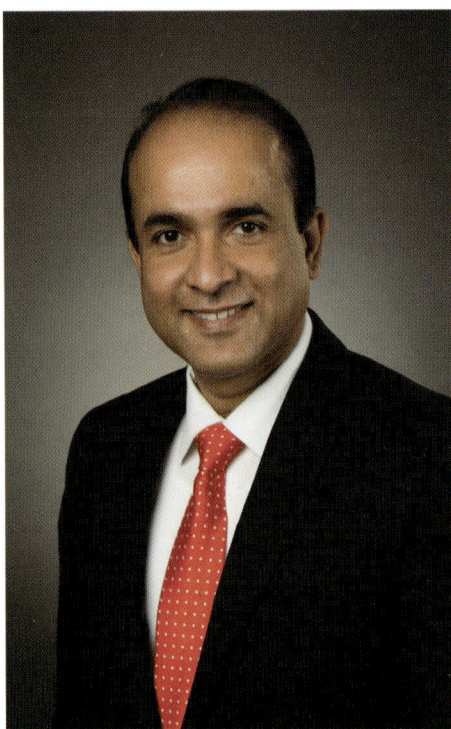

Santhosh Koshy, MD, Chair Internal Medicine

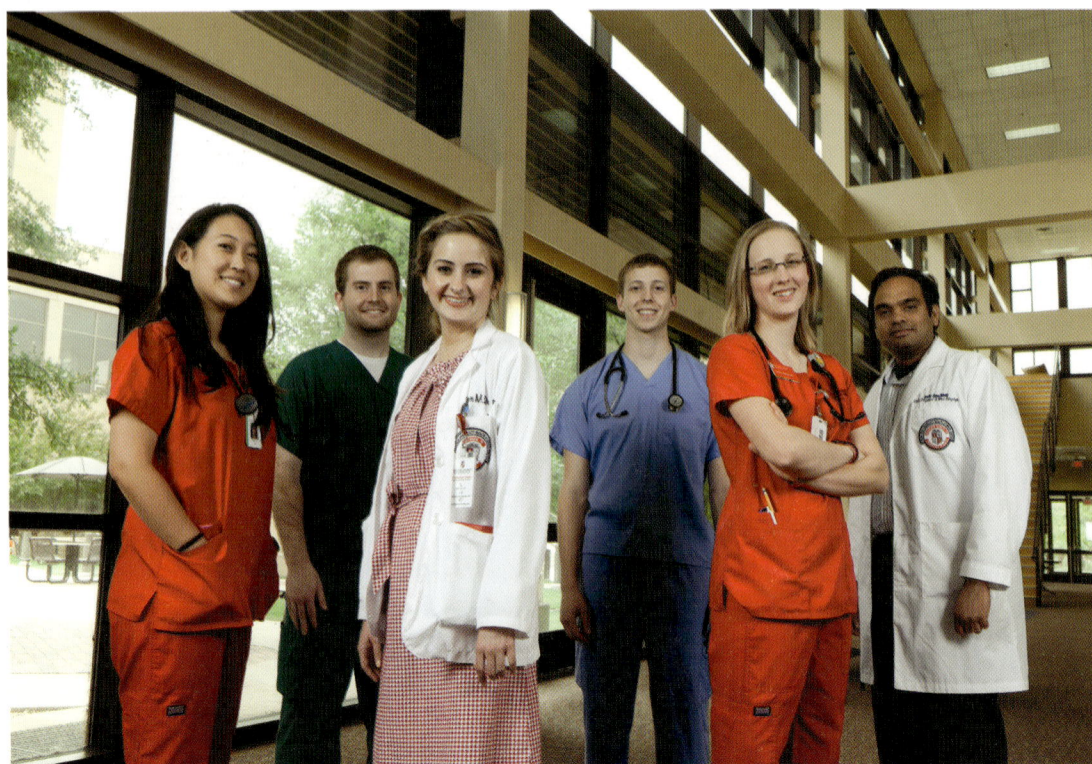

Interprofessional group of students

Dermatology

Barbara Way, MD, was the first chair of dermatology and served from 1976 to 1981. Way and her husband Anthony Way, MD, were founding faculty of the School of Medicine. Craig Urban, MD, who now practices in Abilene, was the first resident in the program and during his first year, 1978–1979, he was the only resident in the program. Between 1977 and 1979, Way built a dermatology faculty with two dermatologists, a dermatopathologist, and a biochemist—some part-time, some full-time. All were involved in teaching, research, and patient care. Way left the department and the School of Medicine near the end of 1981. Without leadership, the department struggled for almost a year and a half and was threatened with loss of both its accreditation and its residency program. In 1983, Kenneth H. Neldner, MD, arrived as chair to put the department back on its feet. Within six months of his arrival, the department was once again accredited and its residency program moving forward. A year later there were 4 faculty members and 4 residents. Beginning in 1983, every full-time chair has been a certified dermatopathologist, including the current chair, Cloyce Stetson, MD, who has led the department since 2005. This allows the department to provide dermatopathology services for biopsies. There are now nine residents and the department sees about 25,000 patients each year.

Obstetrics/Gynecology

The Department of Obstetrics and Gynecology trains physicians and provides high quality obstetric and gynecologic care to its patients. A group of specialists on the faculty serve as role models for students and residents. The subspecialties include maternal fetal medicine, reproductive endocrinology and infertility and gynecologic oncology, and urogynecology. The department also employs an embryologist, a genetic counselor, and a nutritionist for highly specialized needs. The first in vitro fertilization program was established at TTUHSC in 1985 and in 1989 the first "test tube baby" was born. Currently for couples faced with infertility, the state-of-the-art service provided by Drs. Jaou-Chen Huang and Jennifer Phy has enabled hundreds of women to successfully conceive. The program is supported by work in the highly skilled IVF laboratory directed by Sam Prien, PhD, supported by Lindsey Penrose, PhD, and embryologist Khaliq Ahmad.

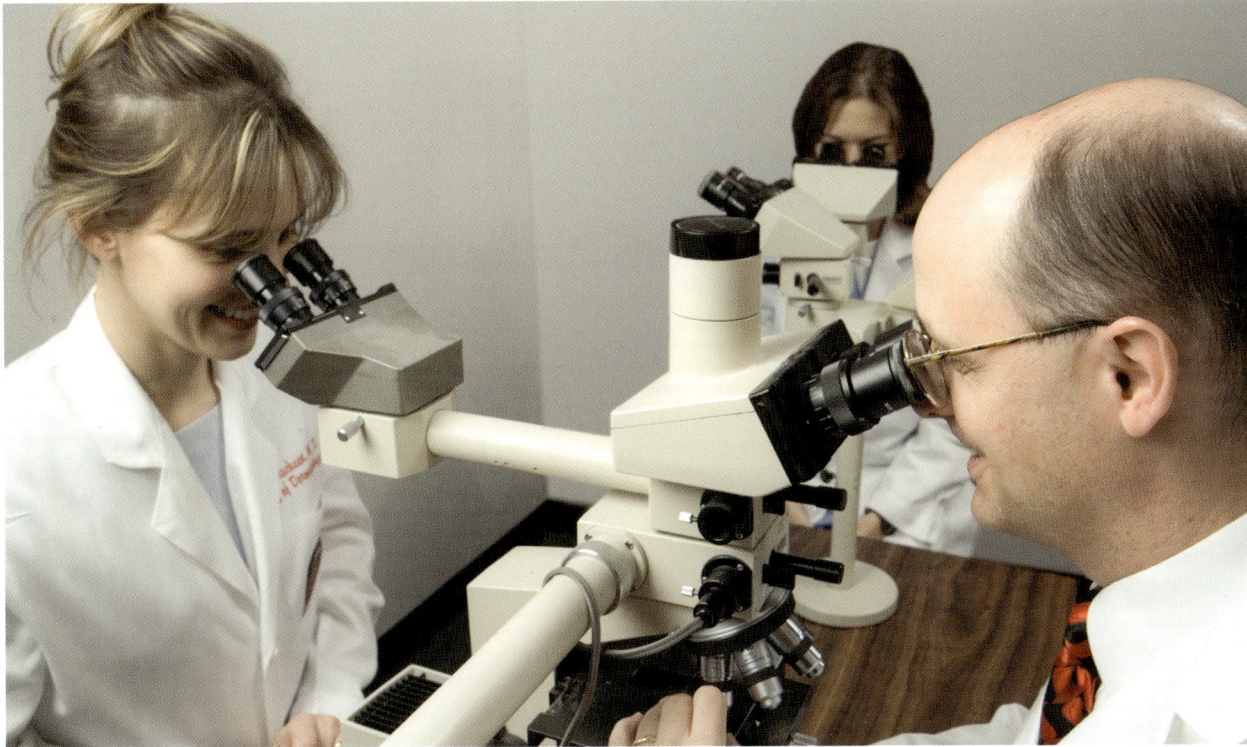

Cloyce Stetson, MD, Chair Department of Dermatology and colleagues

The department has enjoyed significant growth in its clinical teaching and research activities since its inception and this growth has been built on exemplary collaboration between administration, faculty, residents, students, and staff. A succession of chairs, particularly Edward Yeomans, MD, the current chair, has provided excellent support of this growth. Many women have survived high risk pregnancies and delivered healthy babies due to Yeomans' expertise. He has trained many residents who are now sound practicing physicians and represent his legacy.

Surgery

The Department of Surgery has been a vibrant and vital part of the school of medicine. It grew under the nurturing of many chairs, among them Peter Canizaro, MD, and John Griswold, MD, just to name two. It has built one of the strongest trauma, burn, and acute care programs in the country. The current chair is Sharmila Dissanaike, MD. TTUHSC's Level-I trauma center is the most geographically isolated one in the country, with the nearest other centers being in Dallas, Albuquerque, and Tulsa. It is life-saving work because trauma is now the number one killer of children and young adults. In 1985,

a burn center was added. It is the only American Burn Association–accredited burn center in a 300-mile radius, providing essential care to burn patients from West Texas and eastern New Mexico, and extending to Oklahoma, El Paso, and internationally via the Timothy J. Harnar Regional Burn Center. The Surgery Department also has become a designated training center for Robotic Surgery and Fundamentals of Laparoscopic Surgery accreditation. In 2015, the department created the Burn Center of Research Excellence to focus its research primarily on injury, wounds, biofilm, necrotizing soft tissue infections, and other surgical infection, as it collaborates with TTUHSC's Clinical Research Institute. The Department of Surgery is recognized within the medical school for the outstanding teaching it provides for medical students and other healthcare professionals. The encouragement which the faculty and staff provide for young researchers is exemplary and most appreciated.

Pathology

TTUHSC's Pathology Department studies the cause, progression, and indicators of disease—seen by examination and under the microscope. The department's nine

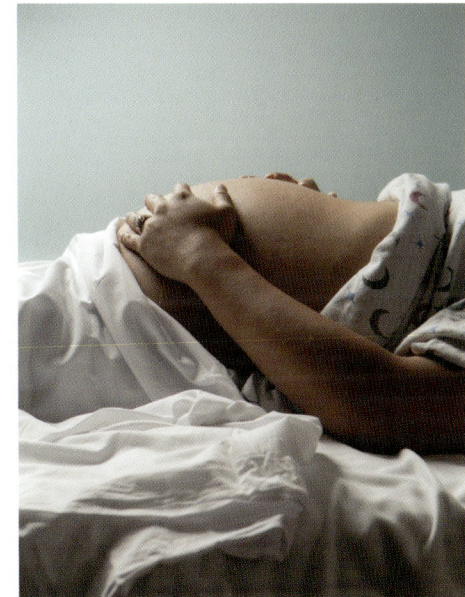

Pregnant mother

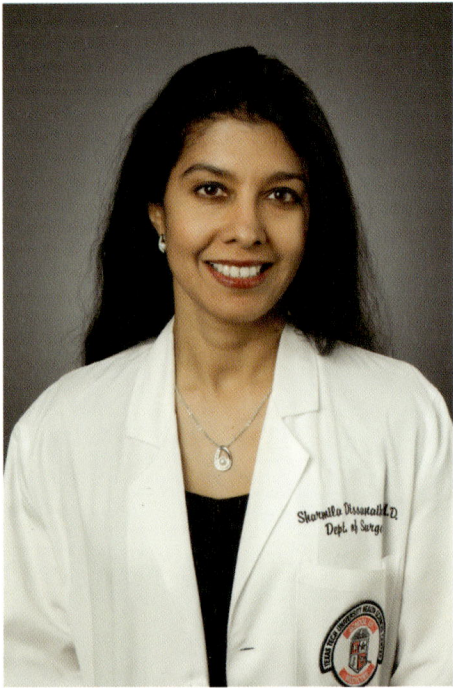

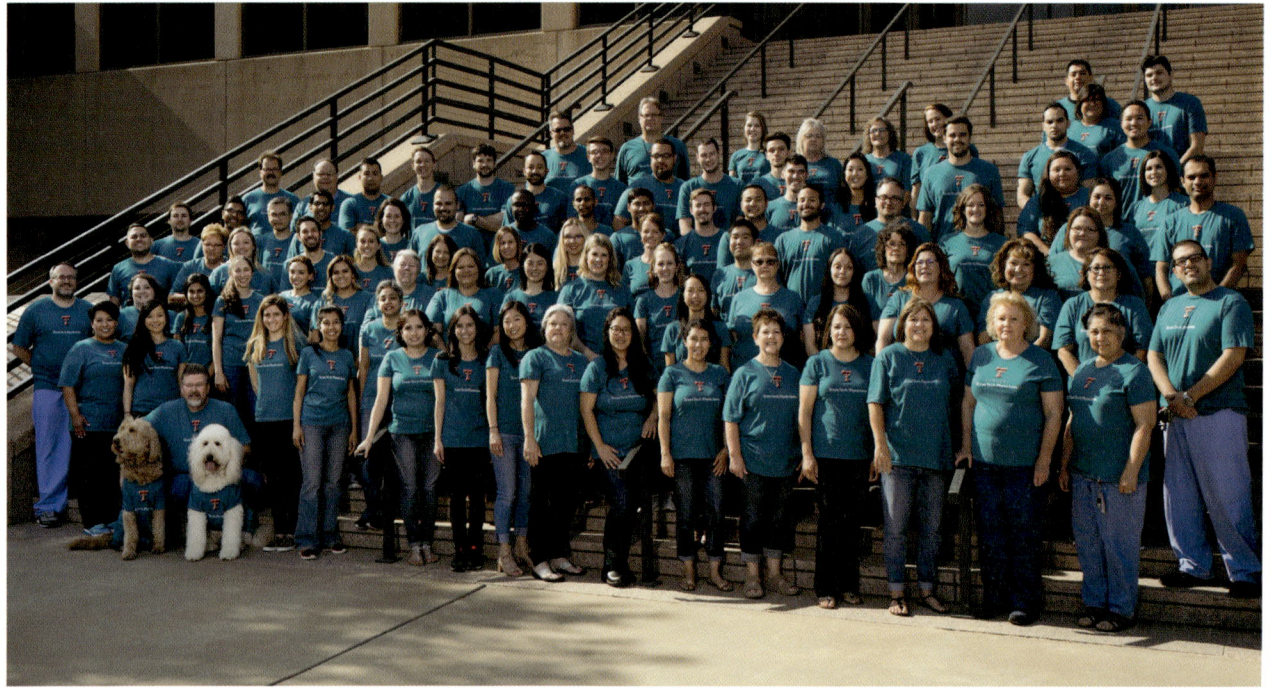

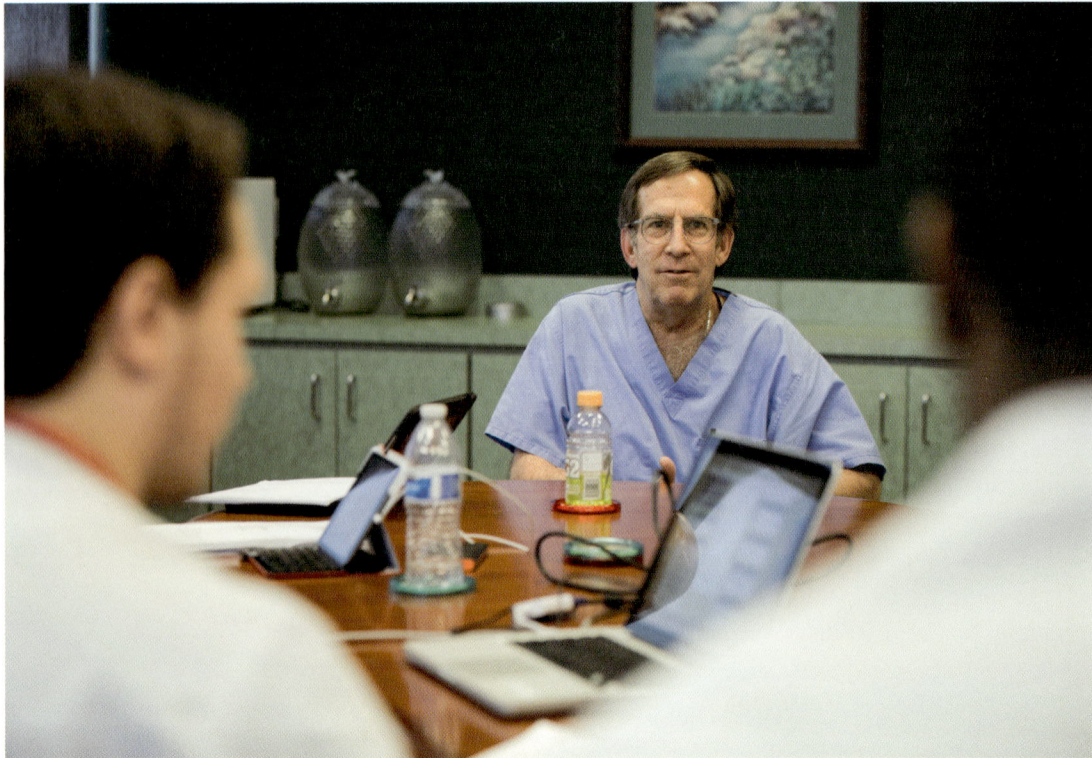

Helicopter bringing in trauma patient.
Margaret Vugrin, Photographer

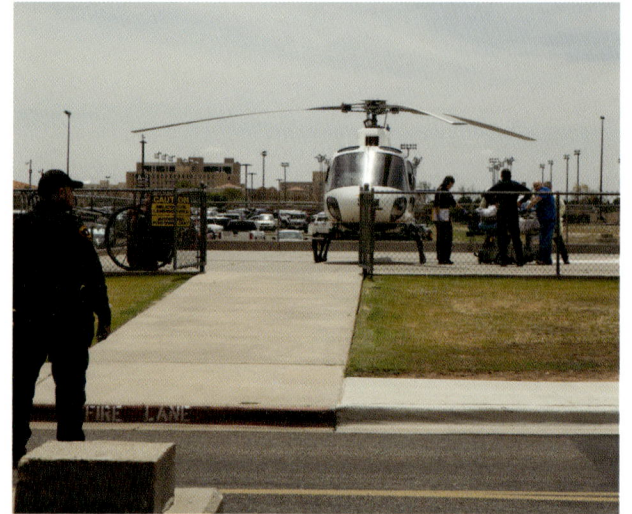

(TOP LEFT) Sharmila Dissanaike, MD,
Chair Department of Surgery

(TOP RIGHT) Department of
Surgery—2018

(BOTTOM LEFT) John Griswold, MD

pathologists are faculty who teach medical students and provide consultation and pathology services to healthcare providers. The pathologists also are actively involved in research. Pathologists are called on to examine tissue samples collected during surgery or other types of procedures and provide valuable diagnostic information to the treating physicians and surgeons to find the most effective, efficient, and timely patient care possible. Pathologists can test peripheral blood and bone marrow aspirates and biopsies under a microscope to determine if there is any problem with the patient's blood such as anemia or leukemia, for example. Clinical microbiology, another division of clinical pathology, identifies any organism that could be causing an infection in a patient such as bacteria, virus, fungus, or parasite. For a bacterial infection, clinical microbiology also tests to determine what would be the best antimicrobial therapy to fight the infection. Dale Dunn, MD has provided outstanding leadership for the department over many years; in addition, Dunn has served with distinction in many leadership positions in the School of Medicine.

Psychiatry

The Department of Psychiatry, part of the medical school since its foundation, addresses the needs of persons and families experiencing mental illness. In addition the department has a long history of dealing with substance use disorders and their consequences. It has enjoyed a close association with St. Mary's Hospital of the Plains, now part of the Covenant Health System. The department has also supported programs addressing the spiritual and religious needs of patients and families, resulting in 2012 in the emergence of the Center for Ethics, Humanities and Spirituality, for which Thomas McGovern, EdD, served in a leadership role. Don Flinn, MD, and Richard Weddige, MD provided excellent direction in the development of the educational, clinical, and community outreach initiatives during their tenure as chairs of the department. Neurology and Psychiatry were combined into one department by David Smith, MD, in 1998 in an effort to strengthen the Department of Neurology. When neurology and psychiatry were again separated in 2008, Terry McMahon, MD, became the chair of the Psychiatry. Over the last decade, he has expanded the department to include 10 faculty members, who train the typical number of five residents. Under McMahon's leadership, new

faculty were recruited in adult and child/adolescent psychiatry. At the same time, the nursing staff in the outpatient clinic, together with other healthcare professionals, physician assistants, nurse practitioners, counselors, and psychologists, enabled the department to meet the needs of patients and their families while enhancing the educational mission of the department. Recently a postgraduate fellowship in psychiatry for advanced practice providers was added under the leadership of McMahon and Phyllis Peterson, PA, and it continues successful growth. Since its beginning, the Department of Psychiatry has housed and supported the Southwest Institute for Addictive Diseases (SWIAD) and the Employee Assistance Program (EAP). It also hosts two ambulatory clinical systems: one devoted to general psychiatry and the other to child and adolescent psychiatry. The department's physicians provide services that include chemical dependency counseling, marriage and family counseling, psychiatry, and psychology.

Neurology

What is currently known as the Department of Neurology had many growing pains. Initially under Paul Meyer, MD, in 1977 it was called the Department of Medical and Surgical Neurology. Joseph Green, MD was the first chair

Terry McMahon, MD, Chair, Department of Psychiatry

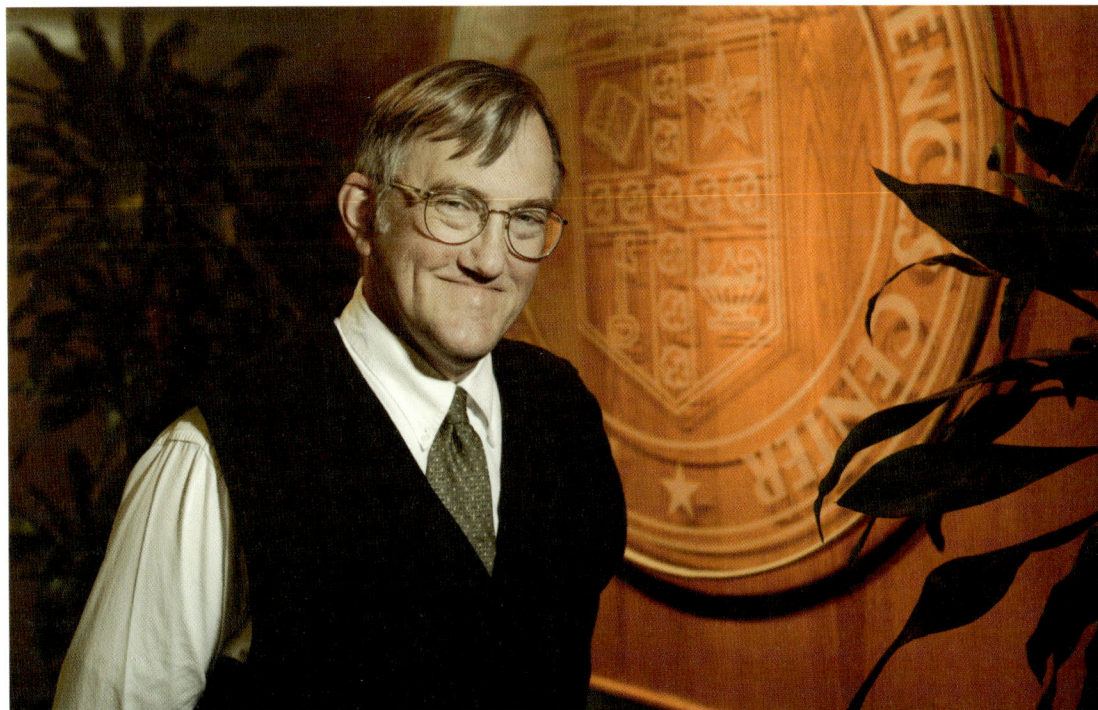

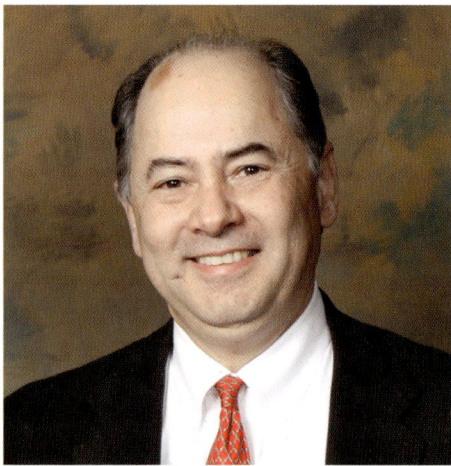

John De Toledo, MD, Chair Department of Neurology

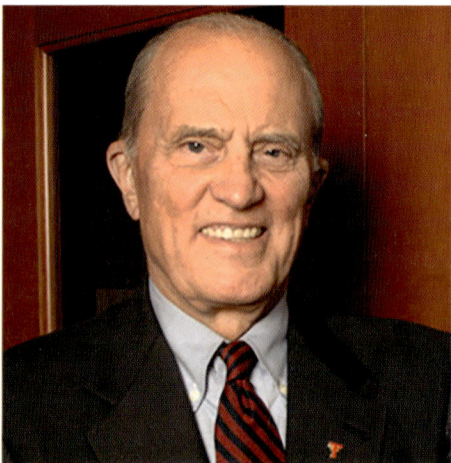

Bernhard T. Mittemeyer, MD

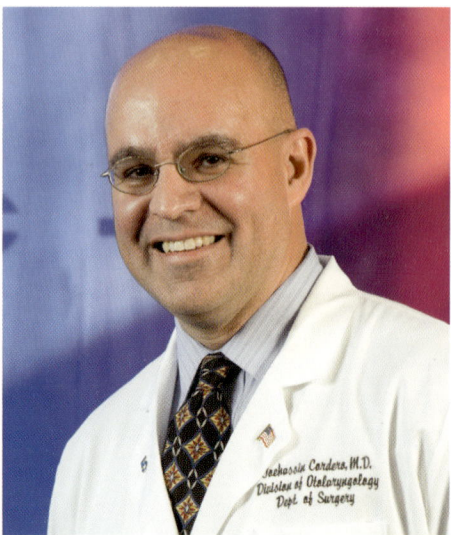

Joehassin Cordero, MD, Chair Department of Otolaryngology

of the Neurology Department at TTUHSC and started the neurology residency program in 1989–1990. He was followed in 1994 by Richard W. Homan, MD. On Dr. Homan's retirement, David Smith, MD, the new president of TTUHSC decided to merge the departments of Neurology and Psychiatry in an effort to strengthen the department of Neurology. They were merged into a new Department of Neuropsychiatry under Randolph Schiffer, MD, the first chair of this department. Upon Dr. Schiffer's departure in 2008, the Board of Regents, the president, and the dean of the medical school approved the reinstatement of a separate Department of Neurology and its own neurology residency program at TTUHSC School of Medicine. Terry McMahon, MD, was appointed chair of the Department of Psychiatry and in 2009 John C. De-Toledo, MD, was recruited from Wake Forest University to become the fourth chair of the newly reconstituted Department of Neurology. Also in 2009, a Texas Tech neurology residency was approved; the program trains three adult-focused neurologists each year. The residency in neurology, a collaboration with Covenant Medical Center, has been another success story for Texas Tech. All trainees have passed their boards and many have gone to work in prestigious institutions, including Harvard, Mayo Clinic, UCSF, Vanderbilt, and the various schools of medicine of the University of Texas System.

Urology

There was no Department of Urology at TTUHSC when Bernhard T. Mittemeyer, MD, a former surgeon general of the U.S. Army, arrived in Lubbock in 1986. As former chief of Urology at Walter Reed Hospital, he recognized the need for urologic care to continue the growth of the medical school and to provide suitable training for students and residents. From 1990 until 2006 urology was a division in the Department of Surgery, with a faculty size that varied from one to four. After serving as TTUHSC's executive vice president, Dr. Mittemeyer returned to urology services in 1996. Mittemeyer and Werner de Riese, MD, who joined the division in 1998, thought that ultimately the school and community would need a separate Department of Urology with a complete residency program to train and attract new urologists. The Board of Regents approved the concept and the Department of Urology was officially established in July 2006. Before year's end, three new faculty members had joined the

team, providing the foundation for the basic science research program. David Van Buren, MD, a renal transplant surgeon, also joined as full-time faculty. Under the leadership of Dr. de Riese, department chair, and Jonathan Vordermark, MD, as vice chair and program director, the urology residency program was approved by the Urology Residency Review Committee and began in 2007. Since then the program, starting with one resident a year, has now produced seven fully trained graduates in urology who are all in active practice. The department anticipates adding a second resident position in the next few years.

Otolaryngology

In the late 1990s, John Griswold, MD, the then new chair of TTUHSC's Department of Surgery, wanted to expand the practice of otolaryngology, or medical care of the ear, nose, and throat, which then was minimal. He hired Joehassin Cordero, MD, as faculty and chief of the new division of otolaryngology within his department. By September 2015, it was clear that creating departmental status for otolaryngology would enhance the ability to attract faculty of differing subspecialties to the institution, allowing it to advance medical knowledge, to grow and to thrive. Steven Berk, MD, executive vice president and dean, requested departmental status for the specialization. Establishing otolaryngology as a separate department demonstrated TTUHSC's commitment to support for this area for a future residency program. Upon approval in April 2017, Dr. Cordero was named chairman. During the fall of 2017, the department underwent its first interview process for the 2018 otolaryngology residents. Today, every cochlear and bone-anchored hearing aid (BAHA) implant procedure completed in the greater West Texas region is handled by this team. Because TTUHSC is a Level-I Trauma Center, this department provides care for all maxillofacial trauma cases in the region. The department performs dozens of different surgeries from tonsillectomies to trans-oral robotic surgery.

Ophthalmology

The School of Medicine's Department of Ophthalmology was established in 1971 along with other medical specialties at the school's founding. Early on, James Price, MD, PhD, was recruited from Tufts Medical School to serve as the chair of ophthalmology. During his 14 years at the

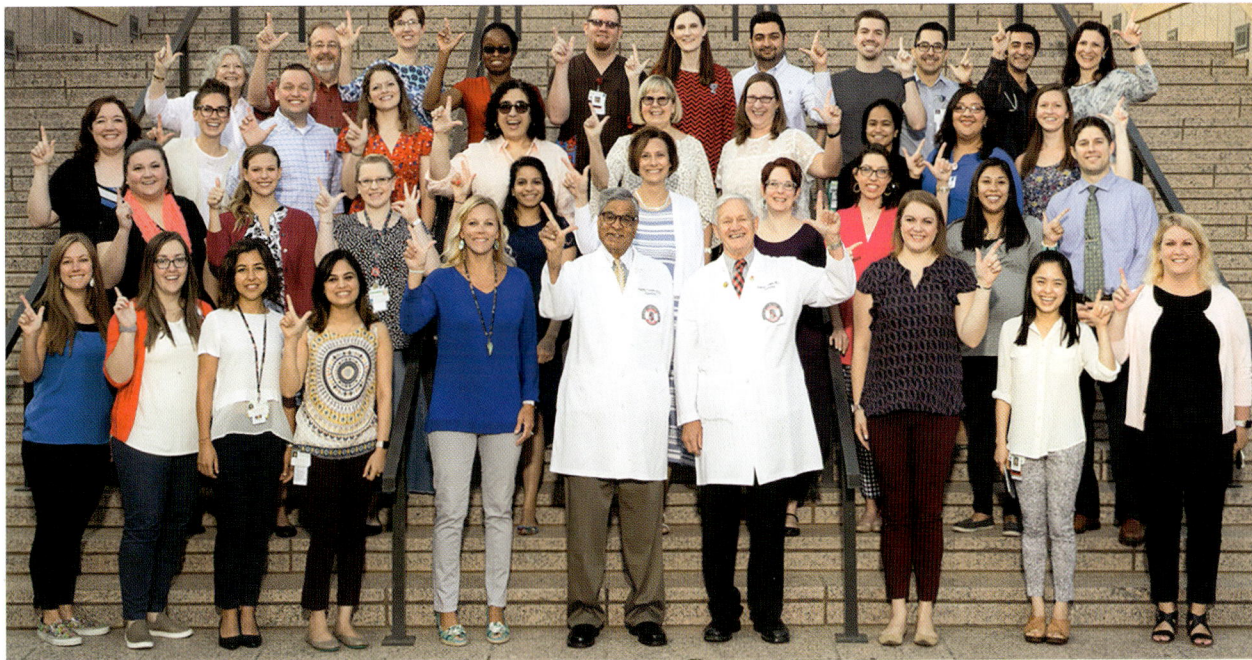

Surendra Varma, MD, and Richard Lampe, MD, Chair Department of Pediatrics (center) surrounded by departmental faculty and staff

helm, Price created the residency training program and built the clinical and research faculty. Another legacy of Price's leadership includes the Great Plains Lions Eye Bank, created in cooperation with regional Lions Clubs. The Eye Bank aids residents' training by providing tissue samples for microsurgery practice. In 1989, Donald R. May, MD, was appointed chairman. He prioritized research, increased the number of basic science faculty members, and advocated successfully to upgrade surgical equipment at UMC. In 1994, David McCartney, MD, succeeded May as chairman. At the time, the department's clinical faculty members had dropped to three full-time members; however, an additional five faculty members were recruited in the next two years, providing a teaching faculty with fellowship-trained, faculty members in all the major clinical subspecialties. Today, the department has 108 residents and fellow alumni. It has provided training for thousands of medical students and is well recognized for its tertiary-level, clinical care in a large region bounded by the cities of Tucson, Albuquerque, Denver, Oklahoma City, the Dallas–Ft. Worth metroplex, and San Antonio.

Pediatrics

The Department of Pediatrics is dedicated to the provision of the highest standard of medical care for pediatric patients from birth through adolescence, encompassing primary, subspecialty, and tertiary care. It serves as an advocate for pediatric health issues affecting the infants, children, and adolescents of our region and state. The department offers an interprofessional model of child and family care which encompasses the physical, mental, and spiritual well-being of its patients. It serves all of West Texas and the neighboring counties of New Mexico and Oklahoma with excellent care and support.

The care of children is a challenging undertaking, especially when the well-being of children is compromised by abuse and neglect. The pioneering work of Patti Patterson, MD, MPH, in addressing the needs of these children is exemplary and the Center for Superheroes exemplifies the dedication of the department to the special needs of these children. In addition, the department provides specialty and subspecialty care for neonates thru clinical and hospital services. Fortunato Perez-Benavides, MD, and other team members of the neonatal intensive care unit have saved many babies from disability and untimely death due to the passion and caring that they have for these smallest patients.

Over the years, the department has been ably led by Richard Lampe, MD, chair and succeeded through the integrated efforts of physicians, nurses, psychologists, and other healthcare professionals. Lampe states, "As a Medical School Department of Pediatrics, we practice real world pediatrics in a variety of ambulatory sites and inpatient facilities (Children's Hospitals) with a broad range of pediatric medical and surgical subspecialists."

Orthopaedic Surgery and Rehabilitation

The Department of Orthopaedic Surgery and Rehabilitation (DOSR) was founded in 1971 under the Chairmanship of J. Ted Hartman, MD. Dr. Hartman served as chair until 1982 when he became Dean of the School of Medicine. Since that time the department has been under the leadership of Gerald S. Laros, MD (1984–1989), Eugene J. Dabezies, MD (1991–2004), and Robert J. Schutt, MD (2004–2010); it is presently under the leadership of George W. Brindley, MD. The department has eleven faculty physicians who are fellowship trained in children's orthopaedics, foot and ankle surgery, hand and microvascular surgery, joint reconstruction, musculoskeletal oncology, and sports medicine and trauma. The department serves the populace of the South Plains region of West Texas, Eastern New Mexico, and Western Oklahoma. In addition, the department has an outstanding record of research publications.

The DOSR has been fortunate to be the benefactor of five endowed chairs with financial support for education, research, and patient care, including the Edward L. Haney, MD, and Mabel Faver Haney Endowed Chair, the Underwood Families Endowed Chair in Pediatric Orthopaedic Surgery, the L. Shannon Holloway, MD, PhD, Endowed Chair in Orthopaedic Surgery to be used in support of research within the department, the Ted Hartman, MD, Endowed Chair in Orthopaedic Surgery, and the Eugene Dabezies, MD, Endowed Chair in Orthopaedic Surgery. These endowed chairs have been funded by grateful patients who have benefited from the care provided by the DOSR as well as dedicated faculty who contributed in countless ways to its overall growth and success. We currently have 15 residents in our five-year residency program and are excited to add an additional fourth resident each year beginning in July 2019. The DOSR provides patient care and education at three clinical locations—Orthopaedics at the Medical Pavilion, the Orthopaedic Hand Center in UMC's Medical Office Building II, and Covenant Children's Medical Office Building. These busy practices saw close to 30,000 patient visits in fiscal year 2018. We look forward to serving the growing community in years to come.

Family & Community Medicine

The Department of Family & Community Medicine was a vibrant part of the School of Medicine from the school's inception. Early leadership in the development of the department was provided by Gayle Stephens, MD, Lester Wolcott, MD, and Orene Peddicord, MD. Wolcott made a significant contribution in acquiring federal funding to ensure the growth of the department. From the beginning the department developed a very close relationship with the Lubbock community which expressed itself in a variety of outreach clinics and in a close affiliations with the local hospitals, especially St. Mary's of the Plains. A collaborative spirit continues to inform the relationship between the department and University Medical Center and the Covenant Health System. The department is noted for the excellent academic and clinical training it provides for medical students and residents. As the medical school was reorganized, preventive medicine and occupational medicine were incorporated into the department. Fellowship training programs in sports medicine, geriatrics, and hospice and palliative care also became part of the clinical and academic program. A further responsibility was assigned to the department when it became responsible for the management of the TTU student health service, now housed in a new student health building since 2007. It was the first department to adopt an electronic medical record and pioneered this important addition to the clinical life of the school. The development of the Family Medicine Accelerated Track (FMAT) program has earned the department and the school a national reputation. Its history and achievements are related in other portions of this book. The relationship between the administration, faculty, staff, residents, students, patients, and families is in keeping with the practice of medicine at its best with a spirit of care for body, mind, and spirit. Various chairs have provided excellent leadership for the department from its inception, including Berry N. Squyres, MD, 1978–1987, Theodore Kantner, MD, 1978–1992, Richard Homan, MD, 1994–2001, Mike Ragain, MD, 2001–2011, Ronald L. Cook, DO, 2011–present.

Anesthesiology

The Department of Anesthesiology has made outstanding contributions to the life of the Texas Tech University Health Sciences Center from the very beginning. It is

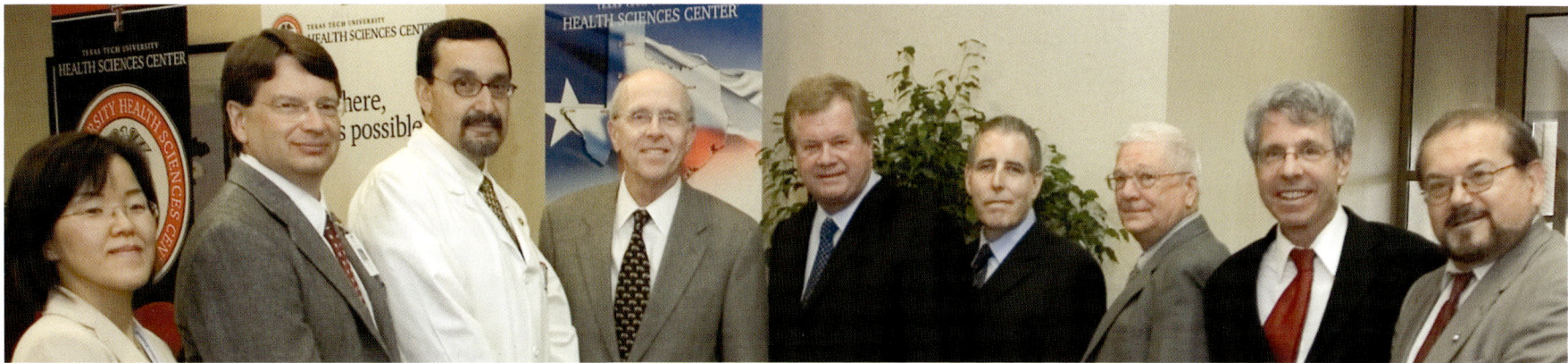

Min Kang, PharmD; Barry Maurer, MD, PhD; Everardo Cobos, MD; Chancellor Hance; John Baldwin, MD, TTUHSC President; Patrick Reynolds, MD, PhD; Harry Weilauf, PhD; Steven Berk, MD, Dean SOM; and Davor Vugrin, MD. Margaret Vugrin, Photographer

recognized as a top ranked general and subspecialty service and a regional leader in anesthesiology education and perioperative scientific research. The Department includes anesthesiologists, certified registered anesthetists, anesthesiology residents, and anesthetists in training. The department provides specialty care in cardiac anesthesia, pediatric anesthesiologists, critical care medicine, pain medicine, and obstetrical anesthesia service. It maintains active training programs in anesthesia and pain medicine. Members of the department can be found throughout University Medical Center providing care in the endoscopy suite, cardiac catheterization laboratory, the labor and delivery suite, the emergency department, the critical care units, and of course the operating rooms. It contributes to the education of medical students, advanced nurse practitioners, and other health care professionals. The department looks forward to the next fifty years of care for and education of the people of Texas.

Over the years the department has distinguished itself with its outstanding research output, recognized for its excellence at the national and international levels. The international reputation earned by Gabor Racz, MD, and the late James Heavner PhD, DVM, in the areas of interventional pain management merits special recognition. The department fosters a harmonious environment in which to carry out quality clinical care, educational activities, scholarly pursuits, and administrative responsibilities. It supports the training and skills advancement of the administrative staff who coordinate the activities of the department in an excellent fashion. The current Chair, John D. Wasnick, MD, PMH provides excellent leadership for the department.

The Cancer Center—
C. Patrick Reynolds, MD, PhD, Director

The School of Medicine's Cancer Center originated in 2008 to improve cancer research and cancer care in the region. The center is organized into three programs: Cancer Prevention, led by Theresa Byrd, PhD; Developmental Therapeutics, led by Barry J. Maurer, MD, PhD; and Clinical Oncology, led by Sanjay Awasthi, MD. Their research is funded by the National Cancer Institute, the Cancer Prevention and Research Institute of Texas, the Department of Defense, and foundations. The Cancer Prevention program investigators have been instrumental in establishing robust cancer screening programs for breast cancer and colorectal cancer in West Texas. Their collaborative work with the Lubbock Colon Cancer Prevention Taskforce led by Davor Vugrin, MD, has introduced the importance of colon cancer screening in Lubbock and the West Texas region. The Cancer Center also sponsors a clinical consortium, the South Plains Oncology Consortium (SPOC), which also carries out clinical trials on investigational drugs in adults and children with cancer. SPOC clinical trials study both industry-sponsored drugs and investigational drugs developed by TTUHSC faculty. The work by the Cancer Center in bringing clinical trials of novel therapies to West Texas provides an important and not previously available access to cutting-edge clinical trials for cancer patients in our region. The consortium serves as a vehicle for collaboration with more than 20 institutions.

Medical Education—Betsy Jones, EdD, Chair

Betsy Jones, EdD, was appointed first chair of the Department of Medical Education (DOME) in 2013. DOME is

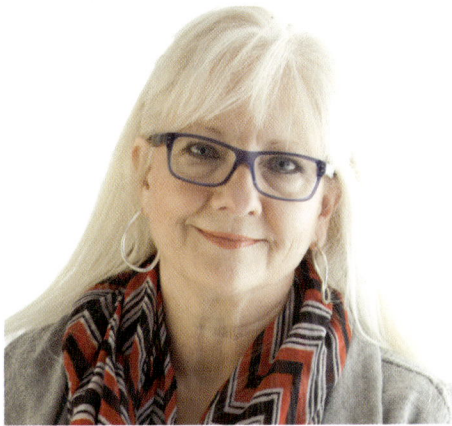

Betsy Jones, EdD, Chair DOME.
Margaret Vugrin, Photographer

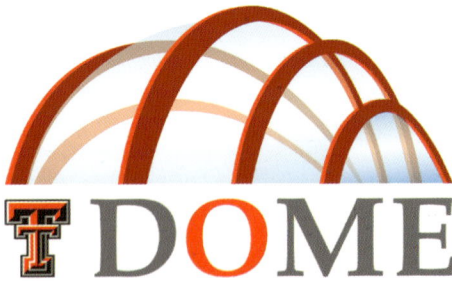

DOME—Department of Medical Education,
Logo

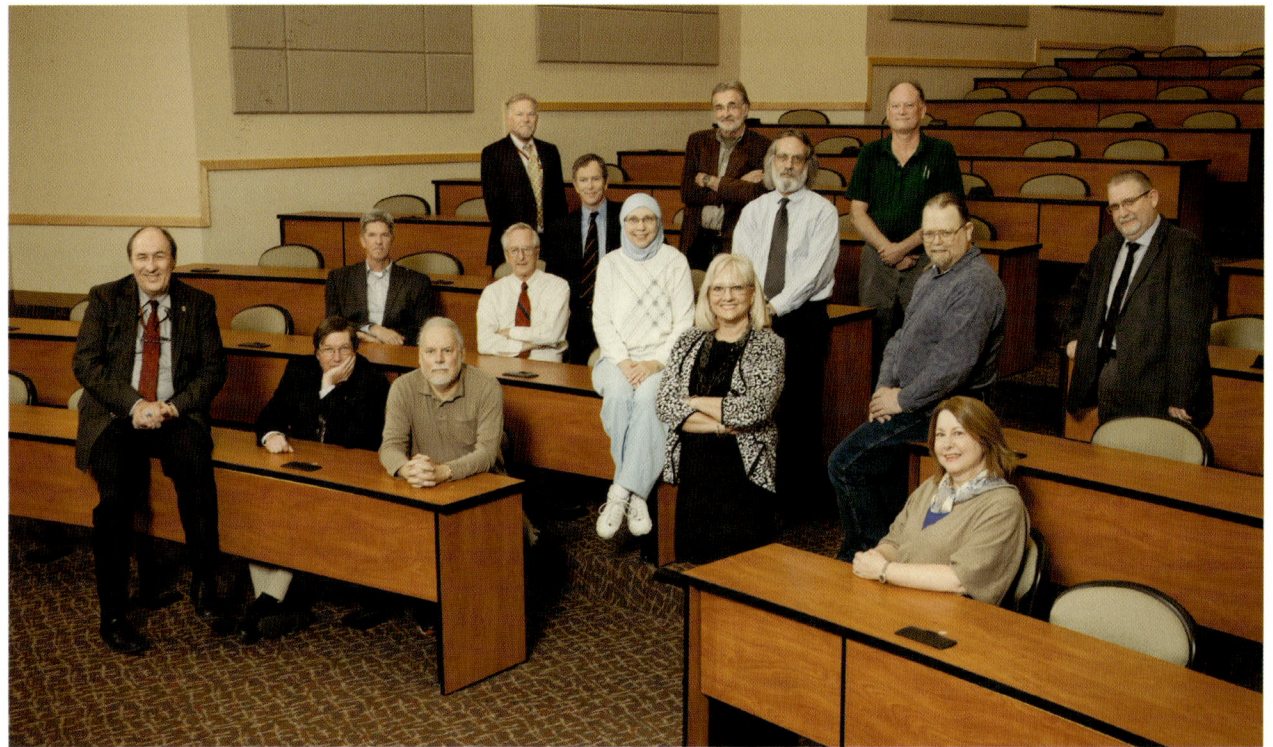

DOME—Department of Medical Education, Faculty

the academic home for faculty with primary responsibility for the first- and second-year curriculum. All current block directors and co-directors have a primary or joint appointment in the DOME. It is also home to the Family Medicine Accelerated Track in the TTUHSC School of Medicine. The department and its faculty members work closely with the Office of Academic Affairs and the Office of Student Affairs within the School of Medicine Academic Affairs and Faculty Affairs and Development, with many members serving on the Educational Policy Committee, the Educational Operating Committee, the Student Affairs Committee, and the Student Promotions and Professional Conduct Committee.

In addition, the Department of Medical Education includes both Educational Media Services and the Division of Anatomical Sciences, which further includes the Willed Body Program. Both of these offices and groups of faculty and staff transitioned to the department from their previous home in the Department of Cell Biology and Biochemistry.

Since the department's creation, it has acquired the nickname "The DOME," as a fond reference to the acronym formed by its name, Department of Medical Education. As the DOME grows and matures, we anticipate living up to our nickname by providing a refuge, a support, a source of inspiration, and an example of aspiration for excellence in medical education, just as do the beloved architectural domes throughout the world.

Betsy Jones, EdD, has been the guiding force behind the P3-C Week. The P3-C course is conducted primarily in one-week sessions before or between basic sciences in the first and second years of medical school. Both years share the final week of the year (P3-C Week) held in March. P3-C Week is designed to mirror an academic conference, with a full menu (around 80 sessions in all) of clinical workshops, breakout sessions, small group discussion sessions, poster sessions, and keynote presentations that allow students to choose sessions that fit their personal and professional interests. In most years, P3-C and Student Research Week are the same week, providing further opportunities for the TTUHSC community to engage with nationally known researchers and to share the fruits of their own scholarly efforts. The overarching goals for the P3-C Week are to prepare students to learn medicine at the bedside and to help students gain the knowledge and skills necessary to understand and influence factors affecting the health of their patients.

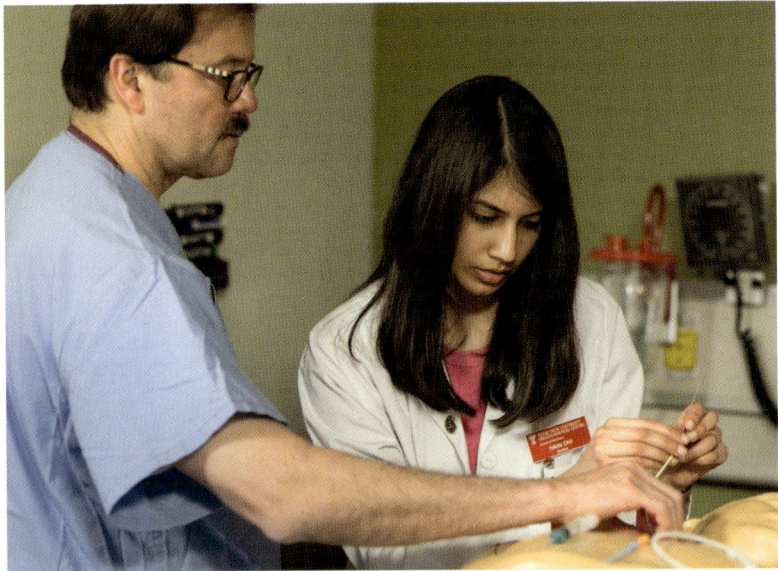

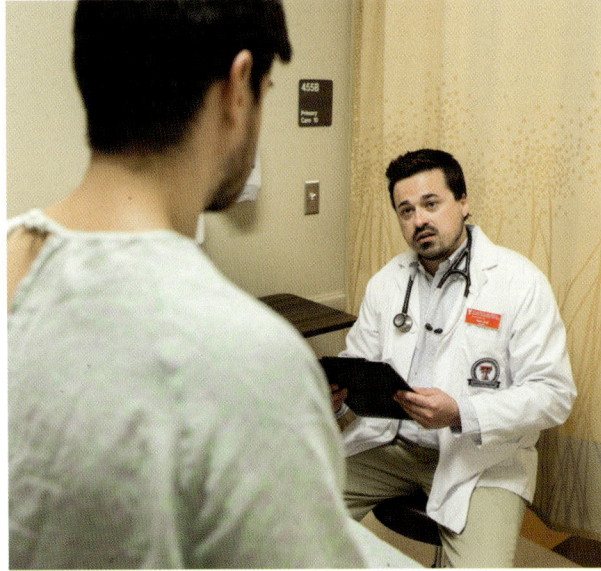

(BELOW) P3 Logo

(FAR LEFT) Dixon Santana, MD, teaching how to insert a central line during P3 week. Margaret Vugrin, Photographer

(LEFT) Student in P3 week interviewing standardized patient

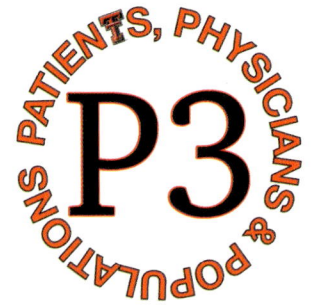

PATIENTS, PHYSICIANS & POPULATIONS

P3

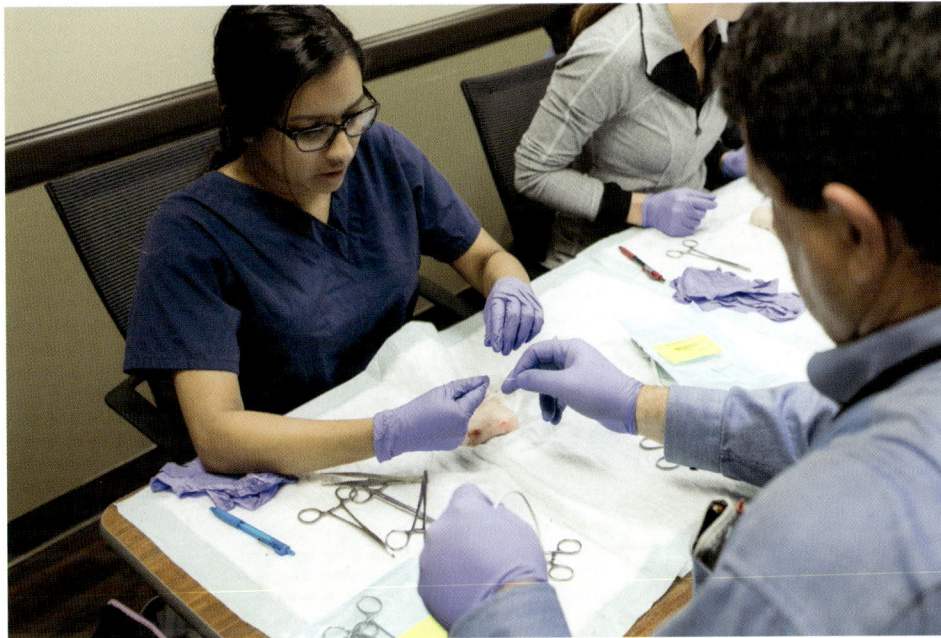

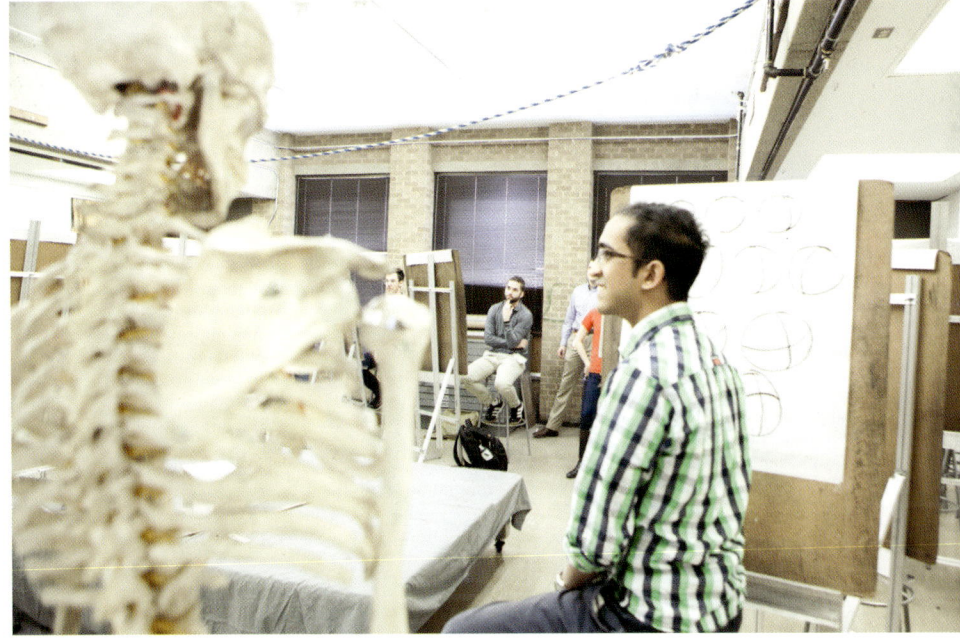

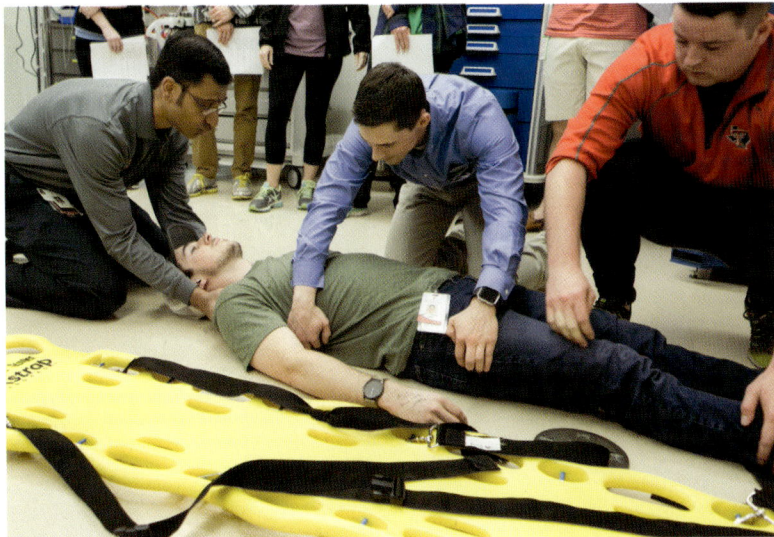

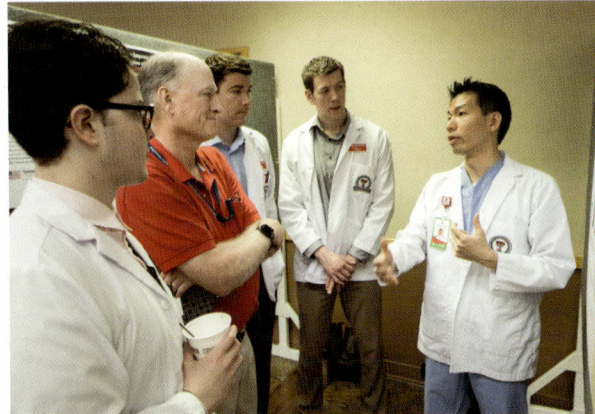

(ABOVE LEFT) Students in P3 week learning suturing techniques

(ABOVE RIGHT) Drawing class in School of Architecture during P3 week. Margaret Vugrin, Photographer

(FAR LEFT) Students in P3 week learning transport maneuvers

(LEFT) Students presenting poster to Dan Webster, PhD

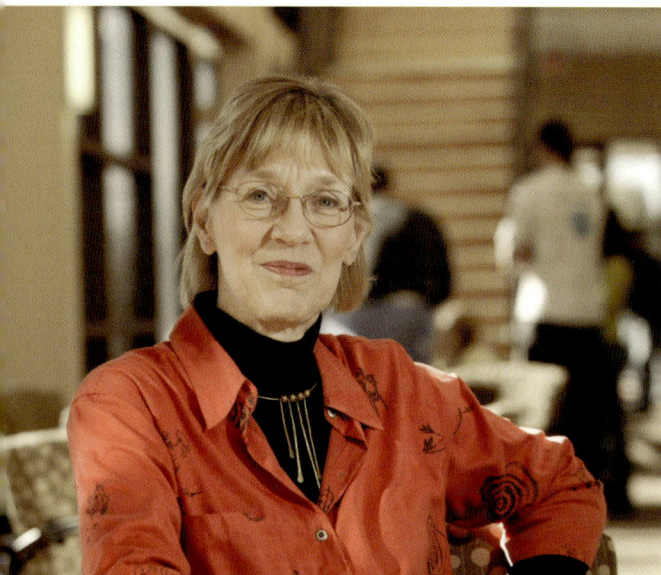
Lynn Bickley, MD

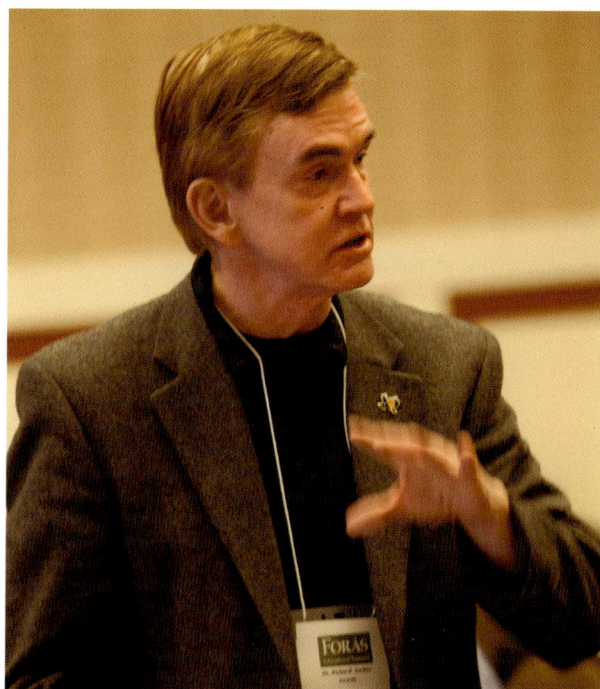
Simon Williams, PhD. Margaret Vugrin, Photographer

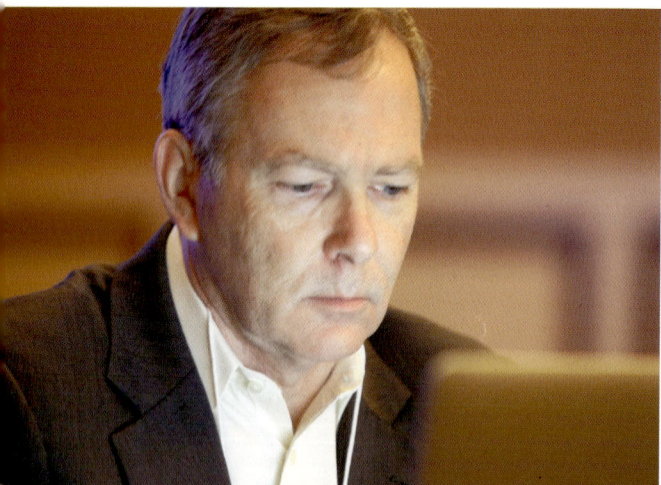
J. Edward Bates, PhD. Margaret Vugrin, Photographer

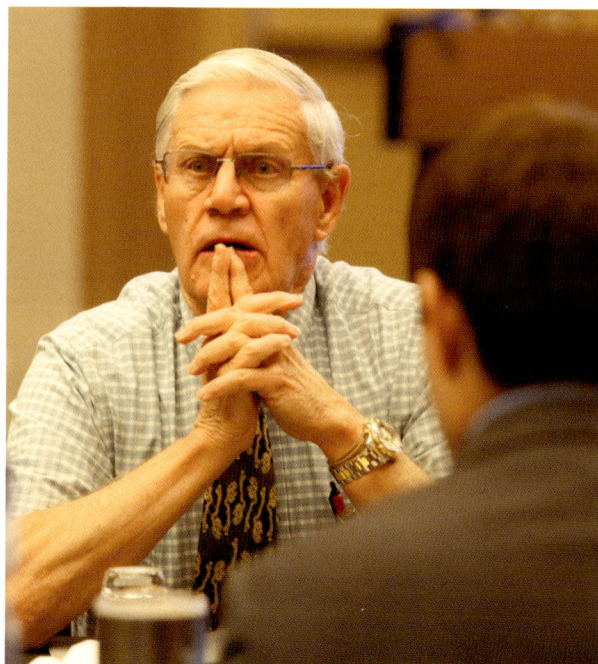
Robert Jordan MD, Regional Dean Amarillo. Margaret Vugrin, Photographer

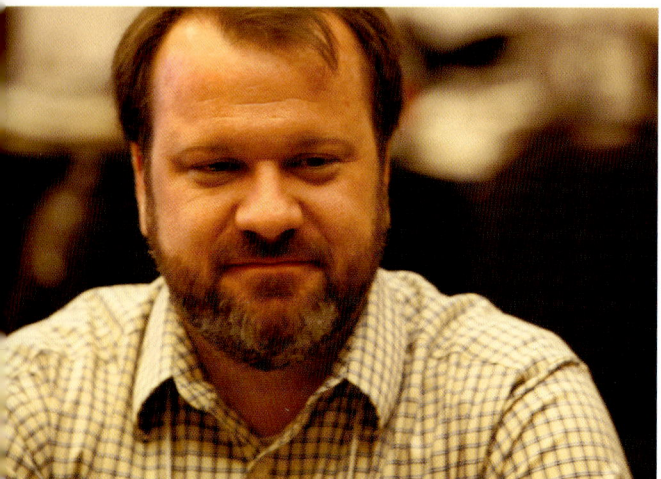
Richard Lampe, MD. Margaret Vugrin, Photographer

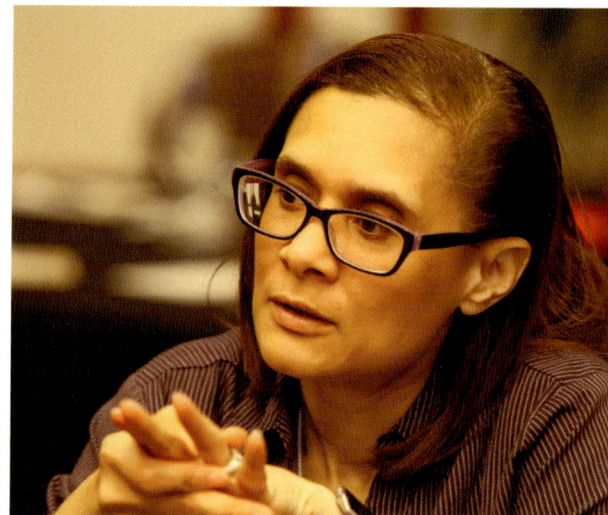
Lauren Cobbs, MD. Margaret Vugrin, Photographer

Educational Summits at TTUHSC School of Medicine

In order to maintain an effective and modern curriculum for our medical students, the School of Medicine has hosted annual educational summits for faculty, staff, and students since 2002. These summits were first organized by Lynn Bickley, MD, associate dean for curriculum, working together with the Educational Policy Committee, the school's main curriculum committee. The first eight summits were named *Renaissance*, signifying the focus of these summits on the redesign (or rebirth) of the medical school curriculum. In 2009, the summits were renamed *Forás*, from the Gaelic word for evolution, to reflect the ongoing development of the redesigned curriculum to incorporate emerging educational methods and technologies. Simon Williams, PhD, leads thought-provoking sessions with collaborations from all departments and all campuses.

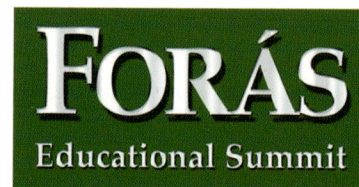
FORAS logo

Longtime Members

Many faculty members have been instrumental in teaching, mentoring, and encouraging our students in all disciplines. We are fortunate to have recruited some wonderful and amazing professors in the course of our 50 years. John Pelley, PhD, MBA, and Joseph Fralick, PhD, began their teaching careers at the School of Medicine as it was being established and they are still active professors. During his tenure at Texas Tech, Dr. Pelley served for a decade in administration of the medical school curriculum. The challenges of helping students with learning issues encouraged him to develop a strong interest in the learning process, thus he has spent the last 30 years working on educational projects in applied metacognition. He has written a book, *Success Types*, that summarizes his experience with learning styles.

Joe Fralick, PhD, works in the Department of Immunology and Molecular Microbiology where his research has produced numerous publications on E. coli; a number of these publications have been cited numerous times. Sam Prien, PhD, joined the faculty shortly thereafter. He has been heavily involved in research and mentoring students both in the TTUHSC Department of Obstetrics and Gynecology and TTU's Department of Animal and Food Science. His work in fertility has brought newborns to life in both the human and animal realms. Surendra Varma, MD, from pediatrics is another strong student mentor. Over his more than 40 years at TTUHSC he has touched the lives of many children as a pediatric endocrinologist. He states that working on creating a state law for "newborn hypothyroid screening was the most gratifying thing for me in academic medicine," and it has saved many children from mental retardation.

Mubariz Naqvi, MD, joined the Department of Pediatrics at the Amarillo campus in 1978. He works full time to provide care to newborn babies born in the Texas panhandle and to teach and mentor our students and residents to provide evidence-based medical care punctuated with respect and compassion to the parents and their babies. This lifelong passion drives him in this field that he loves. Robert S. Urban, MD, also joined the Department of Internal Medicine in Amarillo where he has been a practicing internist for over 40 years. He is board certified in internal medicine and supports clinics that take care of chronic and acute conditions in the adult population in and around Amarillo. In 1978, Thomas Tenner Jr.,

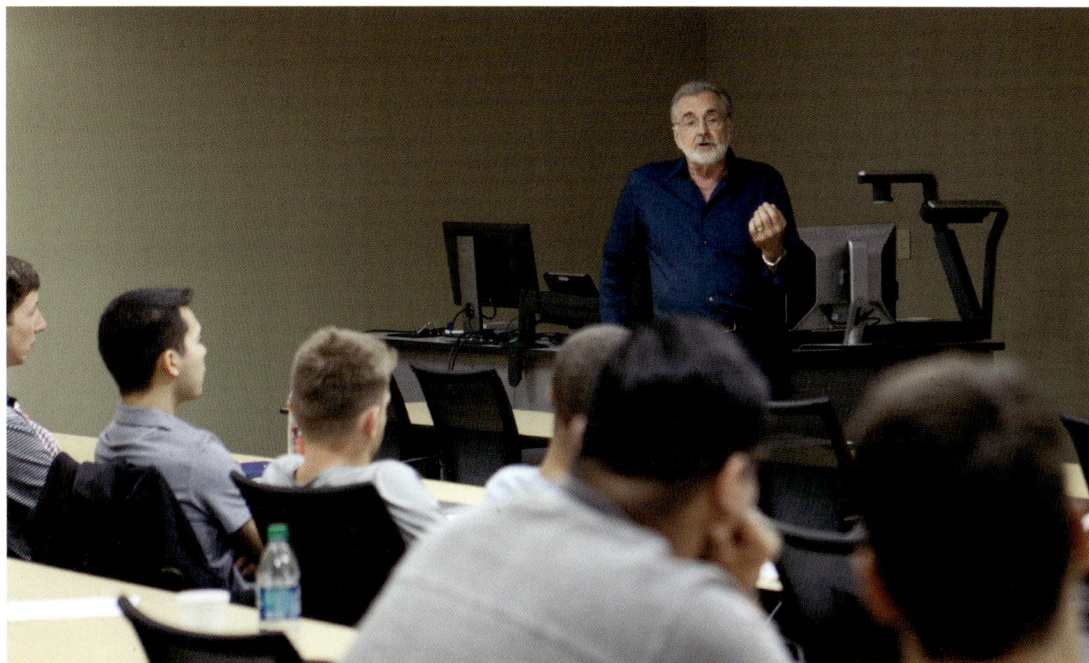

John Pelley, PhD, lecturing Fall 2018. Margaret Vugrin, Photographer

PhD, accepted a position at Texas Tech University Health Sciences Center in the Department of Pharmacology. His research activity concerns studying modulatory effects of chronic drug administration or disease states on cardiovascular function. While fulfilling his teaching duties, he has been an active member of the Texas State American Heart Association and associate dean for Faculty Affairs and Development as well as director of Continuing Medical Education. In this last role he states, "We strive to facilitate the physician's efforts to maintain knowledge currency and to implement changes in practice conducive to improved quality of care and patient safety."

Thomas McGovern, EdD, has been associated with the school since 1978; he has served the entire TTUHSC community in the areas of addiction treatment, ethics, humanities, and spirituality. He is the founder of the Center for Ethics, Humanities, and Spirituality and is constant in his devotion to building communities based on respect and compassion. (Editor's note: His love for TTUHSC was ever so evident as we worked together on the creation of this book.) The care of this center has been competently continued by Cheryl Erwin, JD, PhD.

In the early 1970s, two individuals joined the Department of Physiology and went on to become the longest serving alumni at TTUHSC. Lorenz O. Lutherer, PhD, and Herb Janssen worked together in the Department of

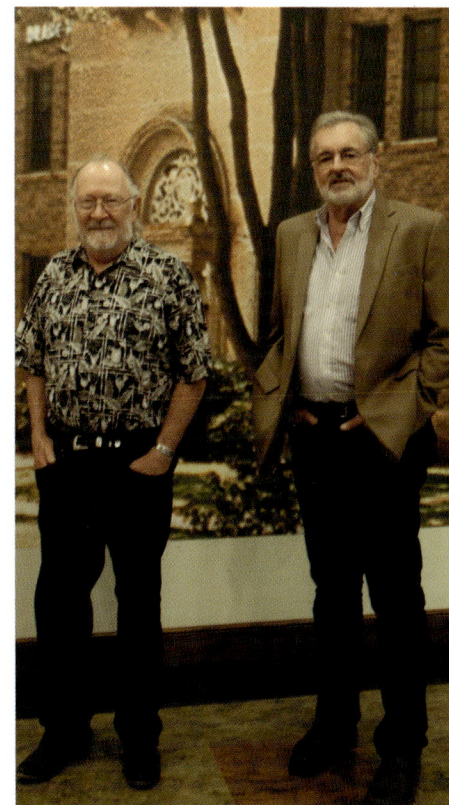

Joseph Fralick, PhD, and John Pelley, PhD. Margaret Vugrin, Photographer

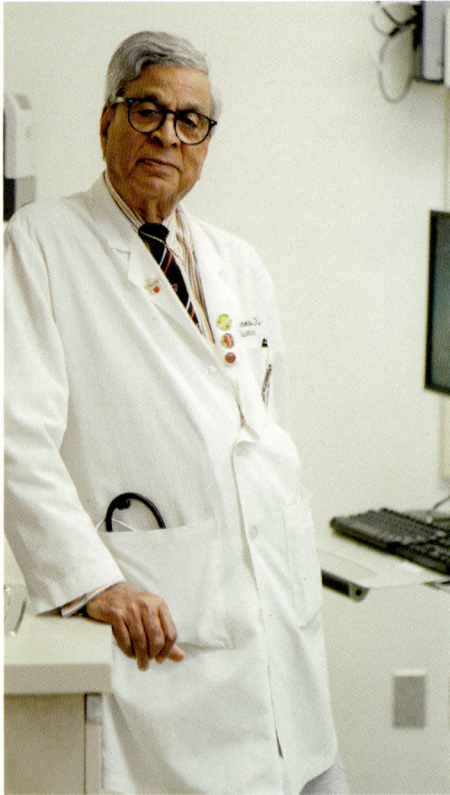

Surendra Varma, MD

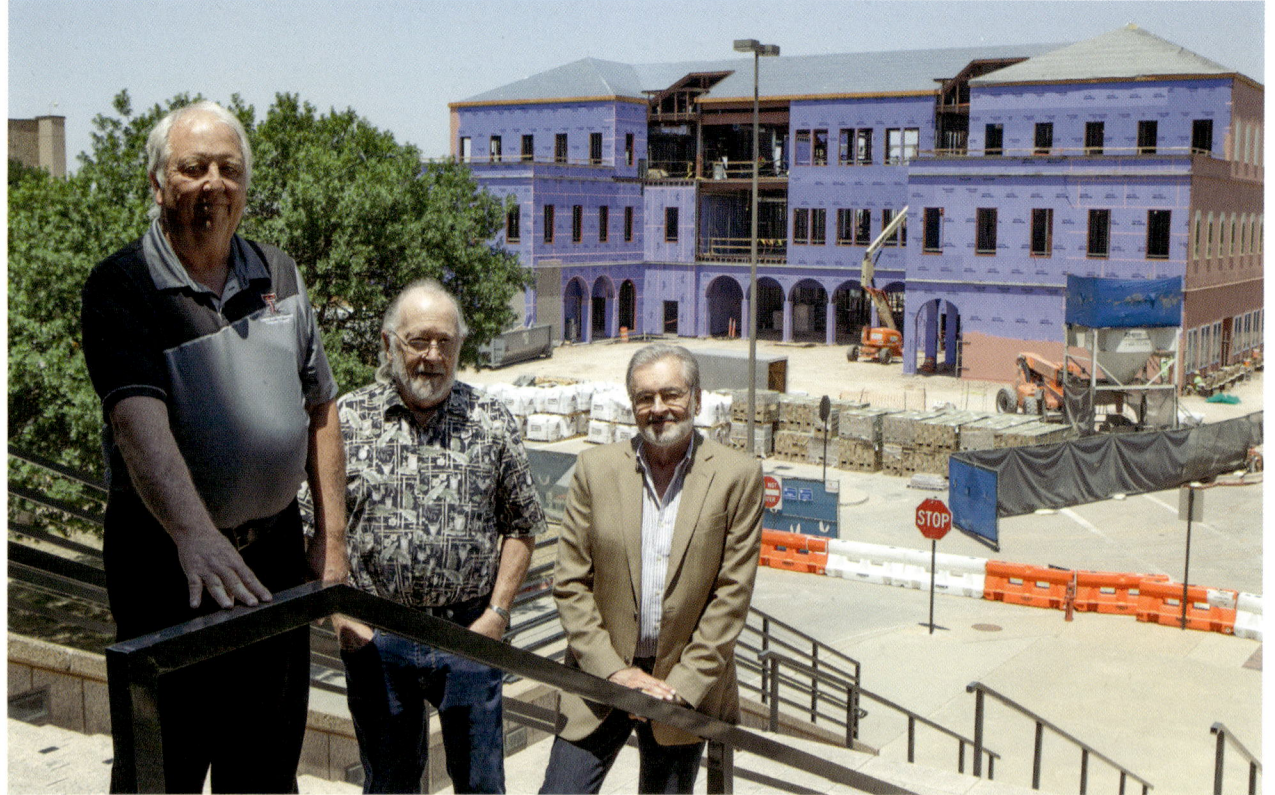

Sam Prien, PhD; Joseph Fralick, PhD; and John Pelley, PhD, with the new Welcome Center construction in the background, Fall 2018. Margaret Vugrin, Photographer

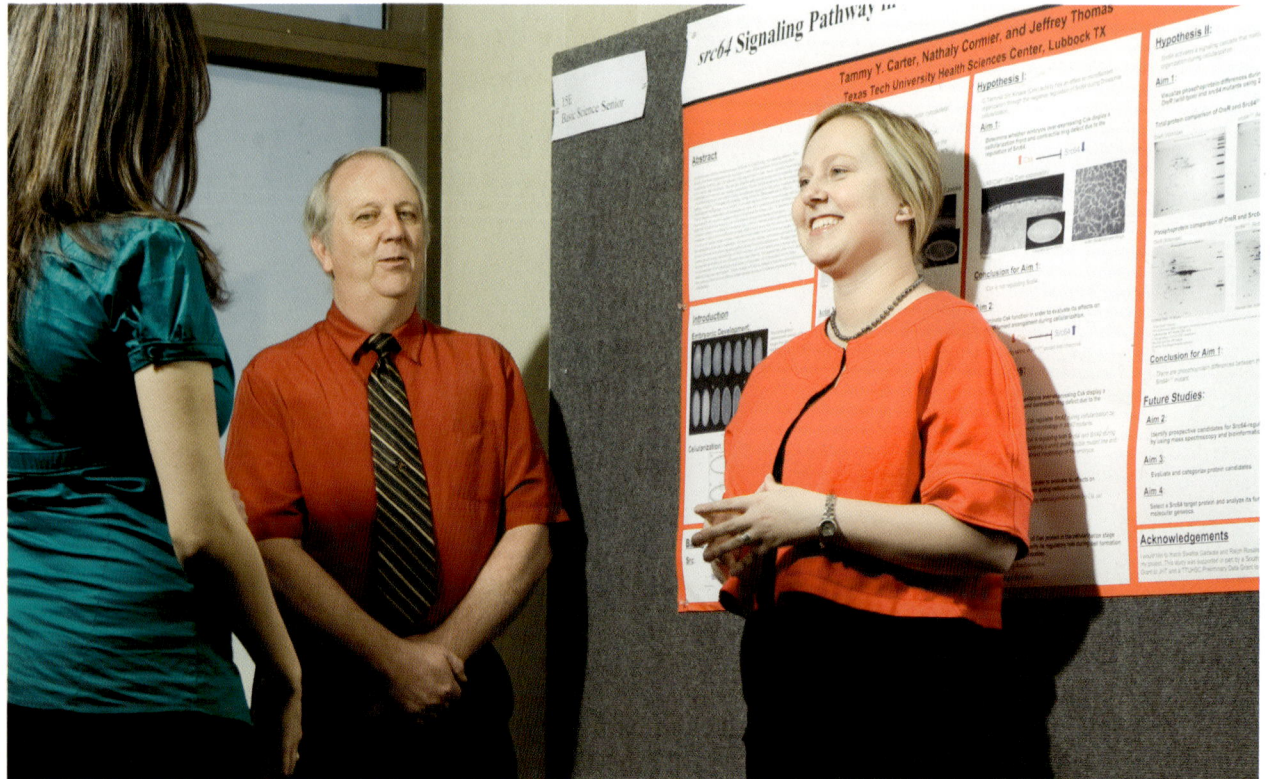

Sam Prien, PhD, reviewing posters during Research Week

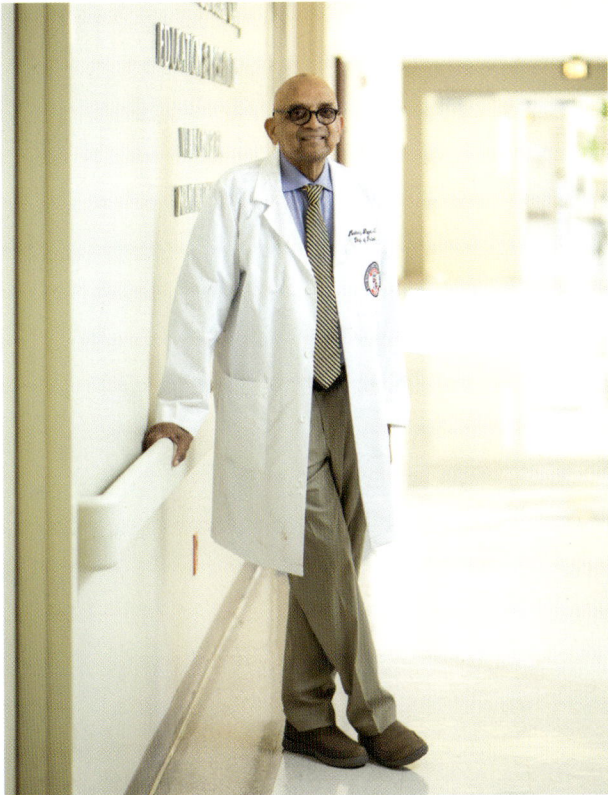

Mubariz Naqvi, MD

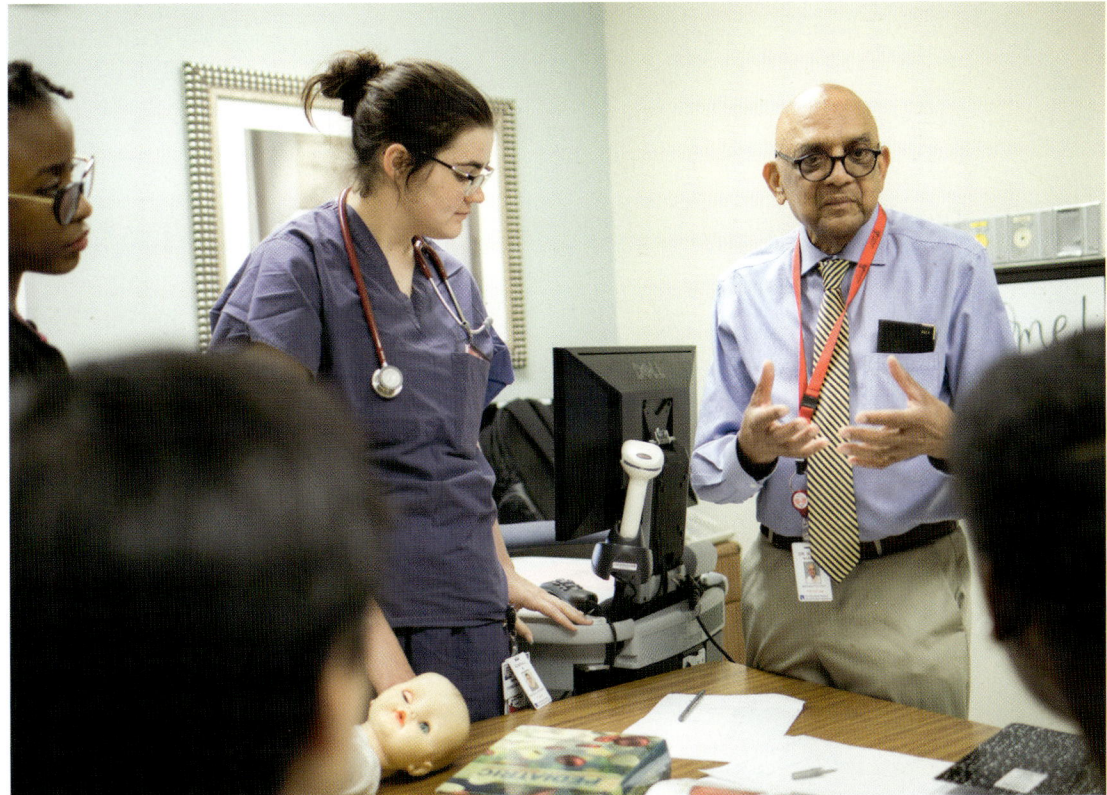

Mubariz Naqvi, MD, with students

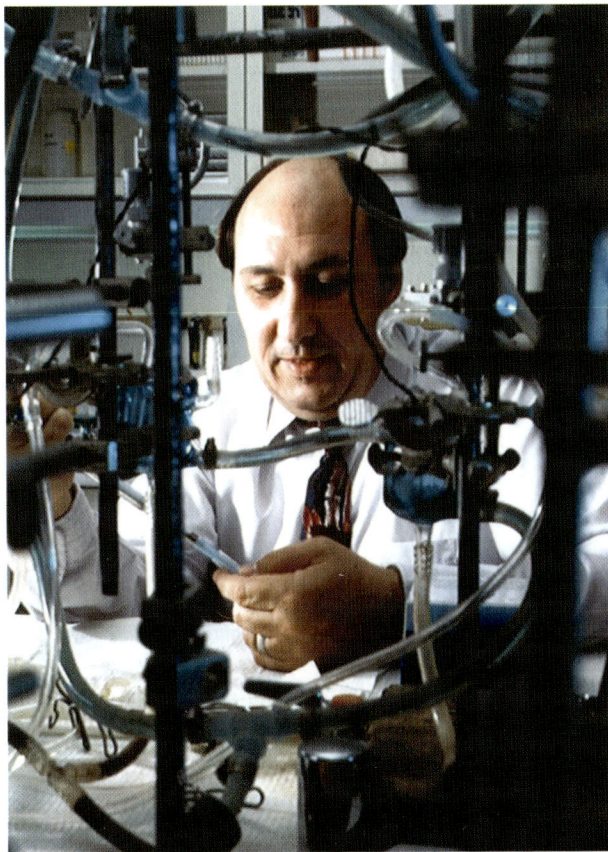

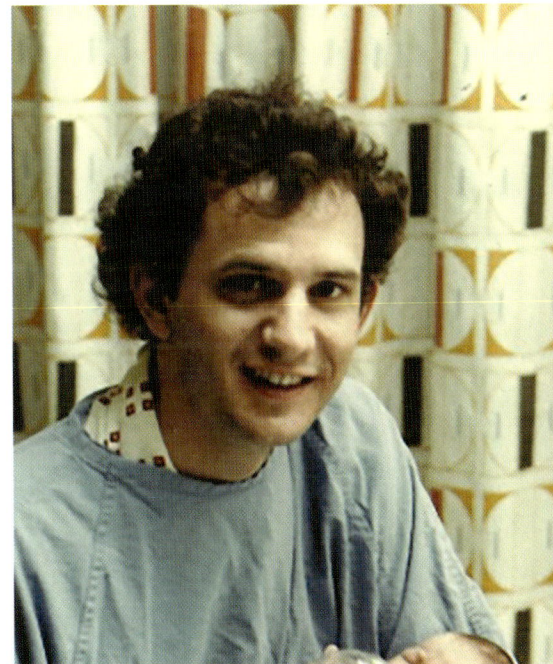

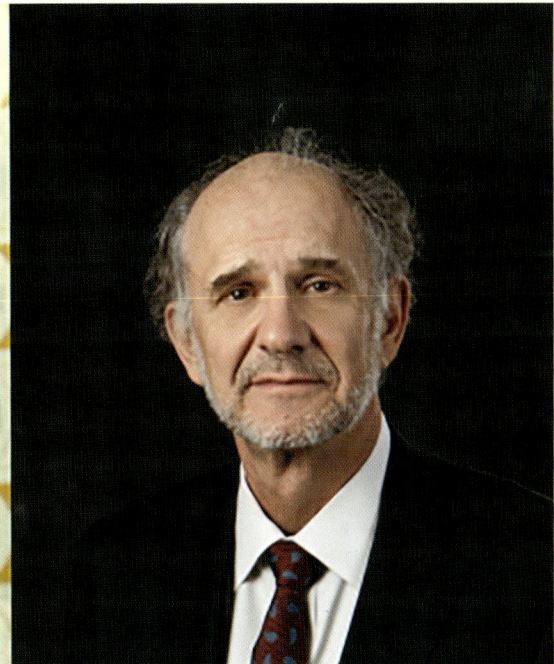

(ABOVE) Robert S. Urban, MD, at 25 years and now

(LEFT) Thomas Tenner, Jr, PhD

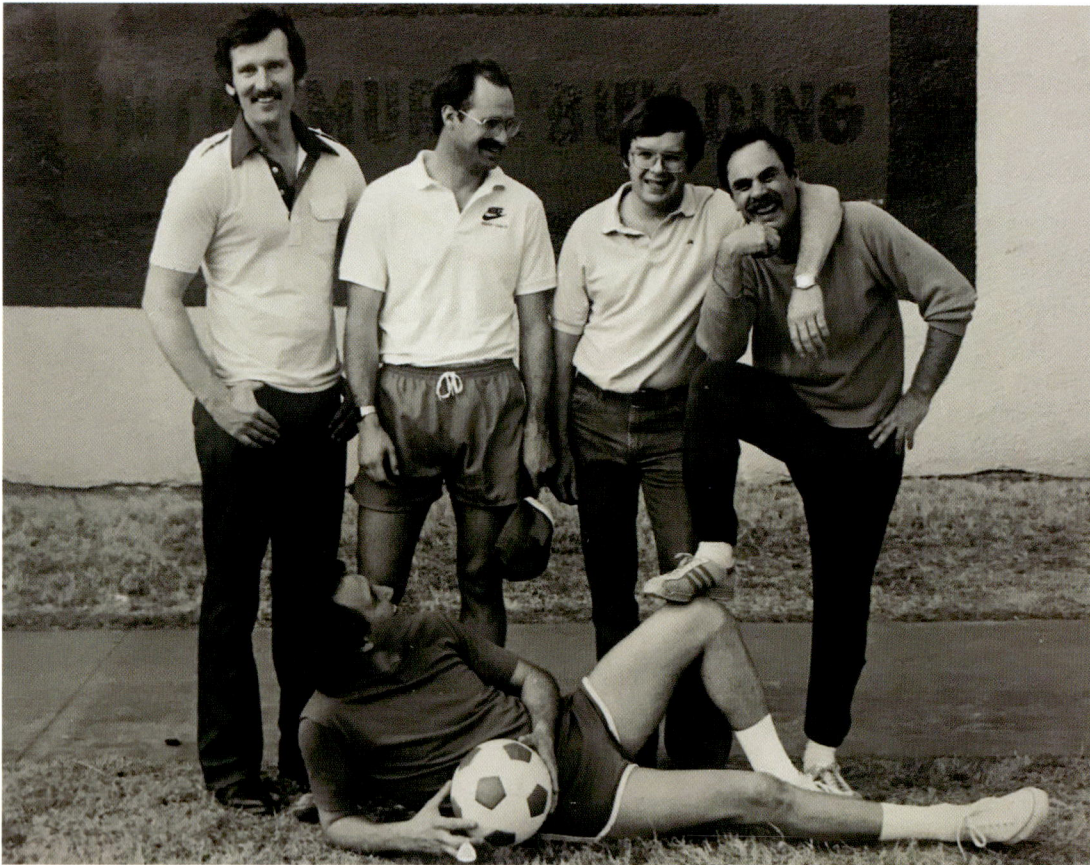

(ABOVE) In their Physiology student days, Herb Janssen, PhD, on left; Lorenz O. Lutherer on the right; Matthew Grisham, PhD, with the ball

(RIGHT) Herb Janssen, PhD on the El Paso Campus

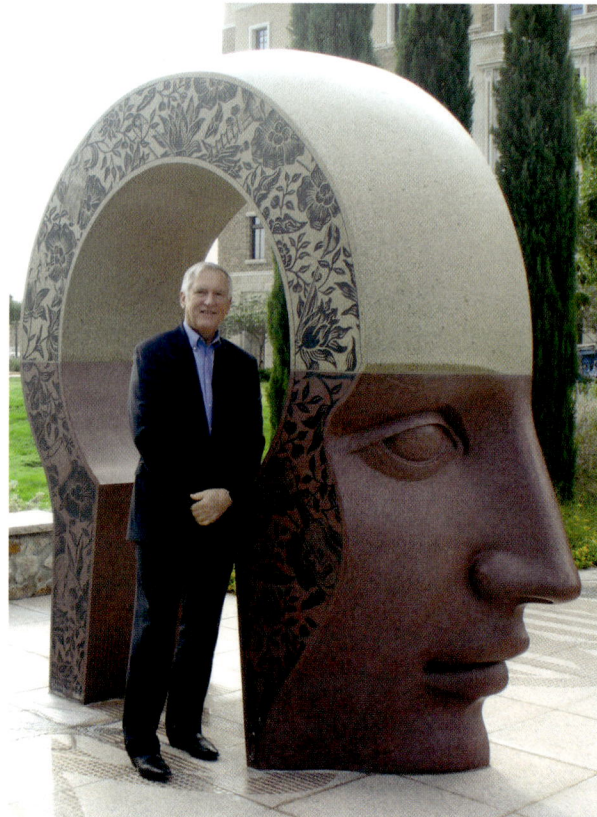

Physiology during the early days and have continued to serve TTUHSC over the subsequent 45-plus years. These two alumni have yet another connection—Dr. Lutherer served as the chair of Janssen's doctoral committee.

Lutherer continued to serve as an assistant professor in the Department of Physiology while he completed his MD degree at TTUHSC. Lutherer published many original research manuscripts and books, mentored countless graduate and medical students, and helped shape the future of TTUHSC by his service on many important committees. During this time, he received numerous awards and was recognized repeatedly for his teaching, research, dedication, and service to the TTUHSC community. He recently retired after serving TTUHSC for over 45 years.

Janssen completed his PhD in 1980 and joined the Department of Orthopedic Surgery as director of research. He went on to become assistant chair and associate chair for research in the Orthopedic Department. In 2008, he accepted a position as professor of physiology in the Paul L. Foster School of Medicine in El Paso. He continues to serve TTUHSC as a professor and college master in the Department of Medical Education. In 2012 Janssen received the Master Teacher Award from the International Association of Medical Science Educators and in 2014 he was awarded the Arthur C. Guyton Educator of the Year Award from the American Physiological Society.

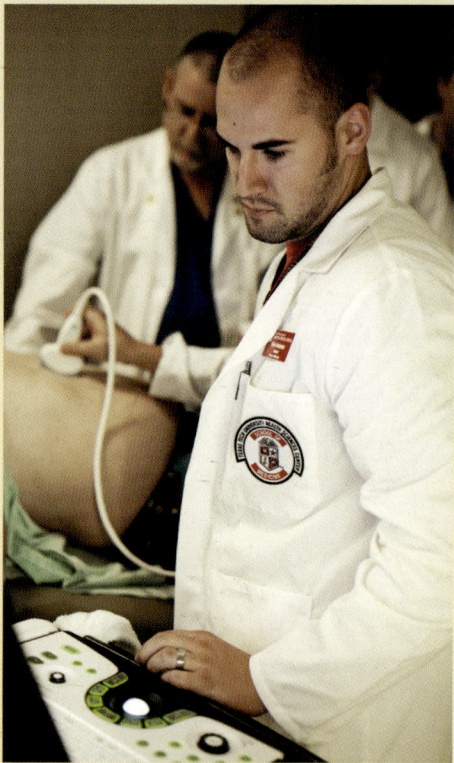
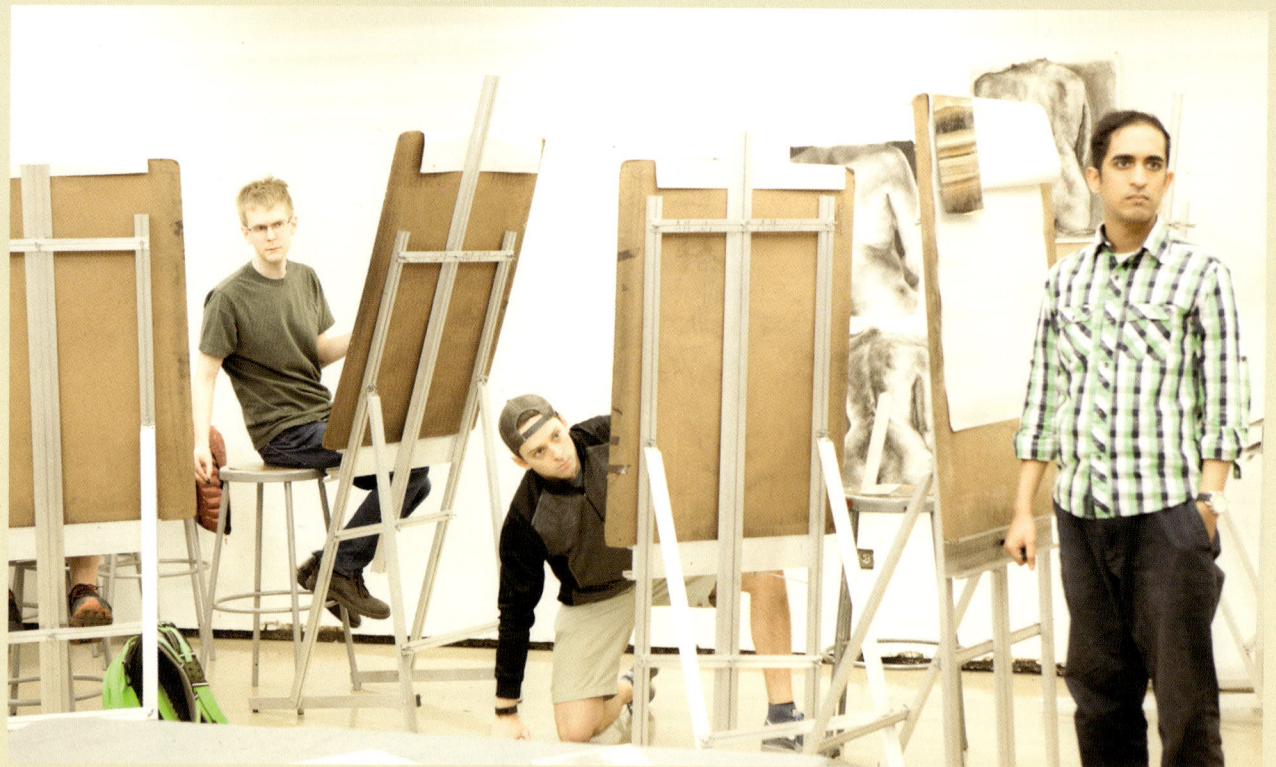
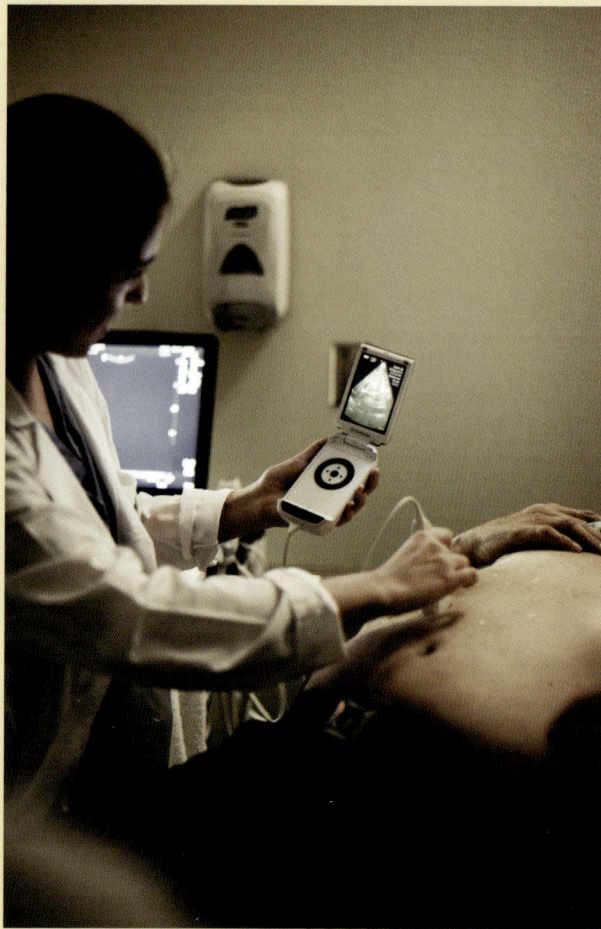
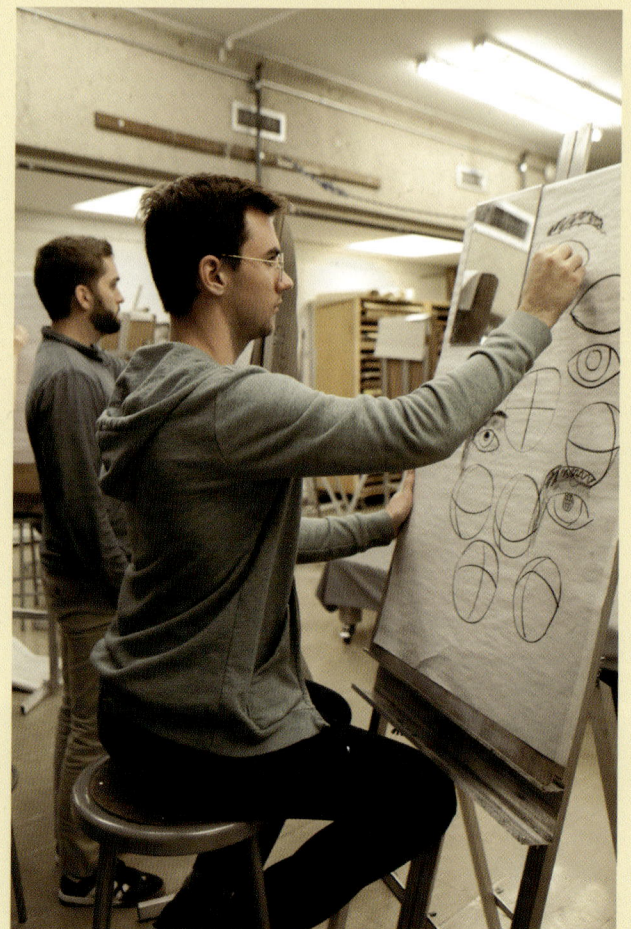

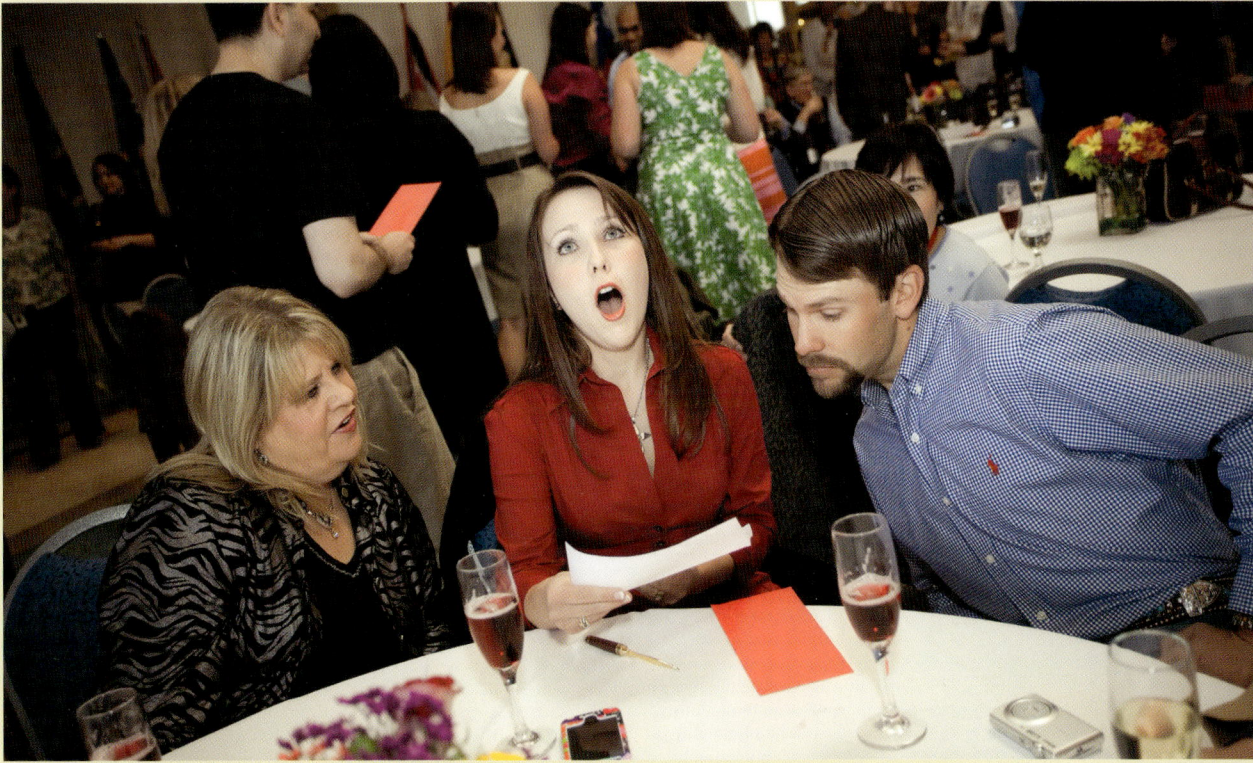
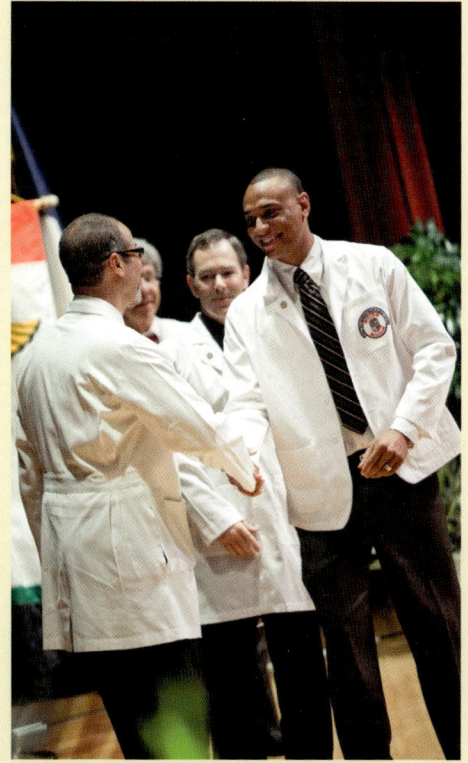
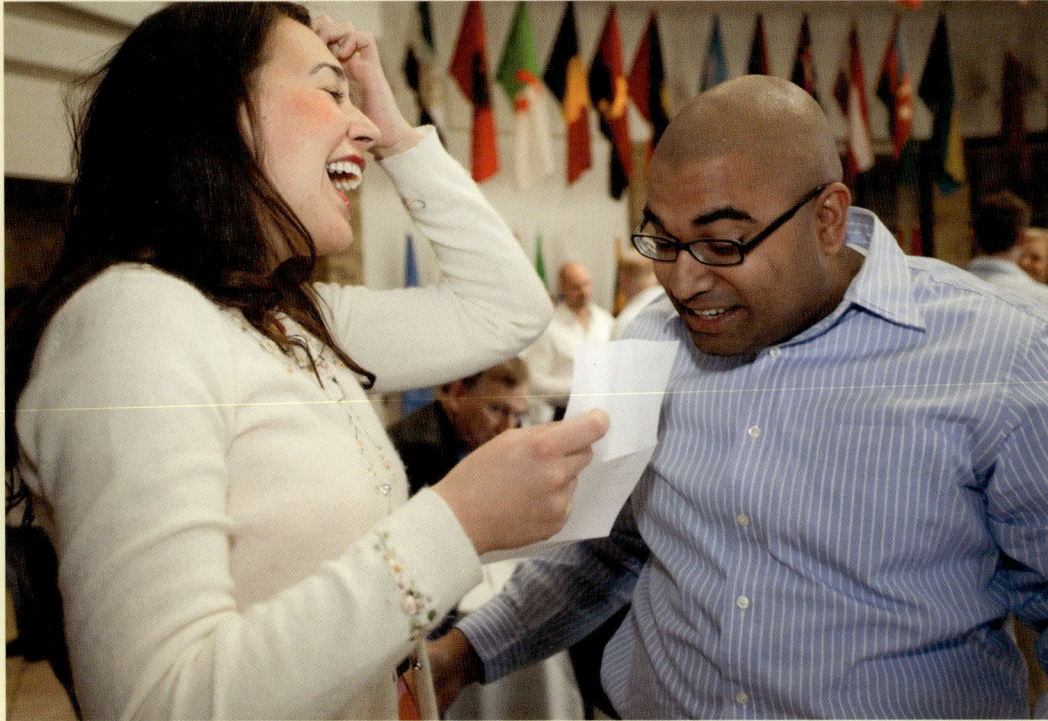
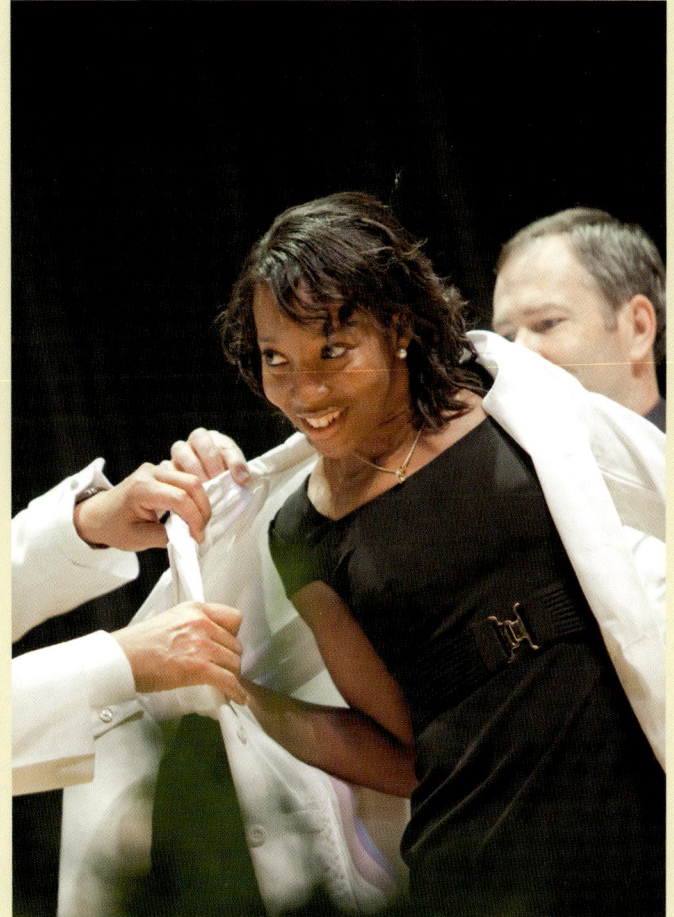

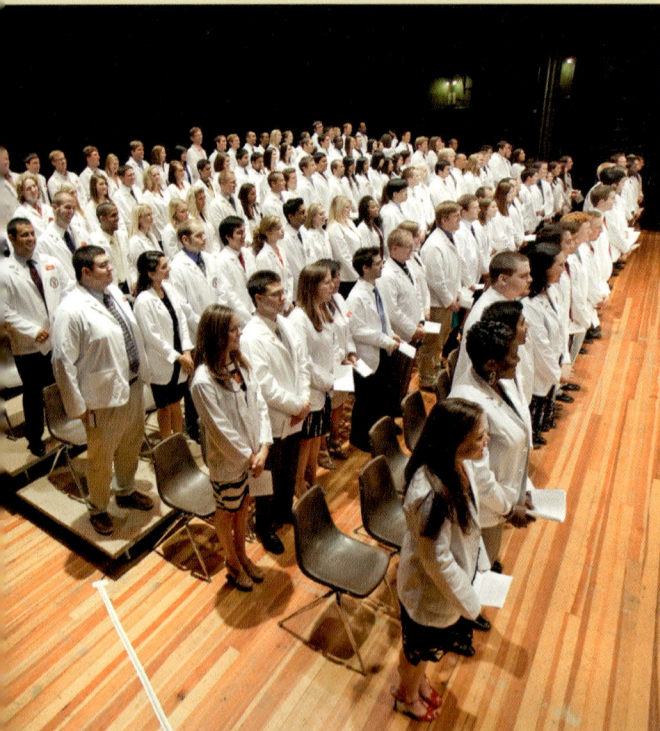
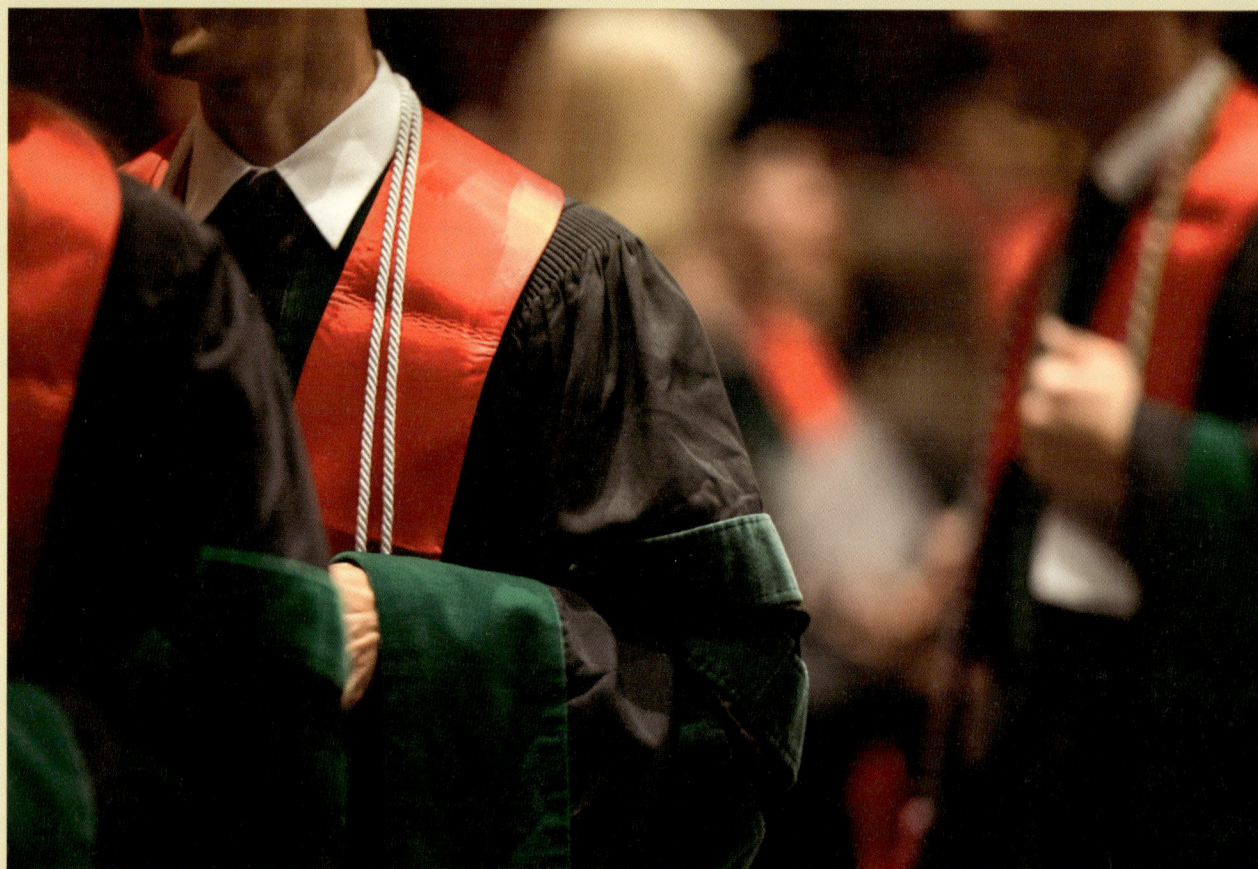
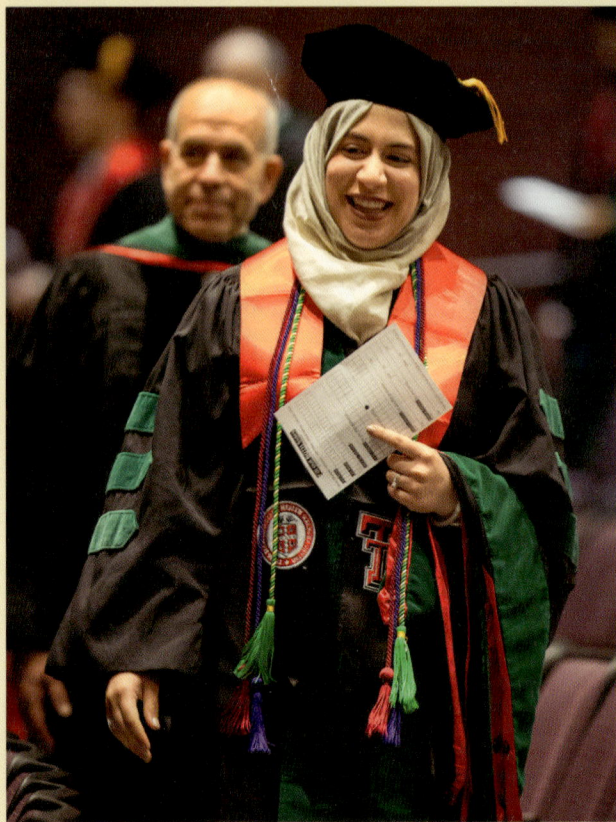
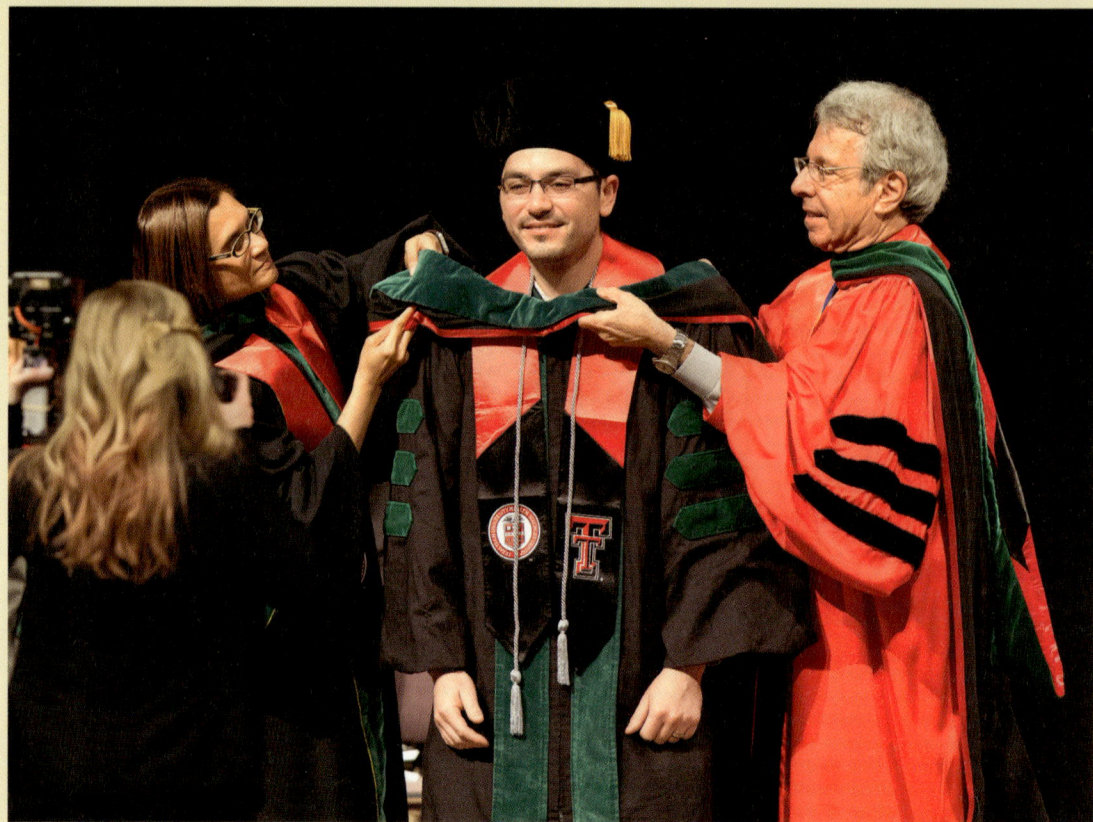

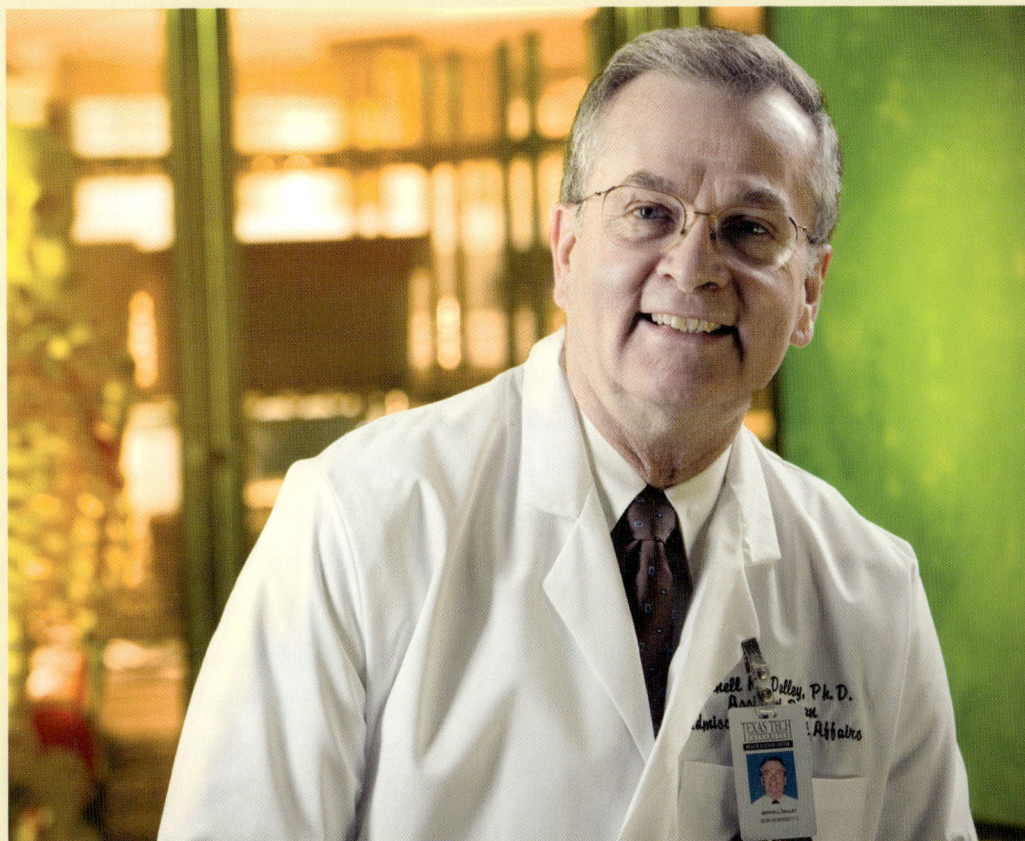
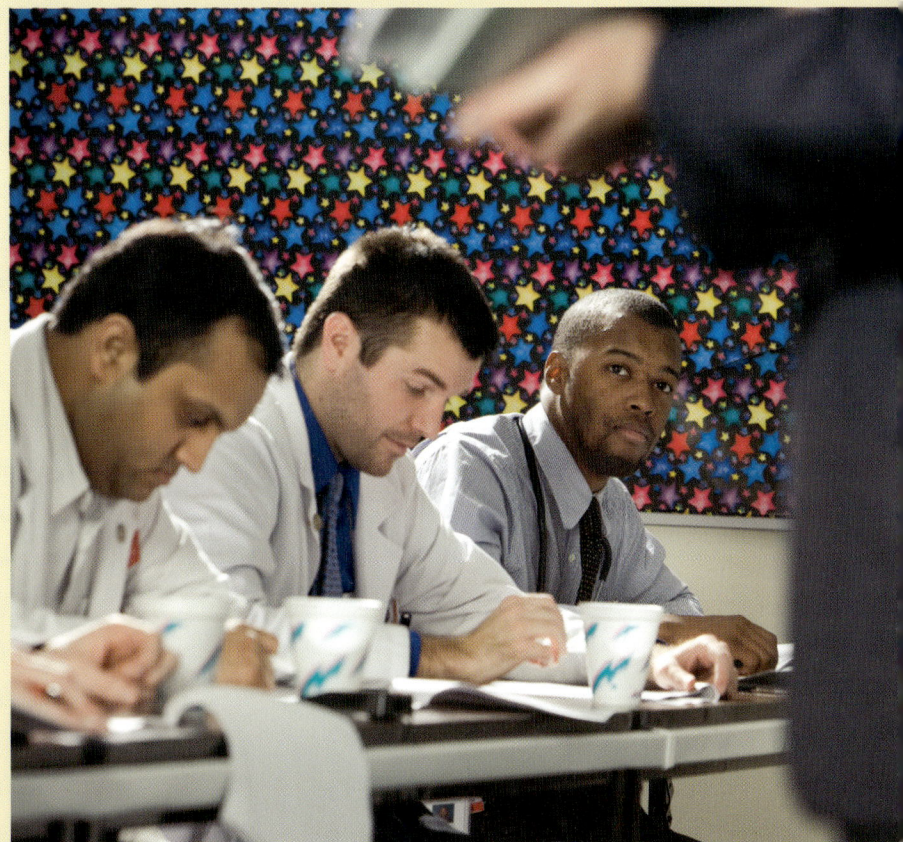
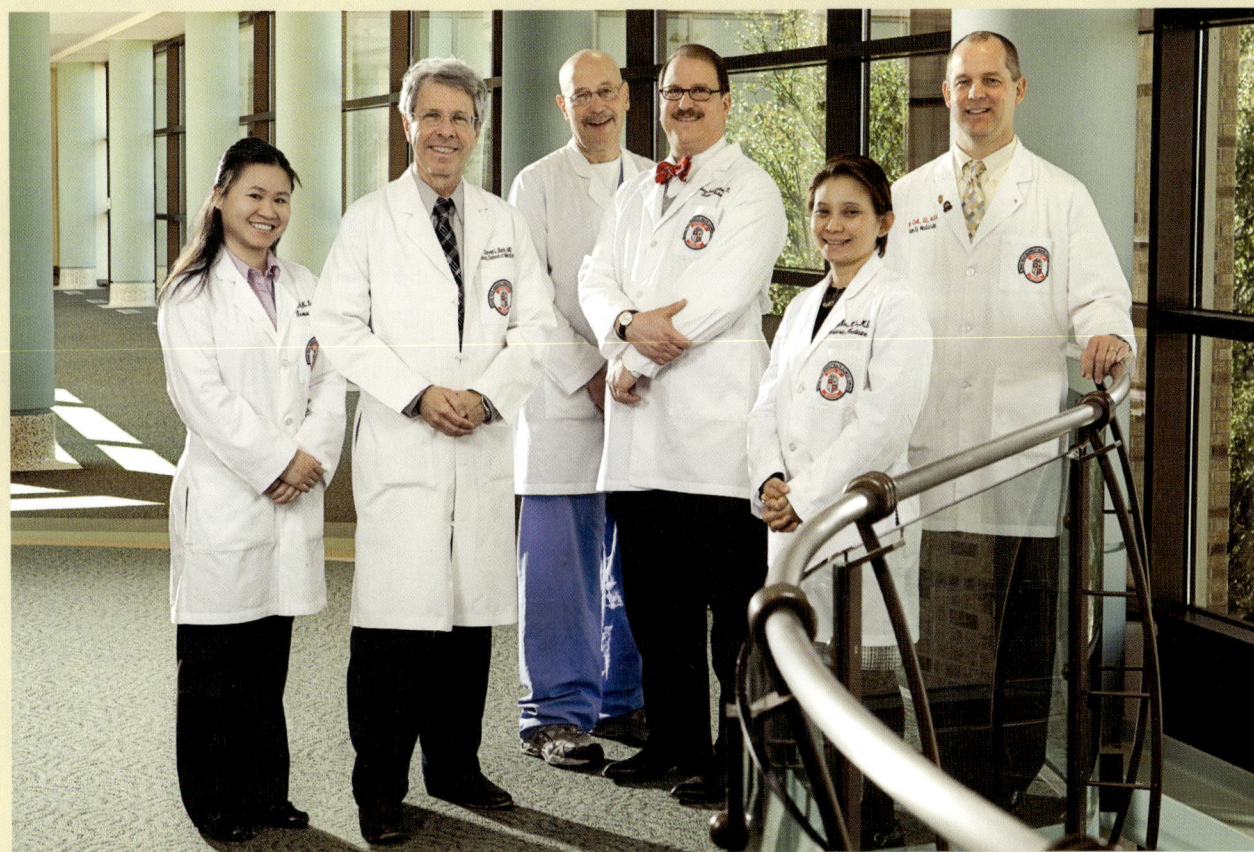

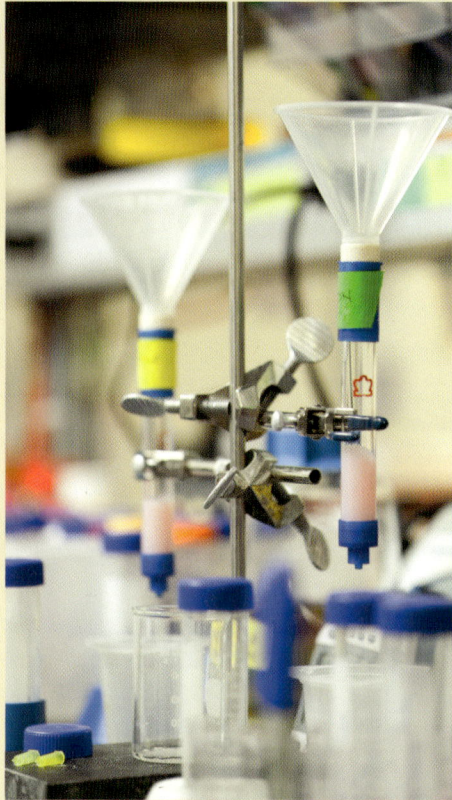

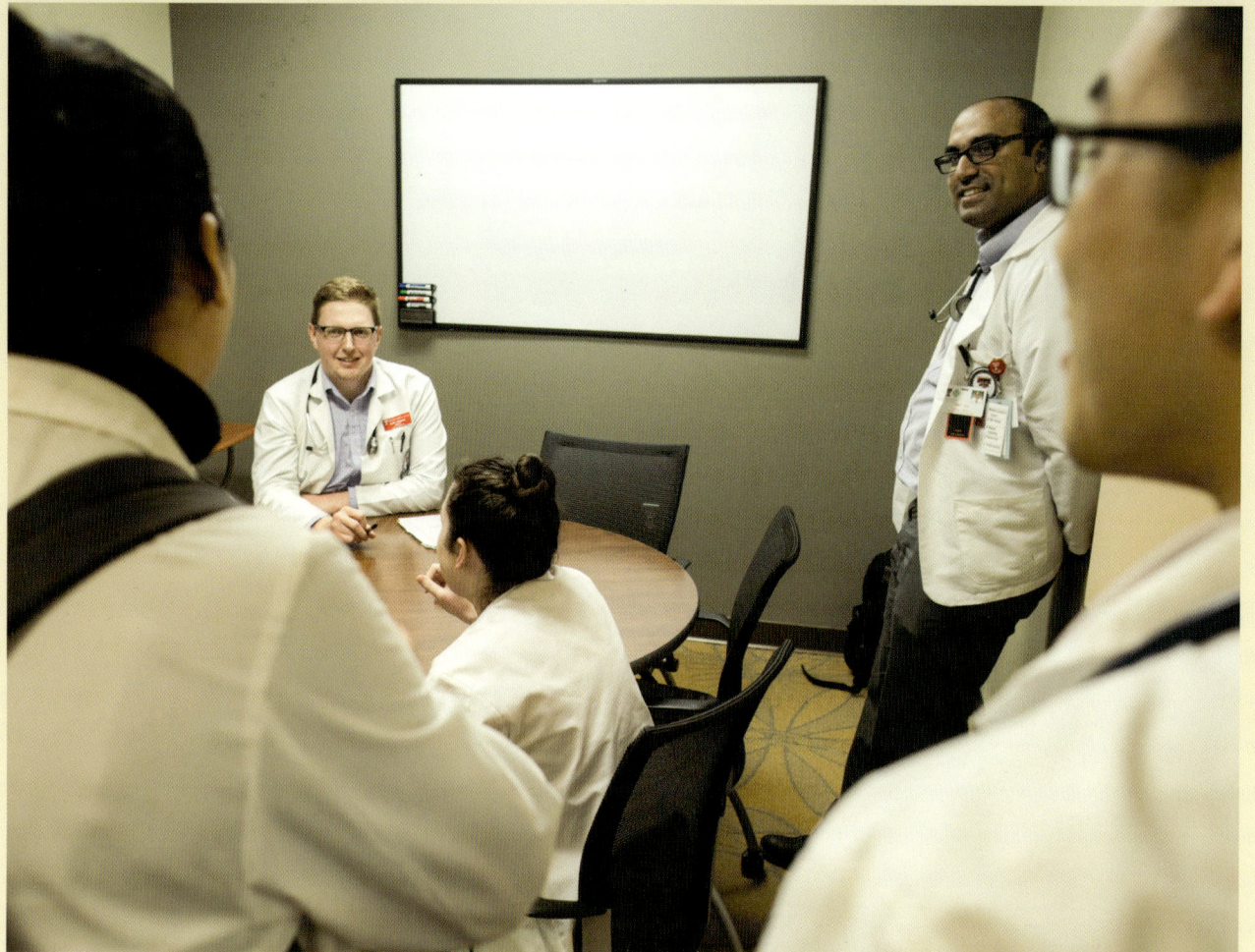

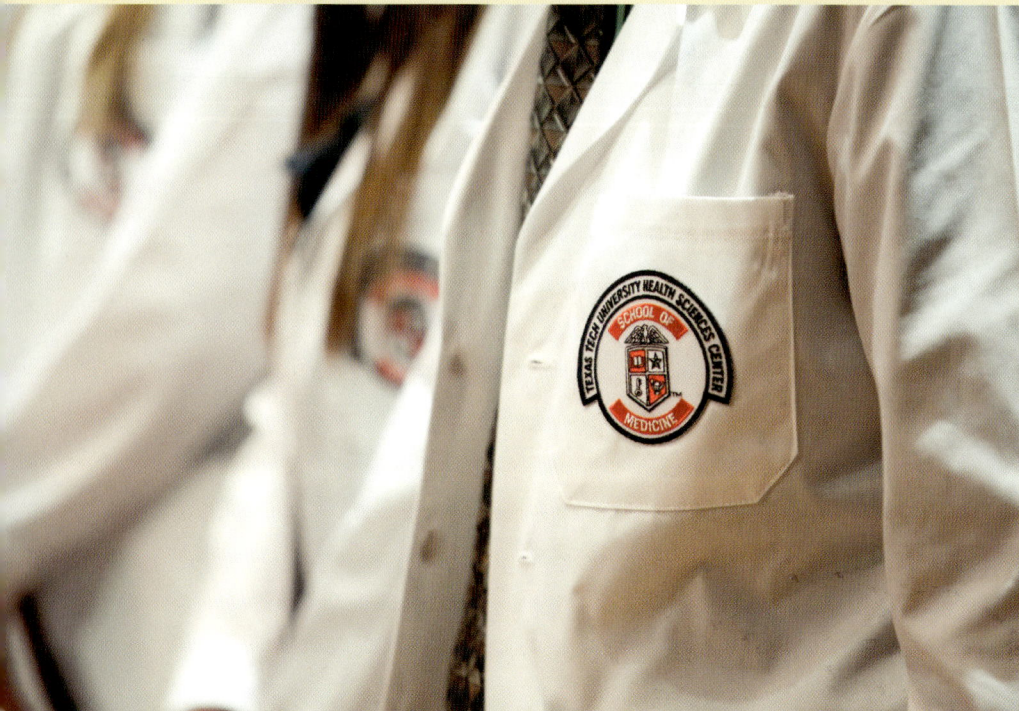

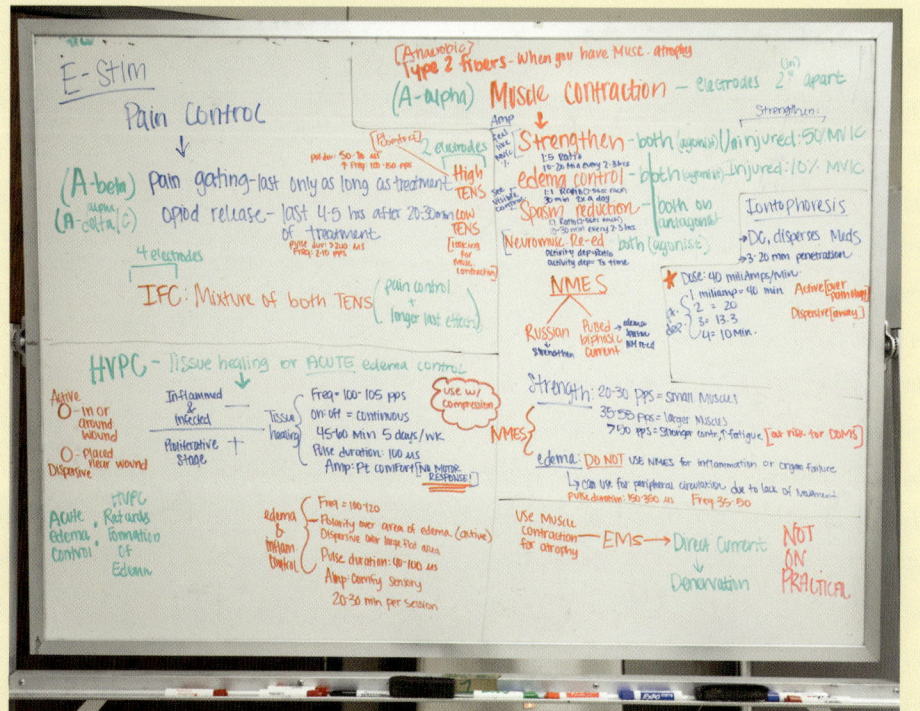

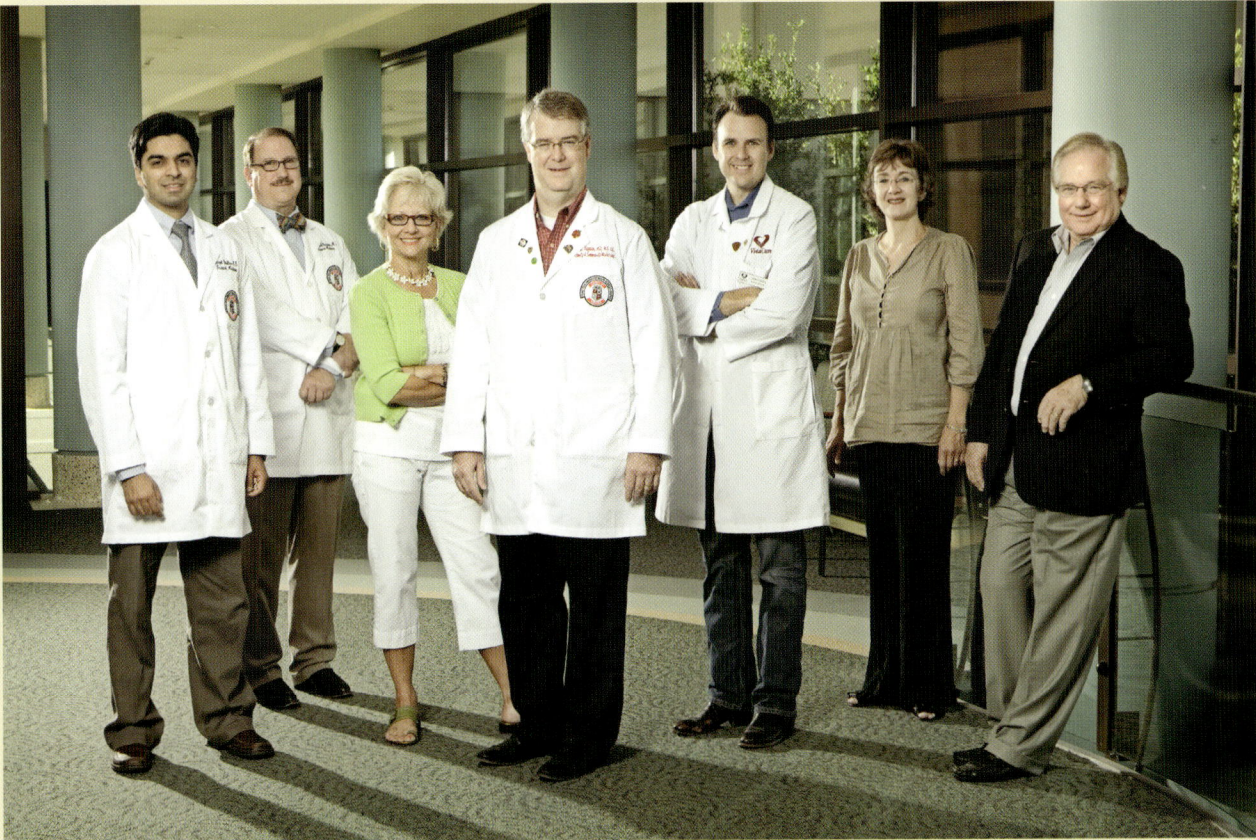
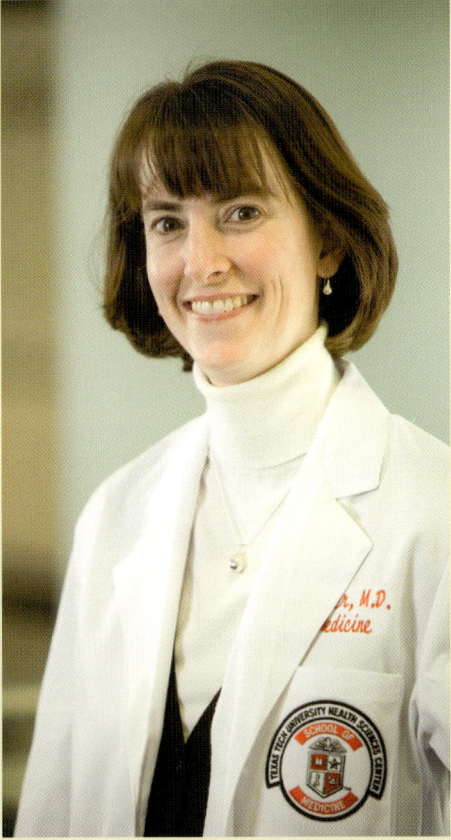
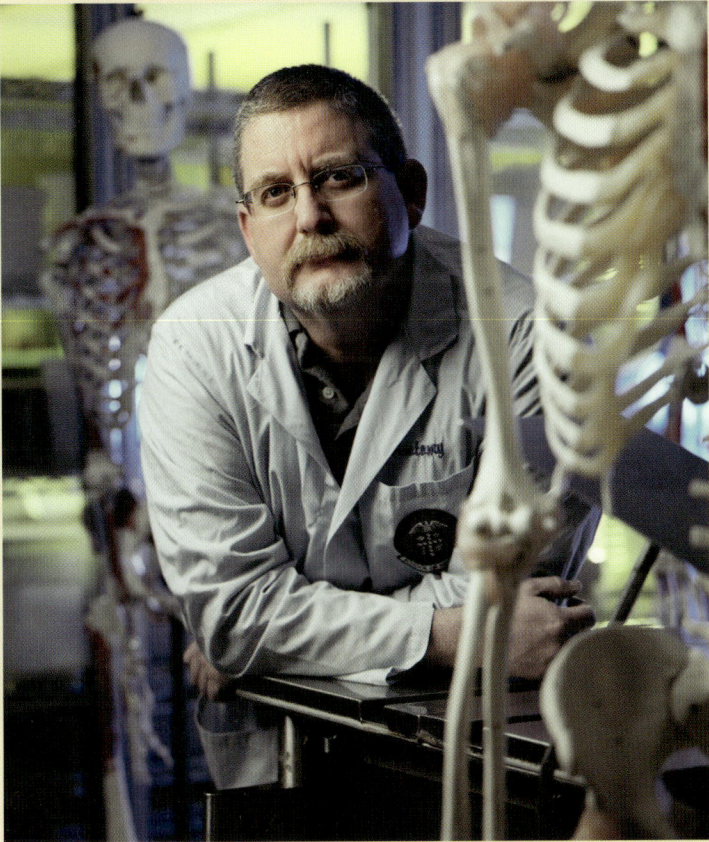
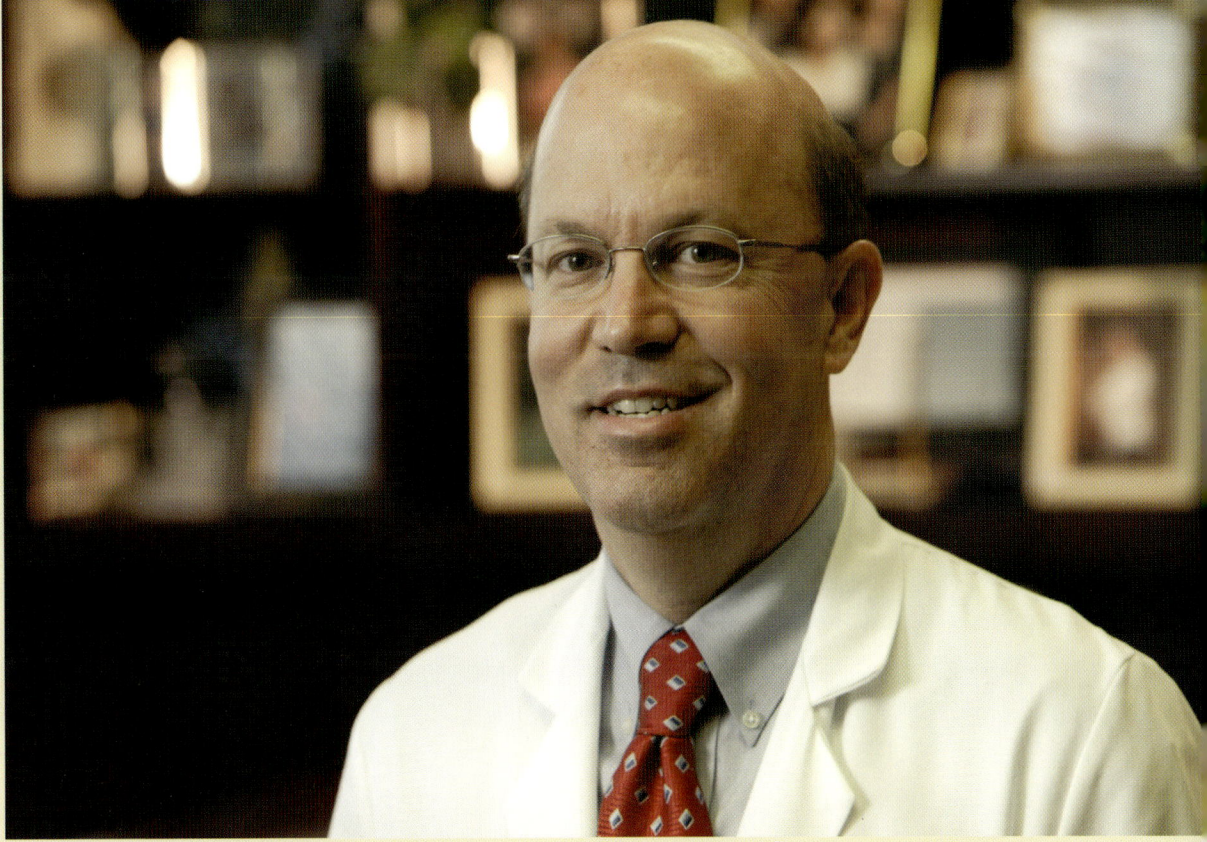

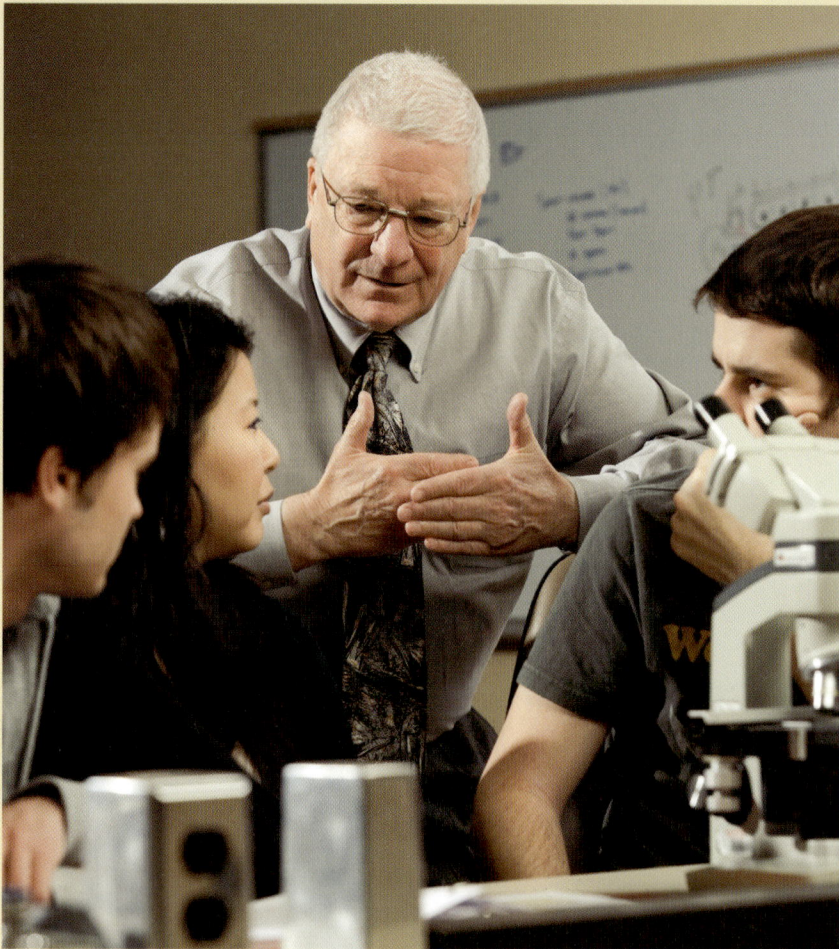

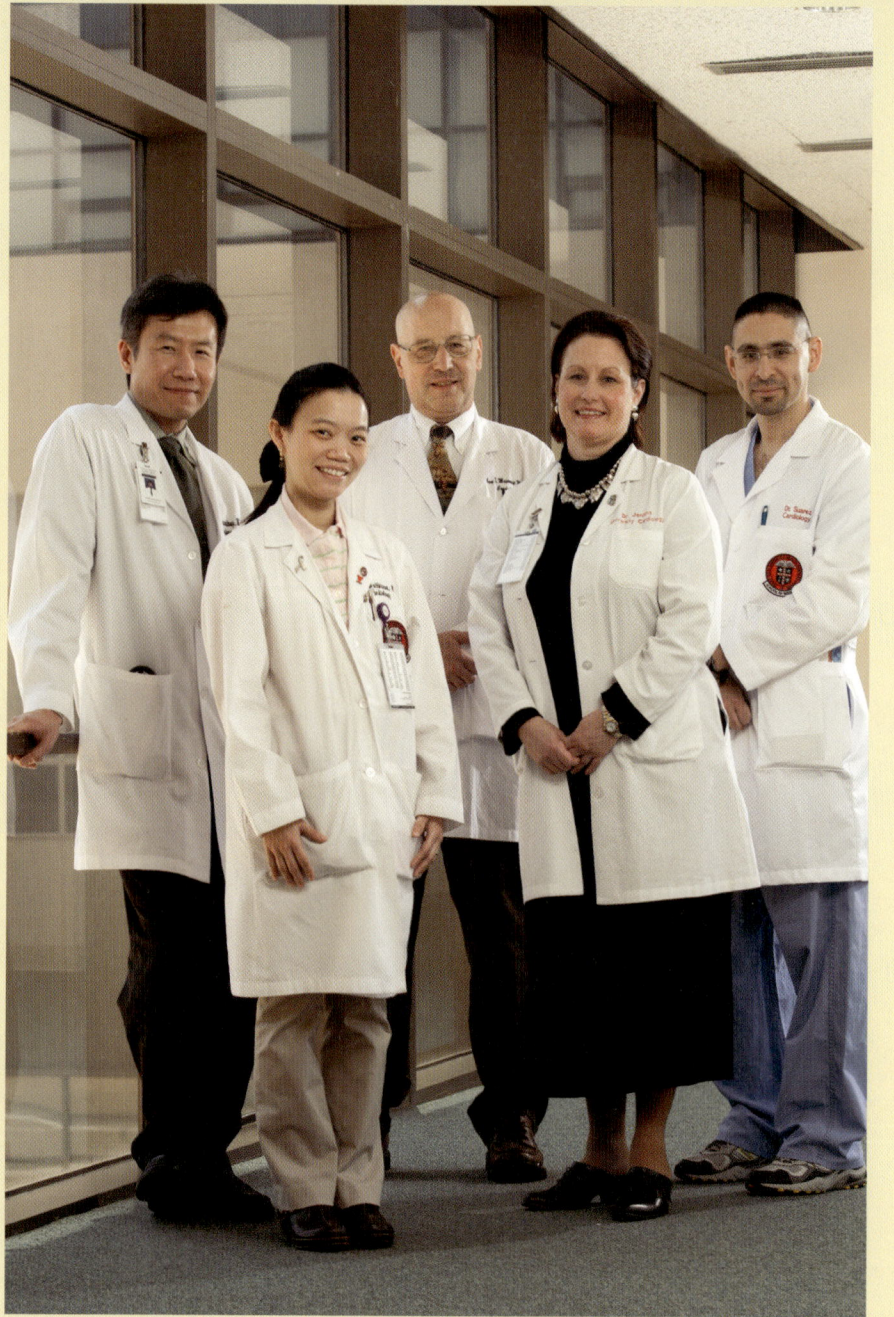

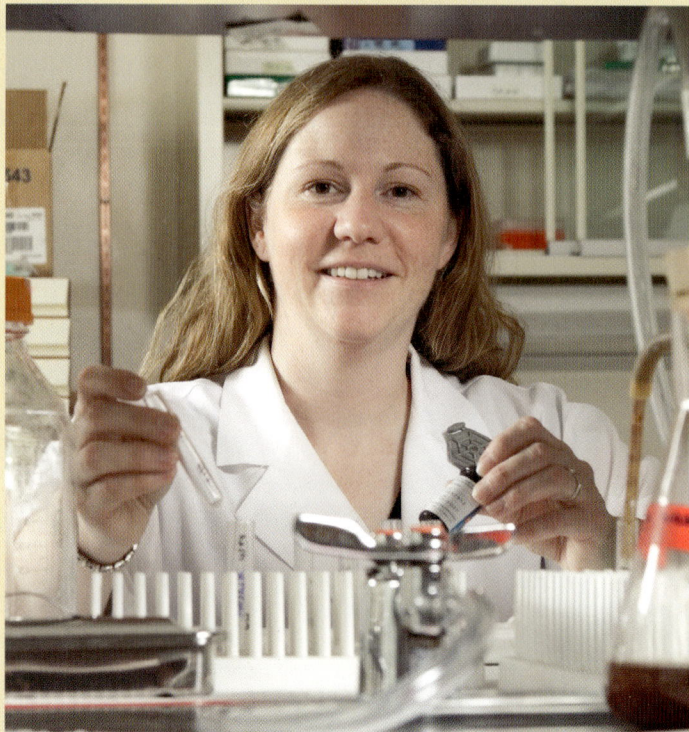

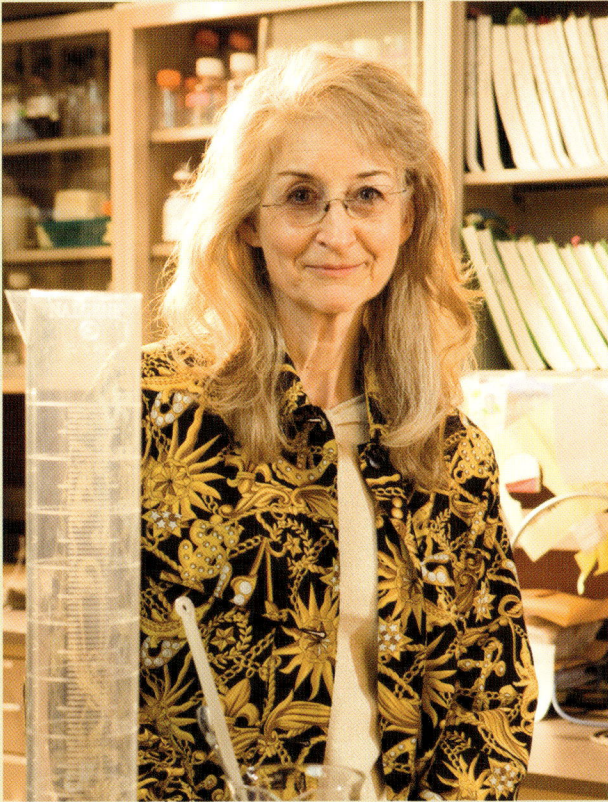

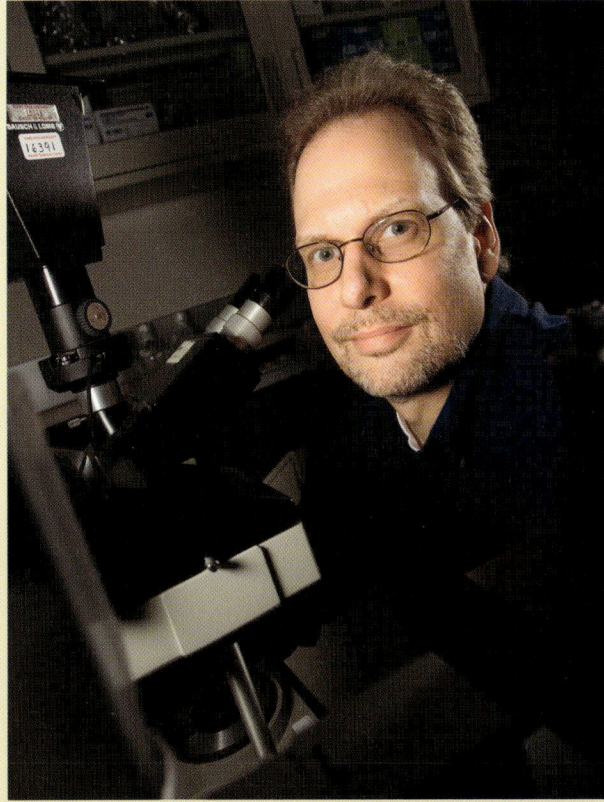

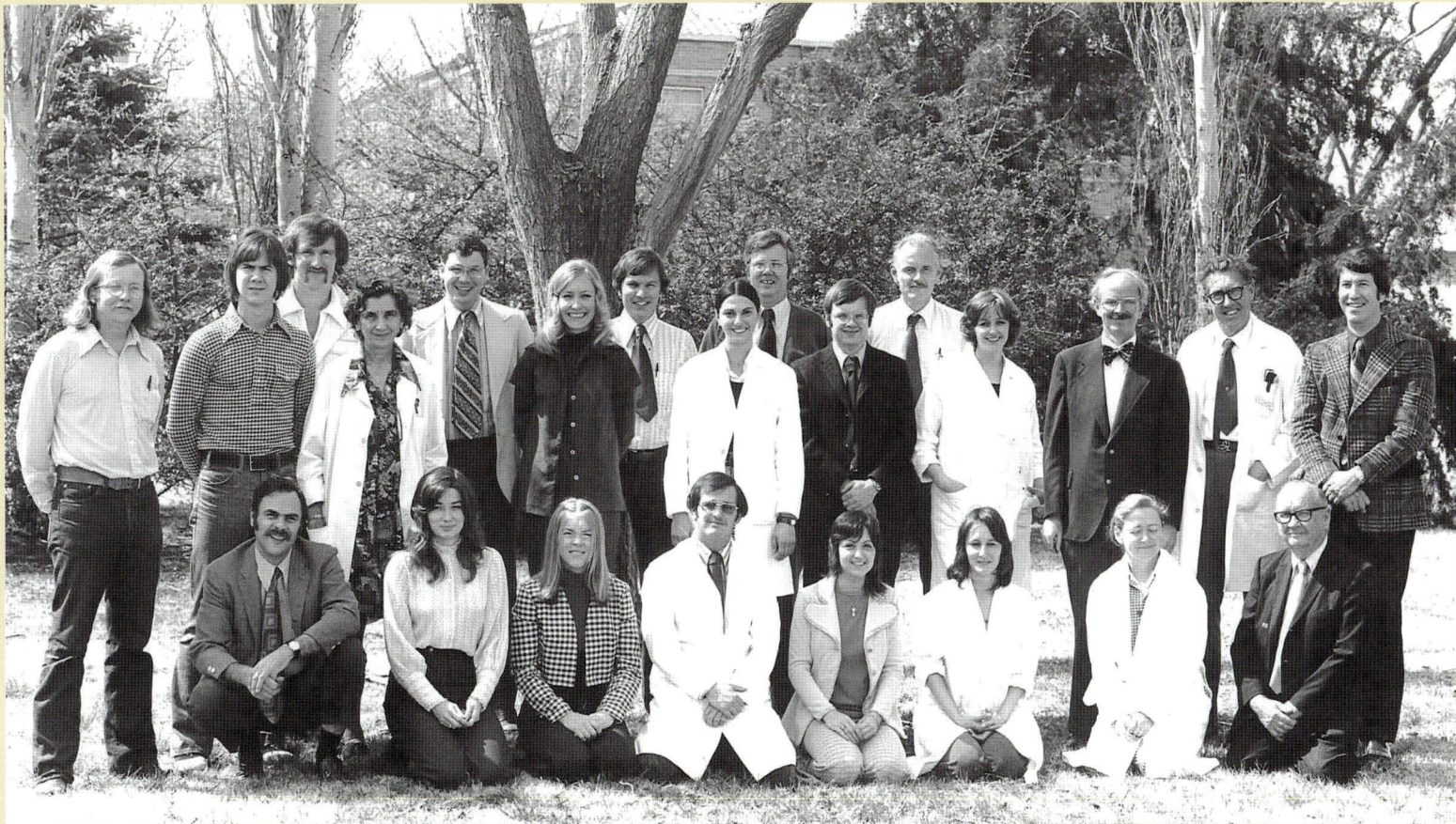

CHAPTER THREE

SCHOOL OF NURSING

Michael Evans, PhD, RN, Dean

The School of Nursing was established at Texas Tech University Health Sciences Center in 1981 when the Sixty-seventh Texas Legislature and Governor William P. Clements approved its funding with hopes of alleviating the shortage of nurses in West Texas. It was phenomenally successful in growing enrollment from 75 students the first year to 1,800 students in 2017.

The School of Nursing grew significantly across multiple campuses and online; it now offers bachelors, masters, and doctoral degrees. It manages practice plans to meet the needs of underserved populations, and its graduates hold positions of leadership as clinicians, academicians, administrators, and researchers. The founding dean and faculty shared a vision of a profession where education, practice, service, and the advancement of knowledge were integrated in the student experience. Faculty were not only educators, they were required to be active practitioners—a first among nursing schools in Texas.

Today, the school continues in this vein, educating new nurses, strengthening the careers of experienced nurses, and preparing innovative nurses to become leaders in health care. "That nurturing attitude is really what the school is all about," said 1983 graduate and former faculty member Mary Slater in a spring 1992 article published in *PULSE*, the publication for alumni and friends of Texas Tech University Health Sciences Center.

Teddy Langford Jones, PhD, RN, CNAA, and founding dean, joined Texas Tech University Health Sciences Center in 1979 and worked for two years on program development and faculty recruitment in preparation of the school's opening. In a letter published in the 1988 edition of *Plexus*, the university's yearbook, she wrote, "I believe as you look back at this yearbook sometime in the future, experience will have shown the advantages of an education here." Jones included improved health care in West Texas, collaboration, and inventiveness. As part of her leadership, the School of Nursing emphasized a strong clinical component in its programs, developed opportunities for practicing nurses through the Continuing Nursing Education program, and established the first nurse-led, faculty-practice income plan in Texas.

The school added an innovative, multiple-entry feature to its undergraduate program, admitting qualified students with experience as LVNs and RNs as well as those with no nursing experience. The school expanded its undergraduate program to Odessa and collaborated with the University of Texas Health Sciences Center at San Antonio allowing students to earn a PhD. One of the first things the school did early—before admitting the first student—was to create an honor society in 1982, and the first 17 School of Nursing graduates and community leader members were inducted in 1983. When membership had grown to 95, they began a lengthy process to

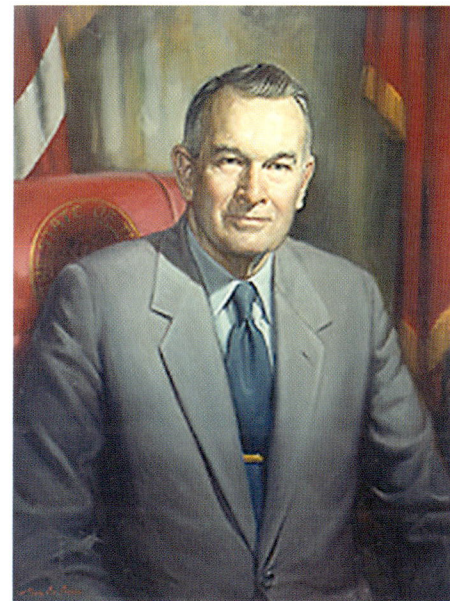

Portrait of William Perry (Bill) Clements, Jr, Governor. Courtesy of the Texas State Library and Archives Commission. Image included in accordance with Title 17 U.S.C. Section 107.

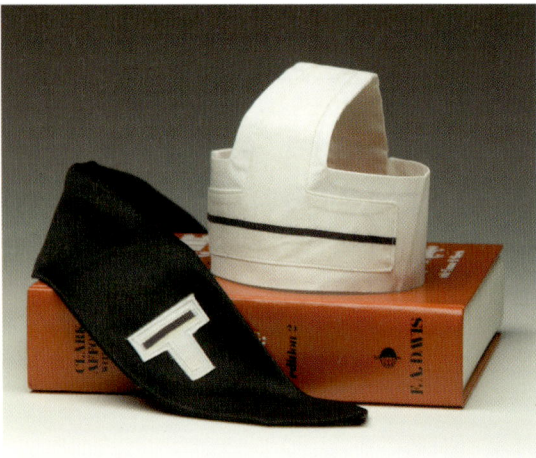

SON Cap and ties

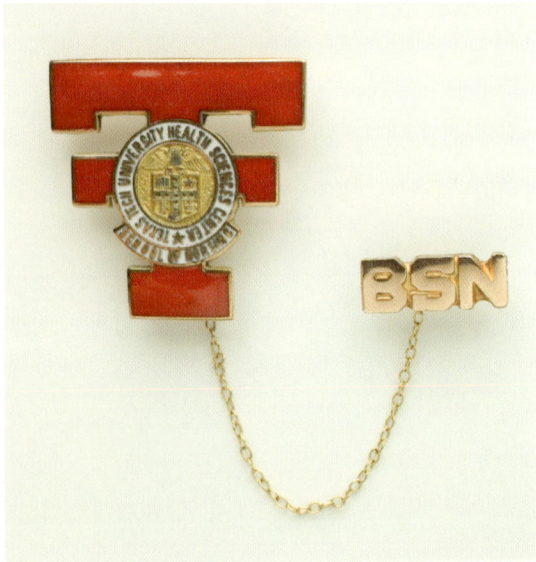

SON Historic nursing pin

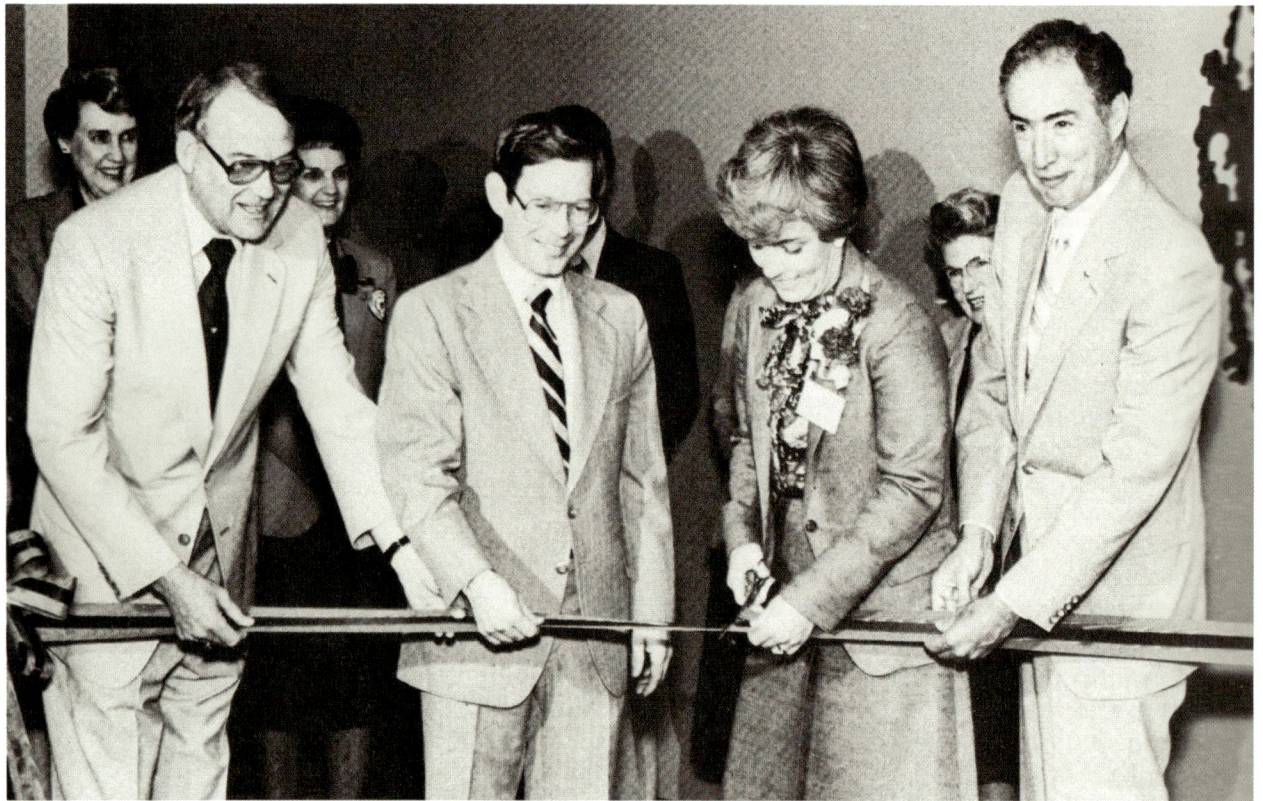

SON Ribbon Cutting Ceremony

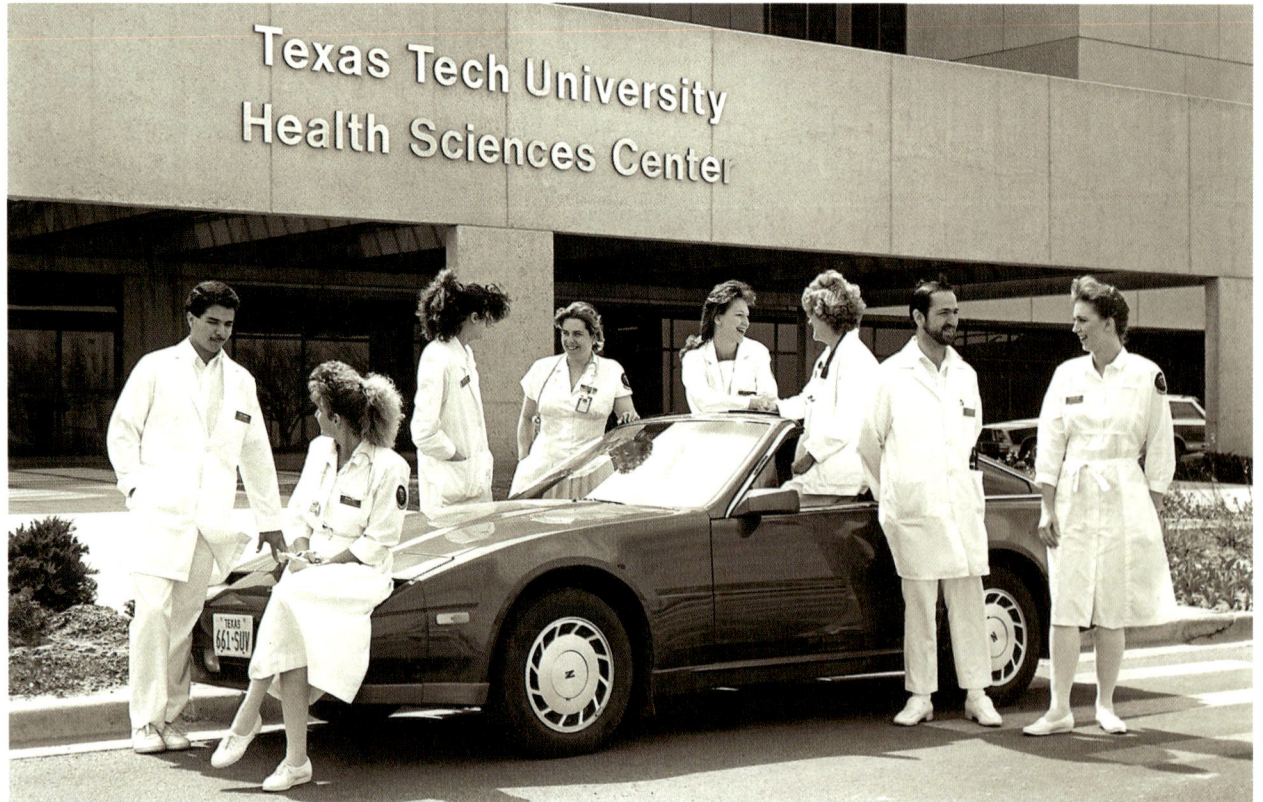

Historic image of SON students

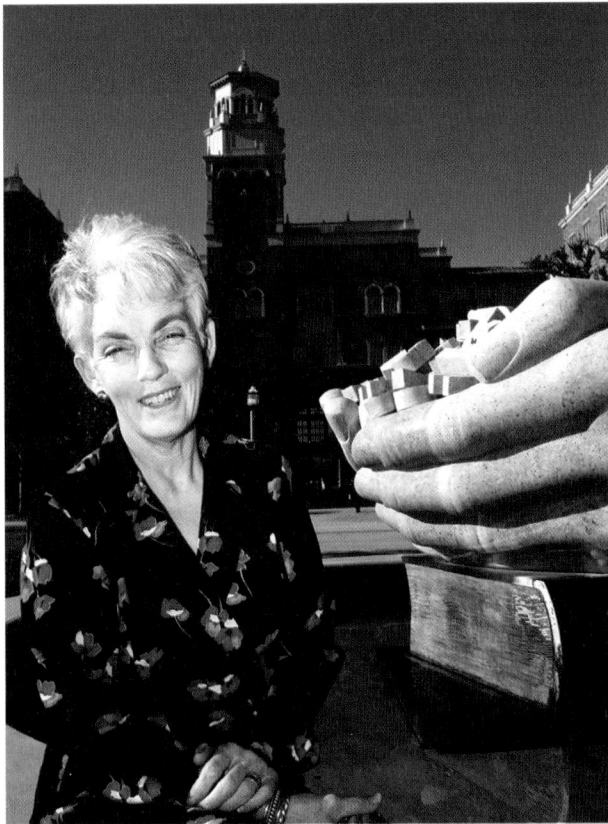

Teddy Langford Jones, Founding Dean

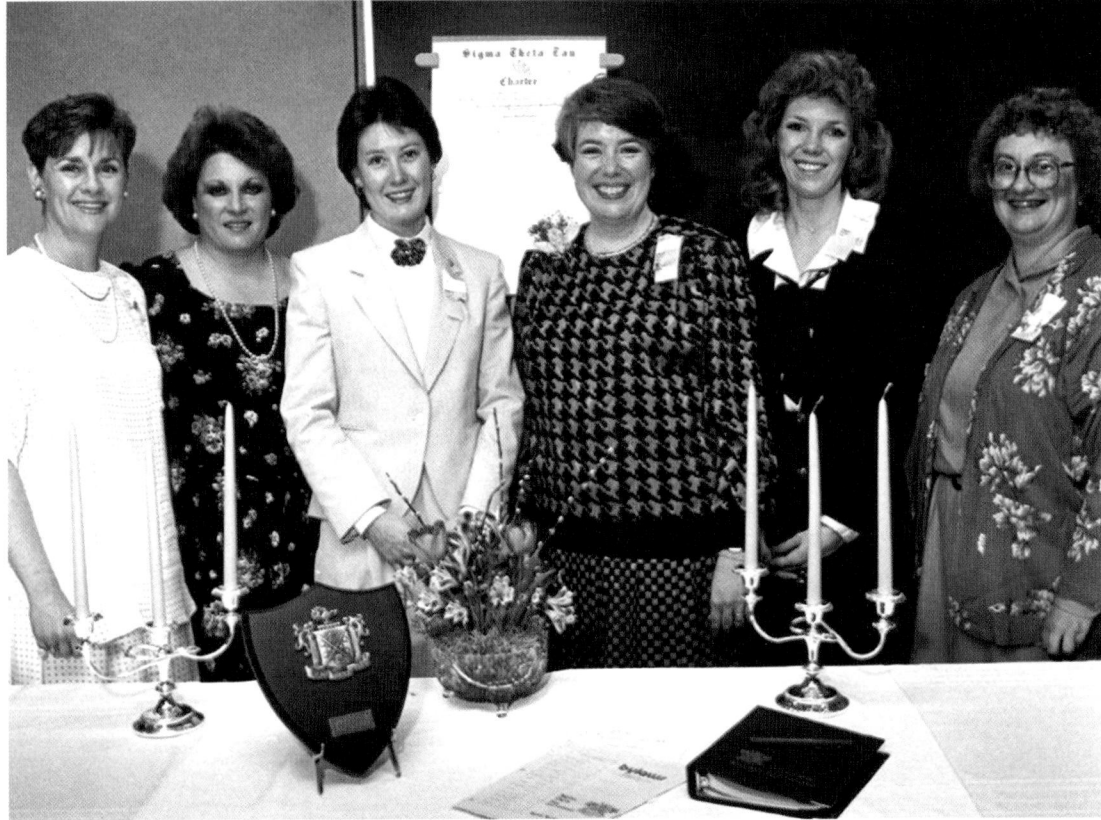

become a chartered chapter of Sigma Theta Tau International Honor Society of Nursing. Faculty members, Suzanne Cooke, RN, as president of the TTUHSC School of Nursing Honor Society, and Karen Dadich, RN, who would become first chapter president, petitioned and received approval to be the 226th chapter in 1988. The chapter, named Iota Mu, holds mentoring sessions, conferences, research days, and has received eight Key Awards, Sigma Theta Tau's recognition of efforts in membership recruitment, programming, professional and leadership development, and collaboration.

When Jones took the position in 1991 as interim director of HealthNet, Patricia S. Yoder-Wise, EdD, RN, FAAN, was named interim dean, a position she held for two years before being named dean. "It only seems like yesterday that Teddy Jones put a business card on my door when we were both in Colorado at a conference," said Yoder-Wise, who was the second faculty member hired for the new school. "The card read, 'Want to join me?' My first question was, 'Where is Lubbock, Texas?' I figure after being here for more than 35 years, I can now share that story because I do think Mac Davis had it right (in

his song), 'happiness is Lubbock, Texas, growing nearer and dearer,'" she said, slightly paraphrasing the song.

As dean, Yoder-Wise focused her attention on the national nursing shortage by expanding the school's resources to grow the undergraduate and graduate programs. She created a Dean's Council comprised of community leaders to advise the school on development activities that would assist with funding for future innovative projects. In addition, Yoder-Wise expanded the school's practice program and focused on recruitment of faculty and students from diverse ethnicities. Under her leadership, the Wellness Center came to fruition and the school broadened its borders by agreeing to collaborate with the University of Texas at Tyler to expand the graduate program's nurse practitioner education, which would benefit rural East Texas students and citizens.

"I was so lucky. My classes were taught by Teddy Langford, Pat Yoder-Wise, Helen Cox, and Nancy Ridenour," said Ruan Reast, FNP ('93, '91), in a 1994 issue of *PULSE*. Reast is now a nurse practitioner in the School of Medicine Department of Family and Community Medicine. "[They] were teaching me not only how to take a pulse or

Iota Mu Chartering Ceremony for Iota Mu, 226th chapter of Sigma Theta Tau International (SSTI), on March 12, 1988. The officers pictured are (left to right): Mary Slater (Chapter Counselor); Joy Ridlehuber (Chapter Counselor); Suzanne Cooke (Chapter Counselor and last President of the SON Honor Society [required precursor to chartering a chapter of SSTI]); Karen Dadich (First Iota Mu Chapter President); Sharon Decker (Iota Mu President-Elect); Nancy Ridenour (Treasurer) Officers not pictured are Dr. Mary Grace Umlauf, Vice President, and Kaye Kendall, Secretary 07-08

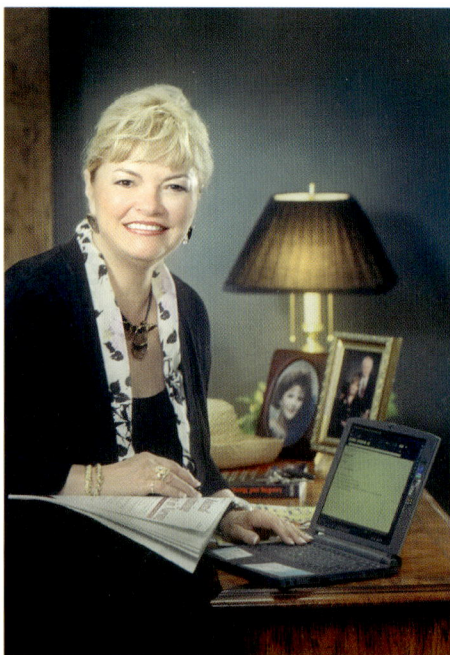

(ABOVE) Pat Yoder-Wise, Dean

(RIGHT) Nurse Faculty—Valerie Gregory
with patient

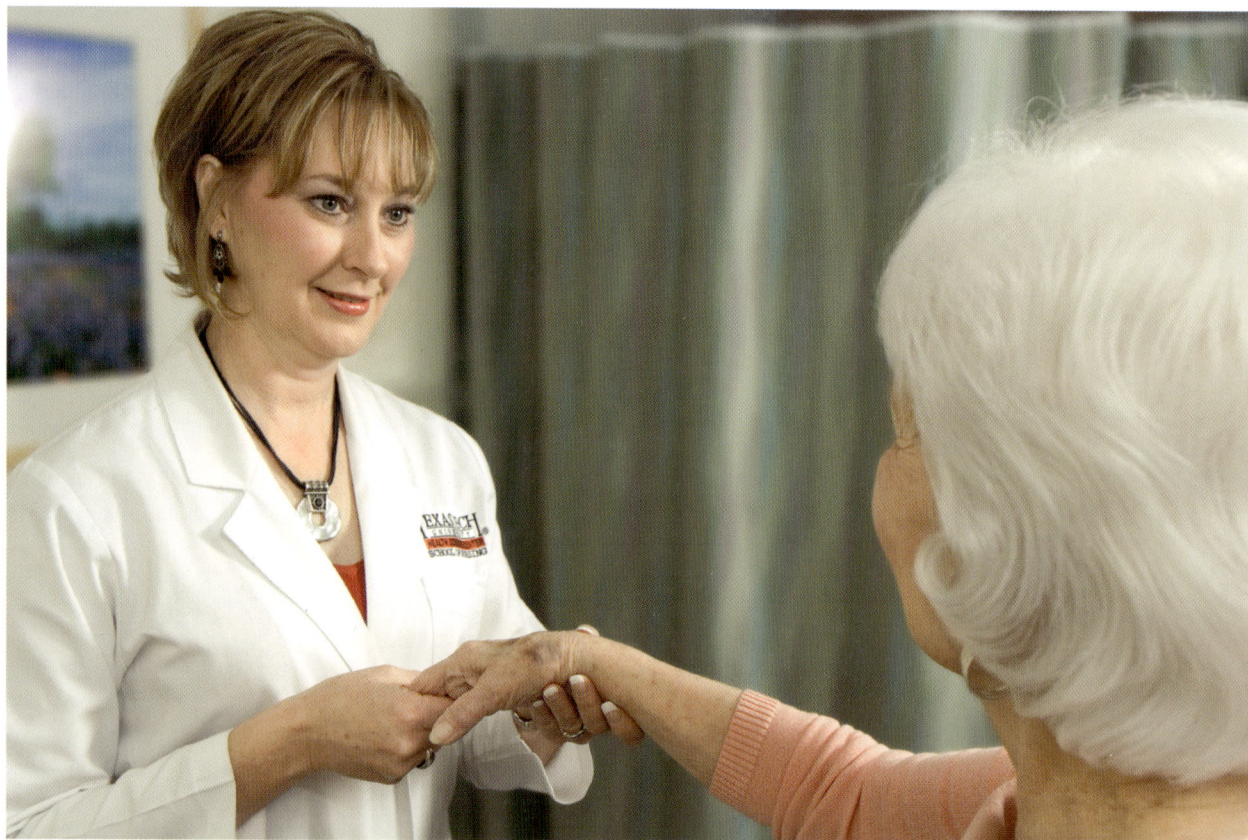

do a blood pressure, but also their philosophy of nursing. They had a vision about what nursing could be."

The School of Nursing continued to expand educational opportunities and has become known for its alternatives to traditional programs, which include the addition of an online program for a registered nurse to obtain a bachelor of science in nursing, an accelerated second-degree bachelor's program, and a veteran to bachelor of science in nursing degree for service members with military medical experience who wish to earn a nursing degree.

"We've grown and yet the growth still allows us to maintain the essence of those very traits that we value," said Kathy Sridaromont, PhD, MSN, RN, traditional undergraduate associate dean and another of the school's founding faculty.

Alexia Green, PhD, RN, FAAN, had served as president of the Texas Nurses Association and long admired the school's nursing students. She succeeded Yoder-Wise as dean, and one of her goals upon taking the helm in 2000 was to establish relationships with students, faculty, and the community. As dean, Green focused on growth in response to the statewide nursing shortage by expanding

the nursing school to Abilene, Austin, and El Paso's Gayle Greve School of Nursing. Green served concurrently as dean and professor within the school and saw student enrollment almost double in the nine years she was dean.

"We were one of the most innovative programs across the state certainly and maybe across the nation at the time," said Jo Ferrer, managing director for the school's education technology services, which were established in 2002. "Technology was being used in some of the schools but because of our service area and serving West Texas we really had to look at new ways to deliver education, new ways to hire and support faculty. We did that through the expertise of a cadre of professionals to help us develop our programs and technology in building a very robust, well-staffed, well-equipped IT team. Our students have some of the best support you can get out there being a distance student. Even if you are a full-time student in class, you are still going to be online. So much education is delivered now online."

It was also during this time that the School of Nursing became increasingly involved in the development of simulation science and the impact it had on healthcare

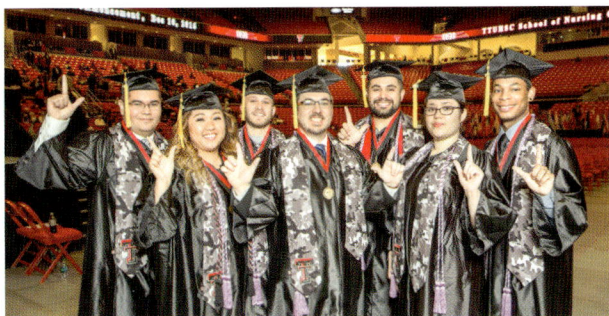
Veterans to Nurse graduates

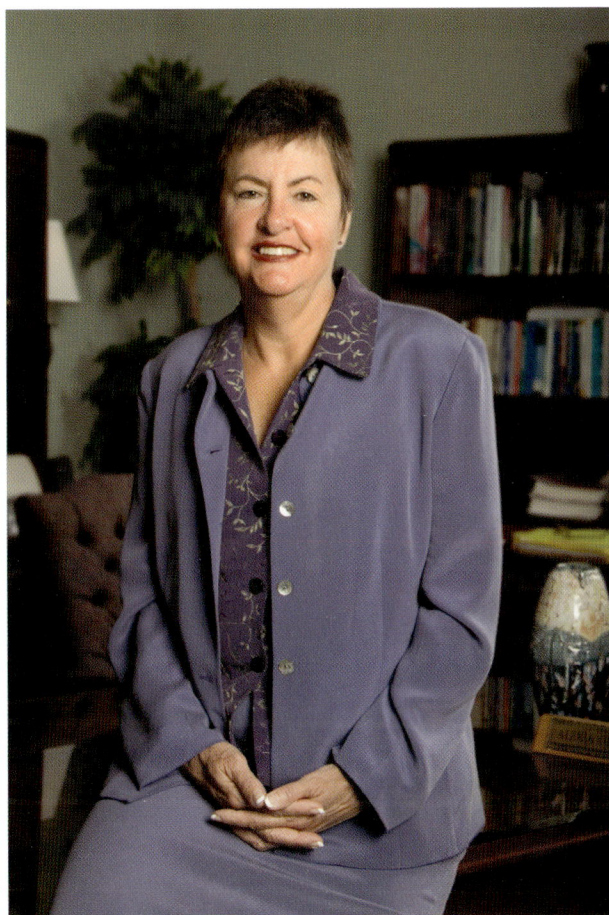
Dean Alexia Green

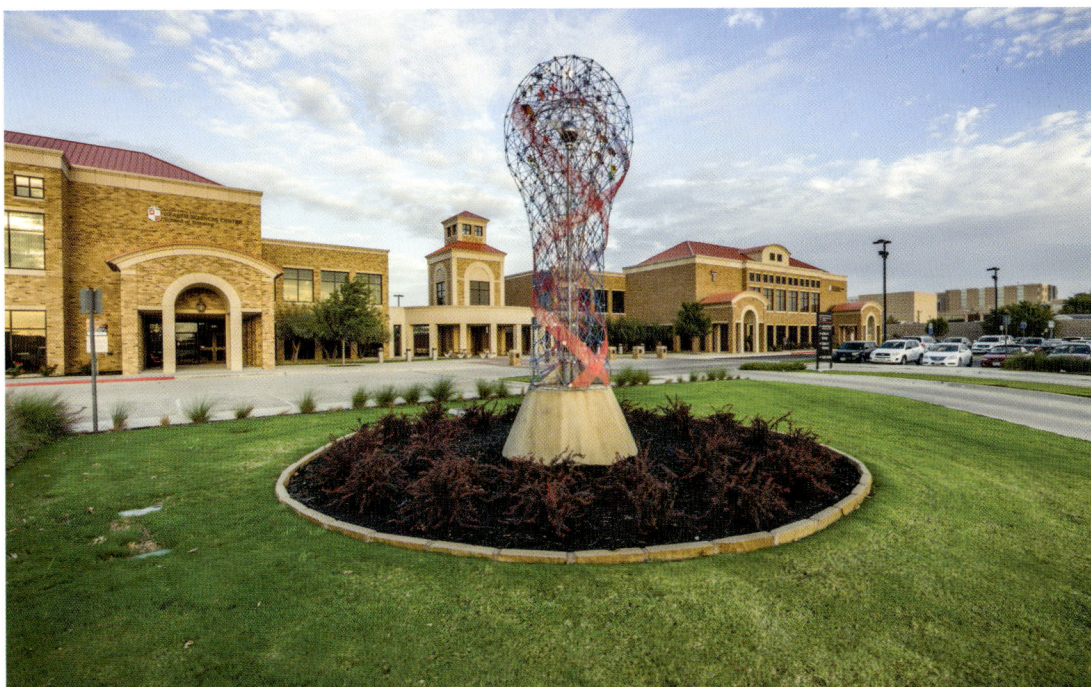

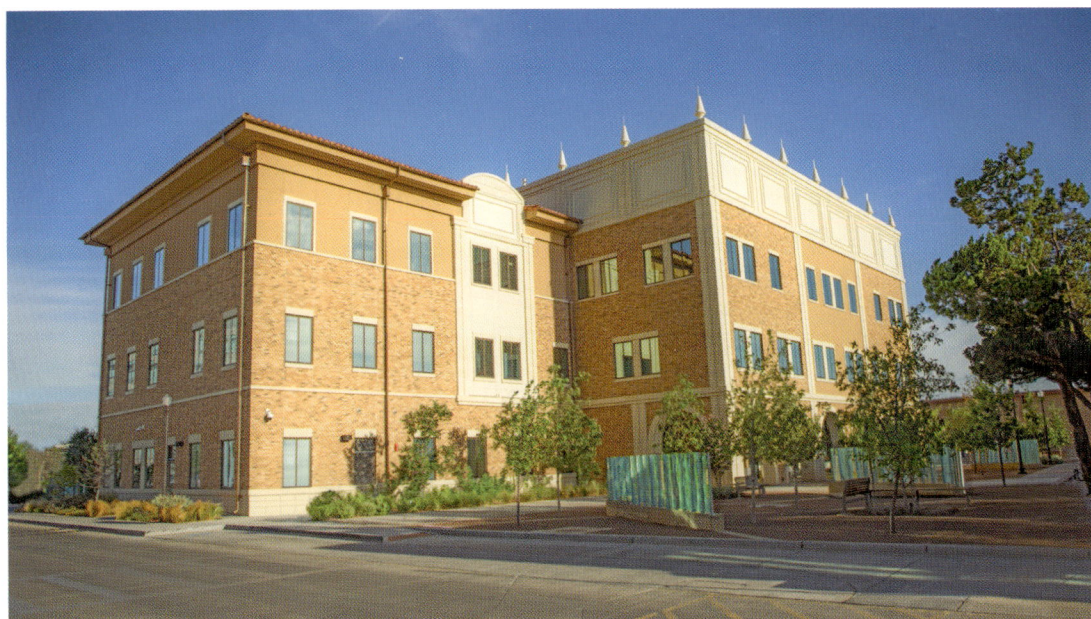

education and patient safety. Since the late 1980s through 2010 the School of Nursing's Clinical Simulation Center was located on the third floor of the Health Sciences Center. It was composed of 8,500 square feet and was predominantly used by the School of Nursing. These computerized simulators had realistic heart, lung, and bowel sounds and could be programmed to respond appropriately to the learner's actions.

At the same time, the School of Nursing was involved in several projects that supported the development of the science of simulation. For example, from 2003 to 2006 the School of Nursing participated as one of the eight national sites for the landmark National League for the Nursing/Laerdal simulation study. The NLN/Jeffries Simulation Theory was an outcome of this study. In the fall of 2009, TTUHSC opened the much larger SimLife Center with

(TOP) SON Abilene. Photographer: Kevin Halliburton, AIA, www.Ice-Imaging.com, Architect: TLP/PSC, www.Team-PSC.com

(BOTTOM) SON Gayle Greve School, El Paso

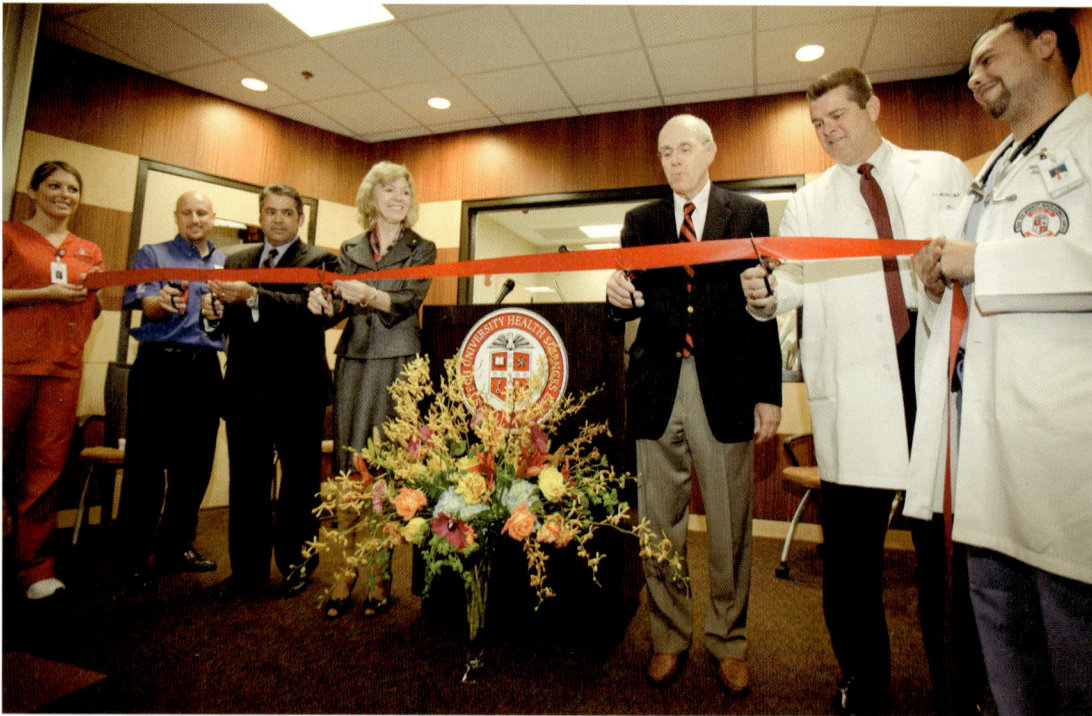
Ribbon cutting with dignitaries and Chancellor Hance

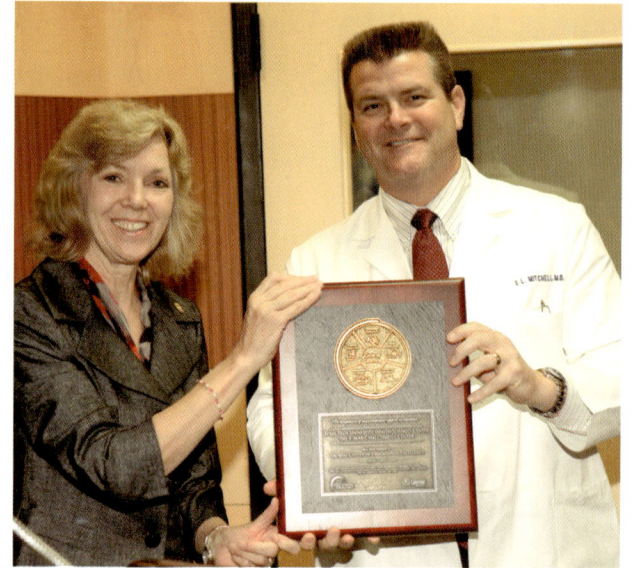
Dedication of SimCenter: Tedd Mitchell, MD with Director Sharon Decker

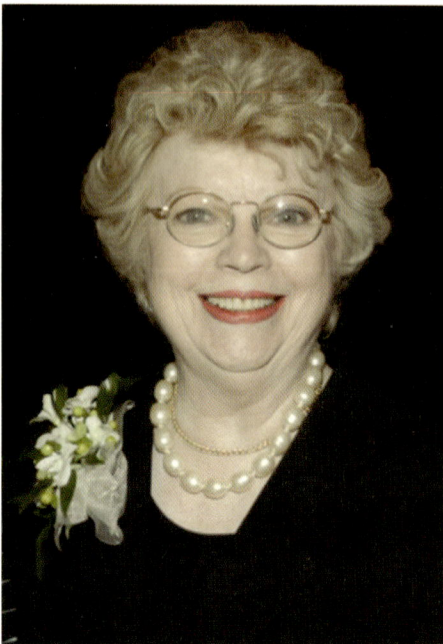
F. Marie Hall, Philantropist

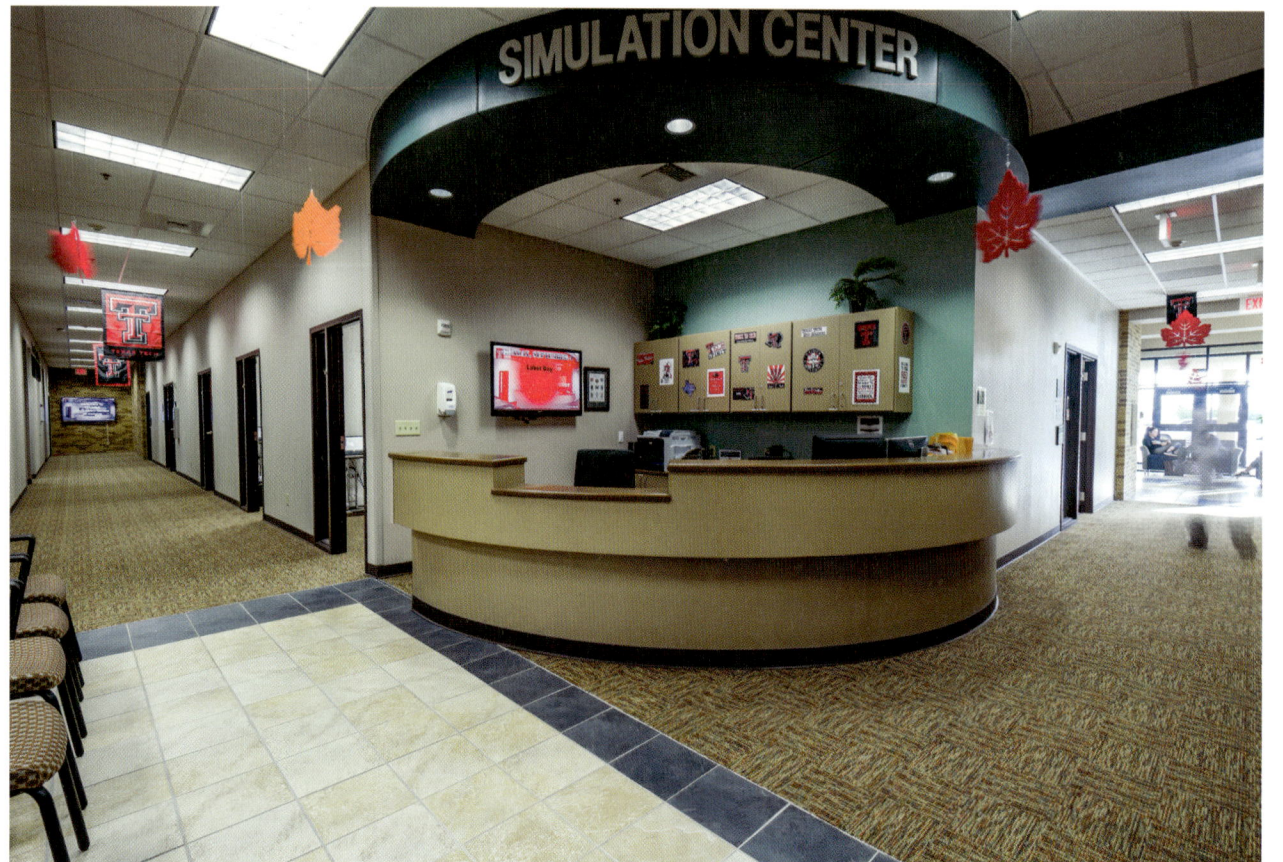
Abilene SimCenter. Photographer: Kevin Halliburton, AIA, www.Ice-Imaging.com, Architect: TLP/PSC, www.Team-PSC.com

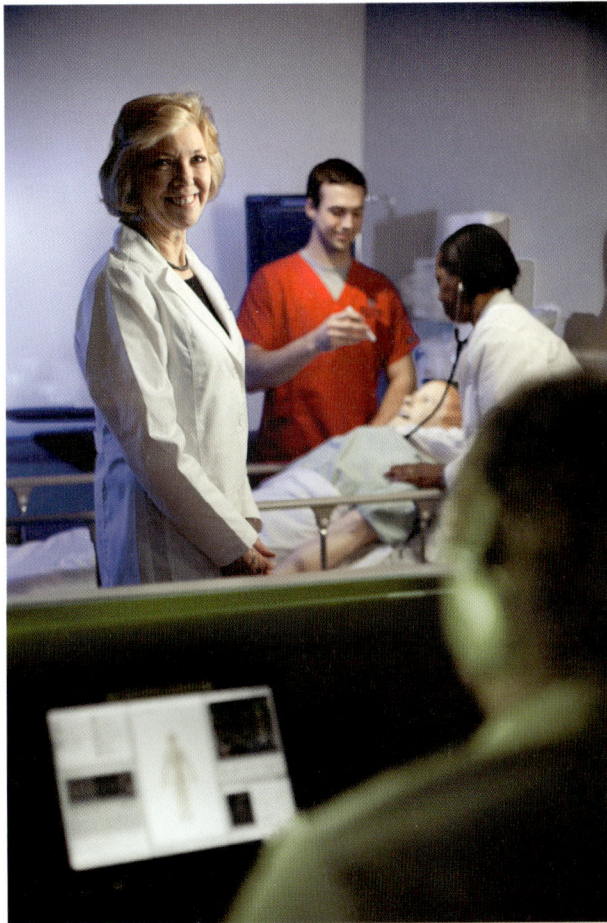

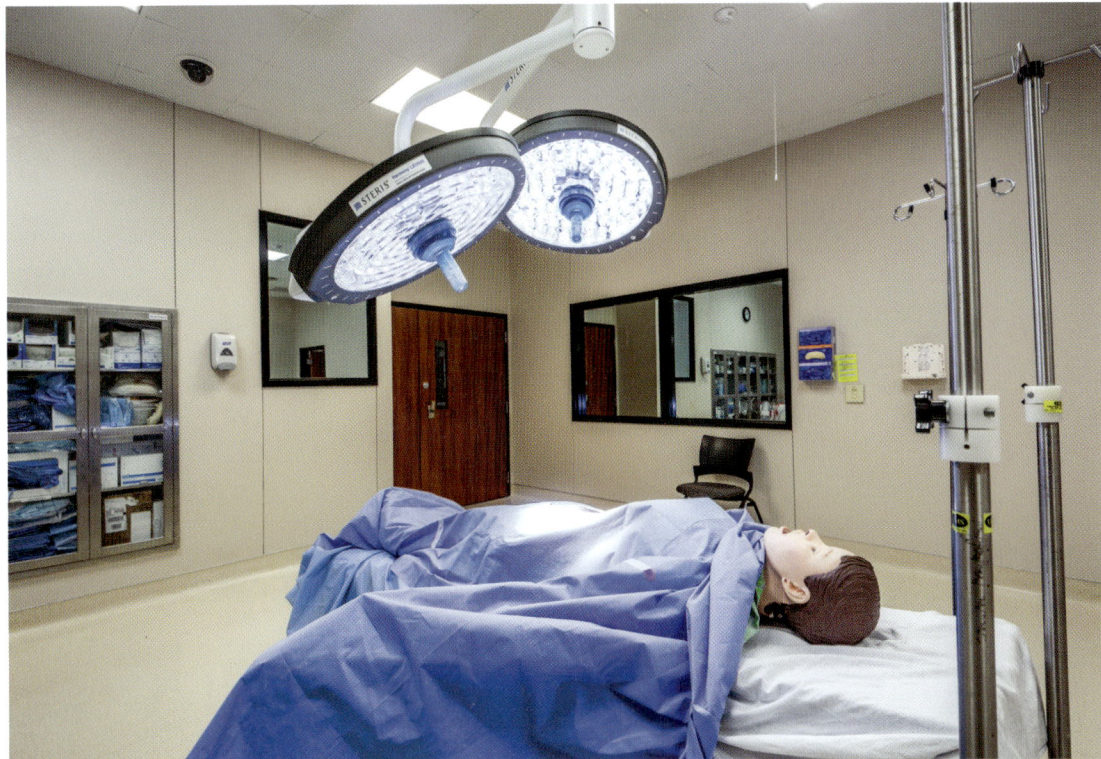

(LEFT) Sharon Decker, Director SimCenter, Lubbock

(ABOVE) Abilene SimCenter. Photographer: Kevin Halliburton, AIA, www.Ice-Imaging.com, Architect: TLP/PSC, www.Team-PSC.com

the support of its namesake, philanthropist F. Marie Hall. As TTUHSC continued to grow, the simulation centers in Abilene and Odessa were proposed and established.

Under Green's leadership, the Larry Combest Community Health and Wellness Center became the state's first nurse-managed, federally qualified health center (FQHC), providing care to those in an underserved area of East Lubbock. These services were later extended to the Abilene community, through a second FQHC. Through these practice plans, the school now provides care to more than 7,000 patients annually in underserved areas. "My time with the school has been one of great pride," said Green. Yondell Masten, PhD, RN, WHNP-BC, served as interim dean from 2010 to 2012. During her tenure, Masten collaborated with the library's Information Literacy modular program. All incoming nursing students were required and still are required to complete these modules before starting their nursing course work.

After being named dean in 2011, Michael Evans, PhD, RN, NEA-BC, FACHE, FAAN, set his sights on

preserving the school's excellent reputation and increasing student and faculty diversity. The Hispanic Outlook in Higher Education has ranked the School of Nursing in the top third for schools conferring the most bachelor's degrees in nursing for Hispanic graduates.

Additionally, the school developed an international program in Jinotega, Nicaragua, where students can earn course and/or clinic credit. The program, begun in 2012, provides training for community health workers to screen for cervical cancer, which is one of the leading causes of death of women under 50 in this mountainous area. They may also do as many as 700 well-child exams per day. The program is part of the school's global health initiative and it expects to expand the program to Peru and Costa Rica and eventually to Thailand, said Amy Moore, DNP, RN, FNP-C, director of TTUHSC School of Nursing's Global Health program.

Longtime faculty in the School of Nursing include Sharon Decker, PhD, Yondell Masten, RN, PhD, and Kathryn Sridaromont, RN, MSN. Sharon Decker, PhD,

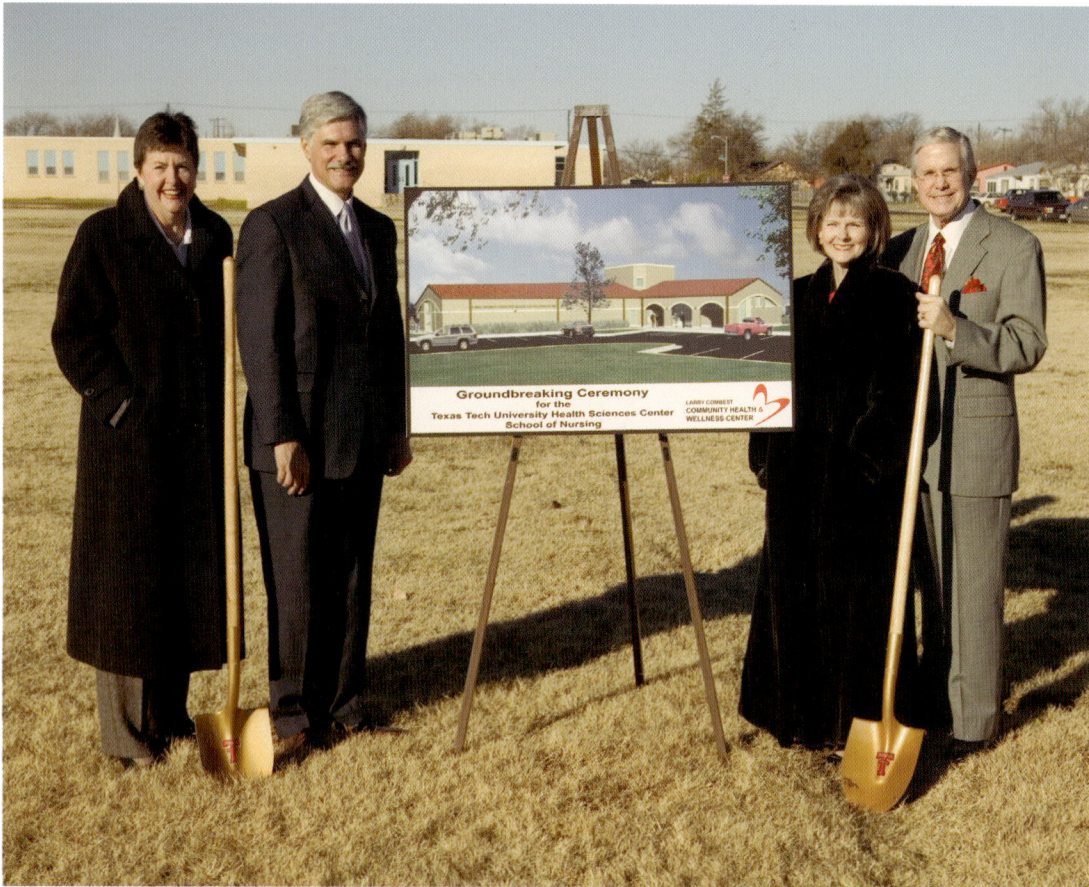

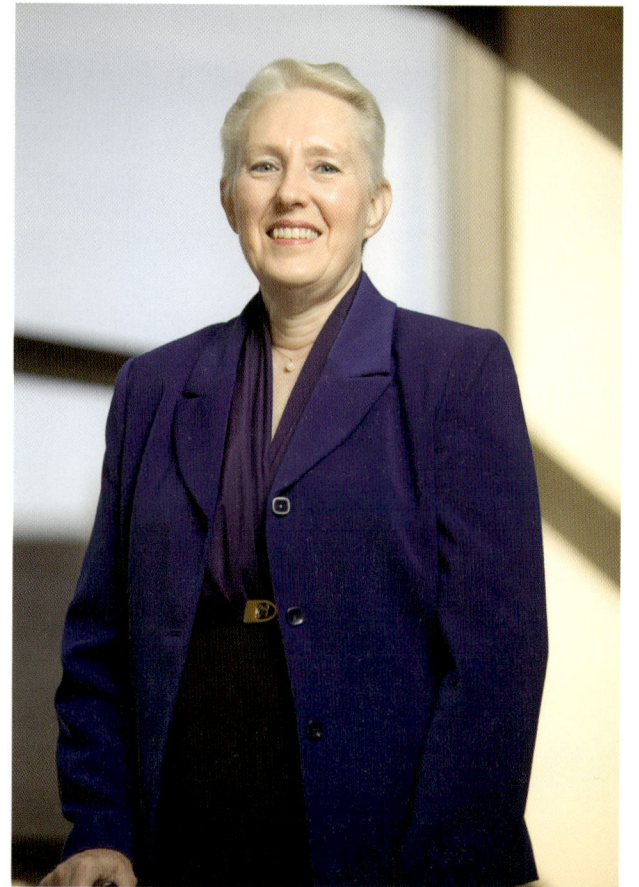

(ABOVE LEFT) Larry Combest Center Dedication. Pictured are Alexa Green, Chancellor David Smith, and Mr. & Mrs. Larry Combest

(ABOVE RIGHT) Yondell Masten, Interim Dean

(RIGHT) Nurse Amy Moore in Nicaragua with student and patient. Michelle Ensminger, Photographer

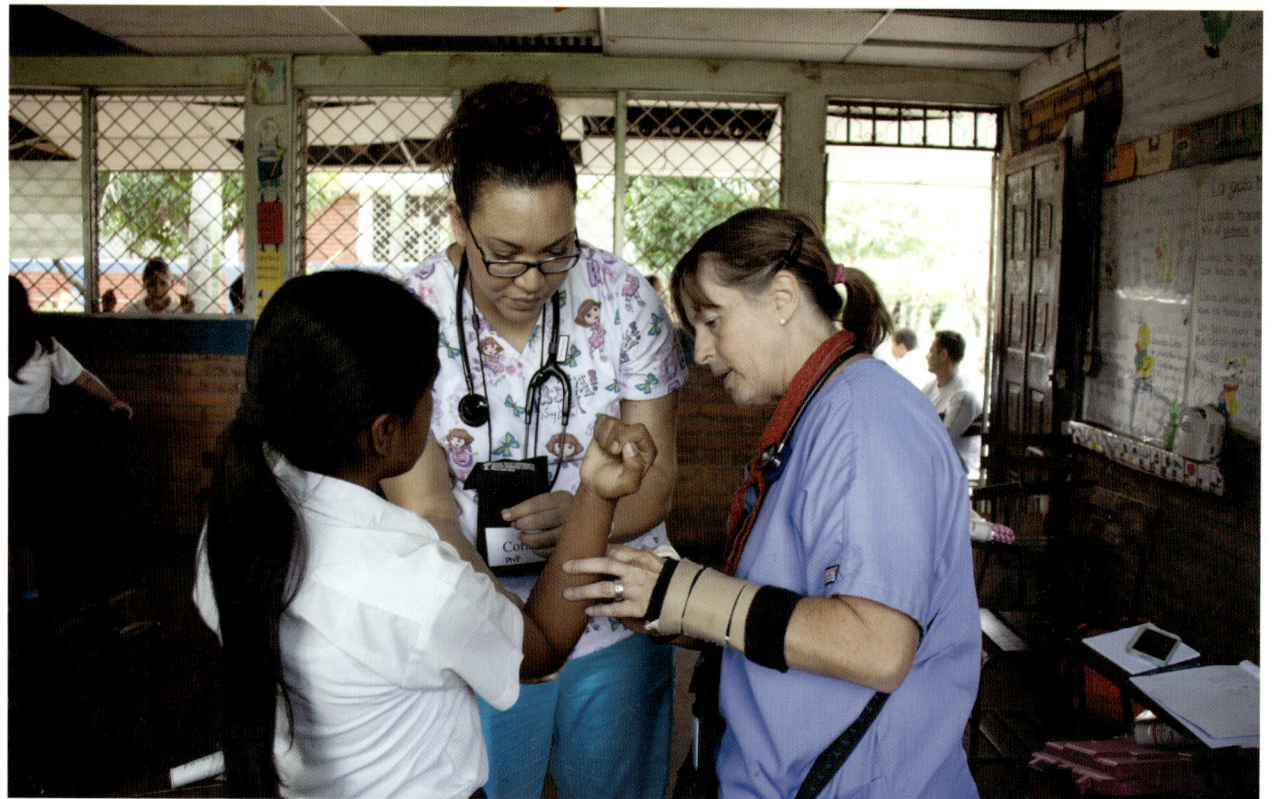

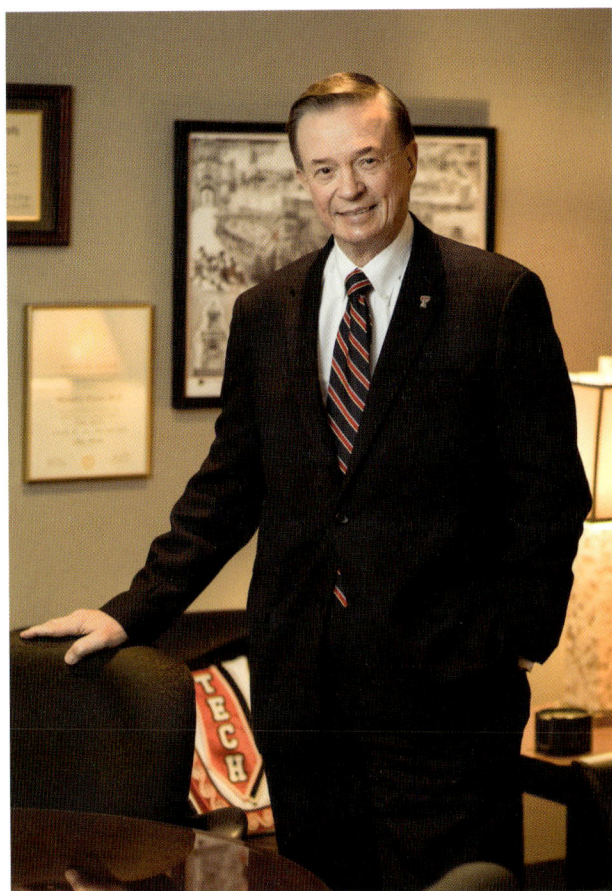

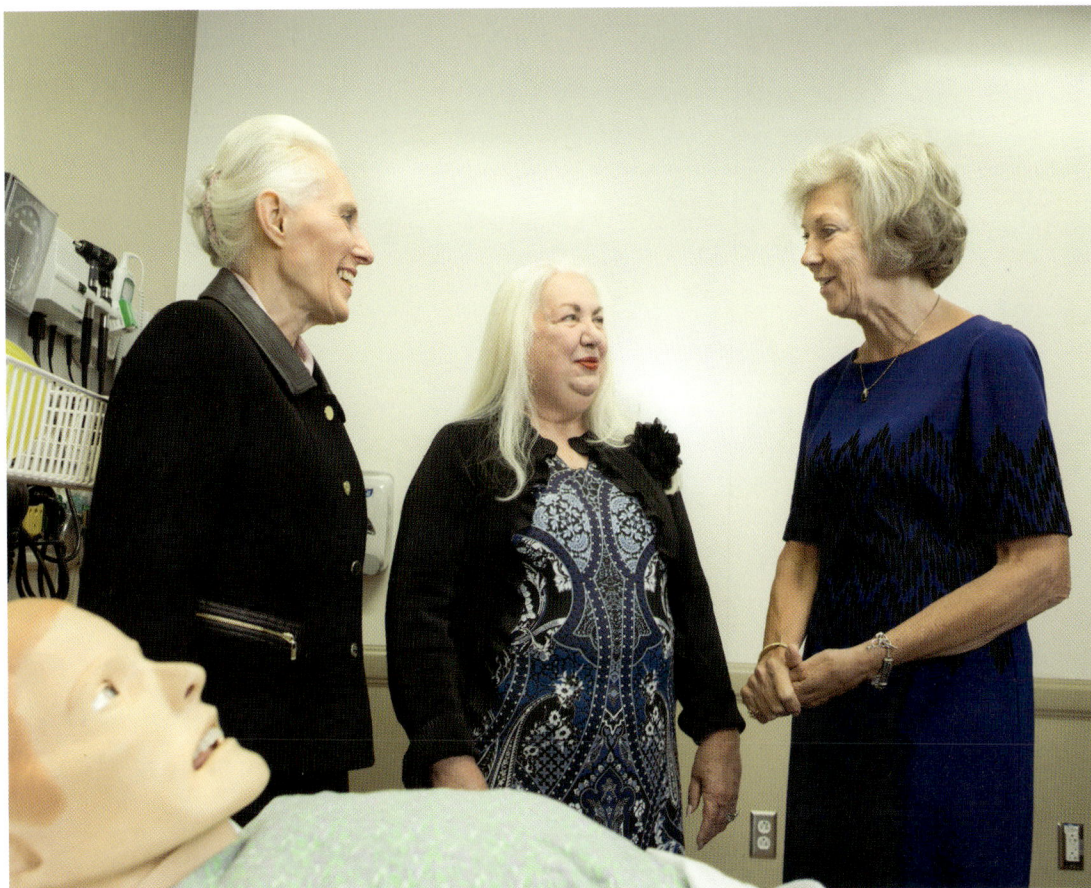

RN, FSSH, ANEF, FAAN is the associate dean for simulation, a professor in the School of Nursing, the executive director of the TTUHSC Simulation Program (Abilene, Dallas, Lubbock, and Odessa), a TTUHSC Grover E. Murray Professor, and holds the Covenant Health System and the Endowed Chair in Simulation and Nursing Education at Texas Tech University Health Science Center in Lubbock, Texas

Dr. Decker's research and scholarship is related to how simulation can be used as an innovative teaching-learning strategy to facilitate the development of critical thinking skills and promote clinical competency. Dr. Decker has presented at conferences and provided consultation for nursing schools throughout the United States related to the integration of simulation into the curriculum and has been recognized numerous times by Texas Tech University Health Sciences Center for her excellence in teaching.

Yondell Masten, RN, PhD, holds the Florence Thelma Hall Endowed Chair for Nursing Excellence in Women's Health and her research focuses on prenatal education, adolescent pregnancy, and women's health. This academic position includes research, clinical, and teaching activities which are in line with Masten's first degree in Engineering. She is the Outcomes Management and Evaluation associate dean for SON and has been an active and innovative instructor. Recent projects include codirecting the Nurse-Family Partnership and the Patient Navigator Program at the Larry Combest Community Health and Wellness Center. Together with Drs. McGovern and Lutherer she was one of the founding members of the TTUHSC Faculty Senate.

Kathryn Sridaromont, RN, MSN, associate professor and department chair of the Traditional Undergraduate Program, has served the School of Nursing as a faculty member, mentor, community connector, and overall outstanding ambassador since 1981. According to her colleagues, she continues to demonstrate an extraordinary love and dedication to nursing, pediatric patients, students, and the School of Nursing in every aspect of her role.

(LEFT) Michael Evans, Ph.D., R.N., NEA-BC, FACHE, FAAN, Dean

(RIGHT) Yondell Masten, Kathy Sridaromont and Sharon Decker

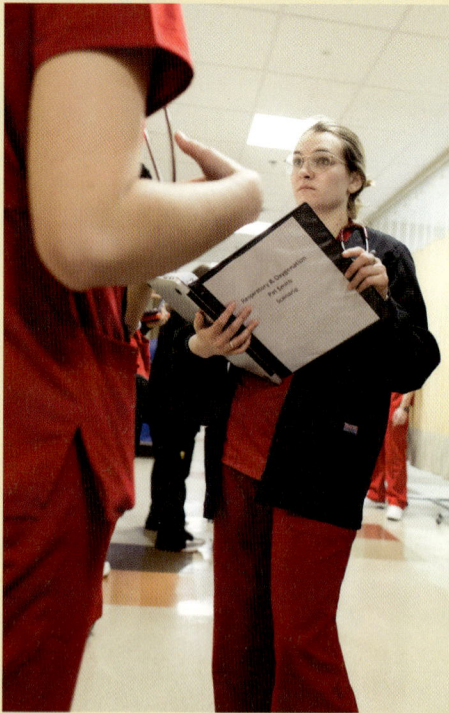
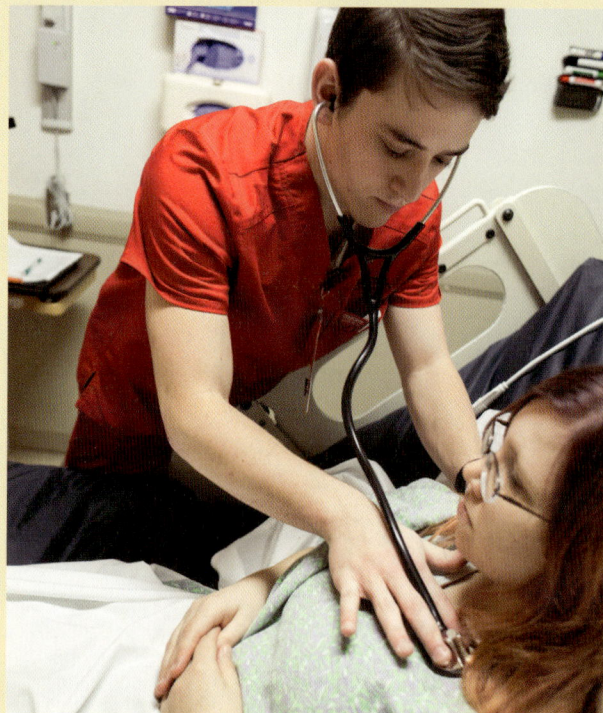
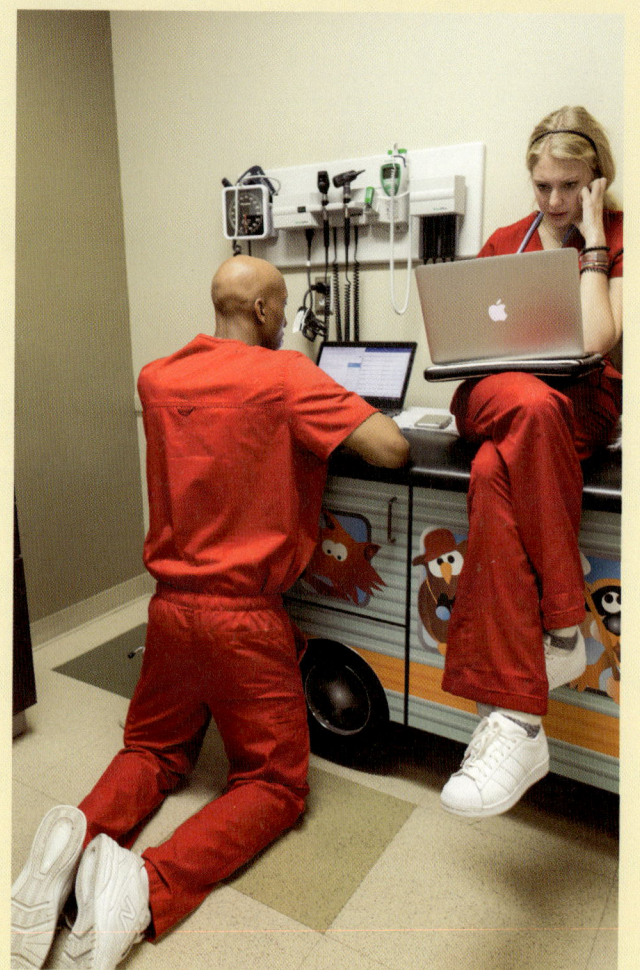
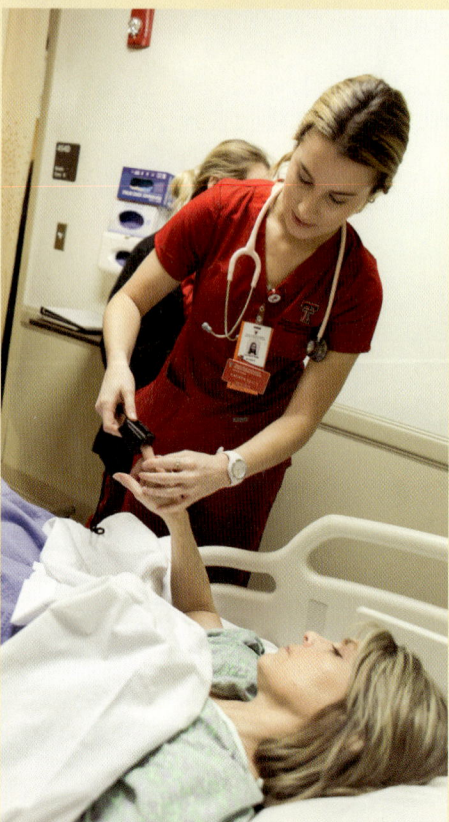
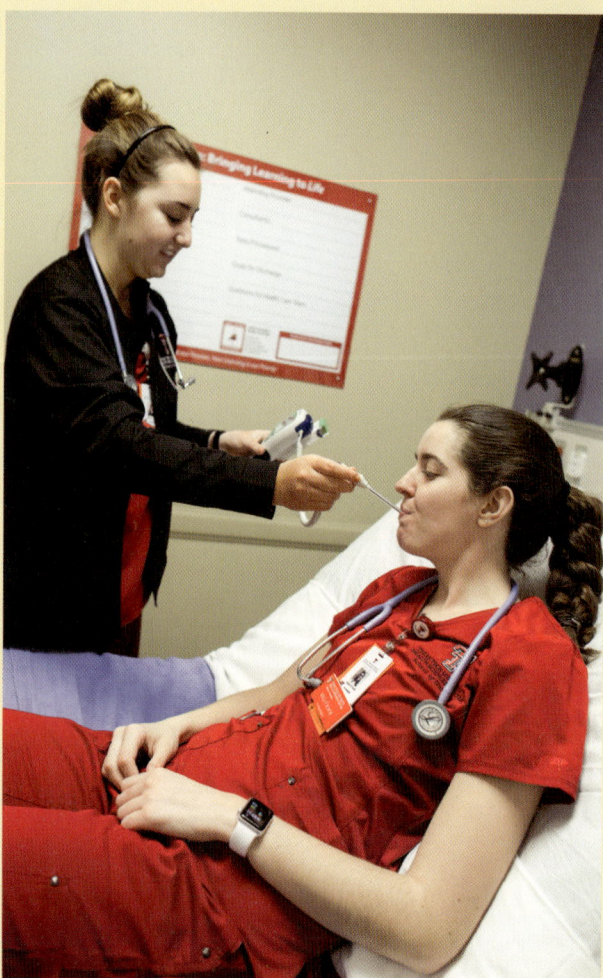
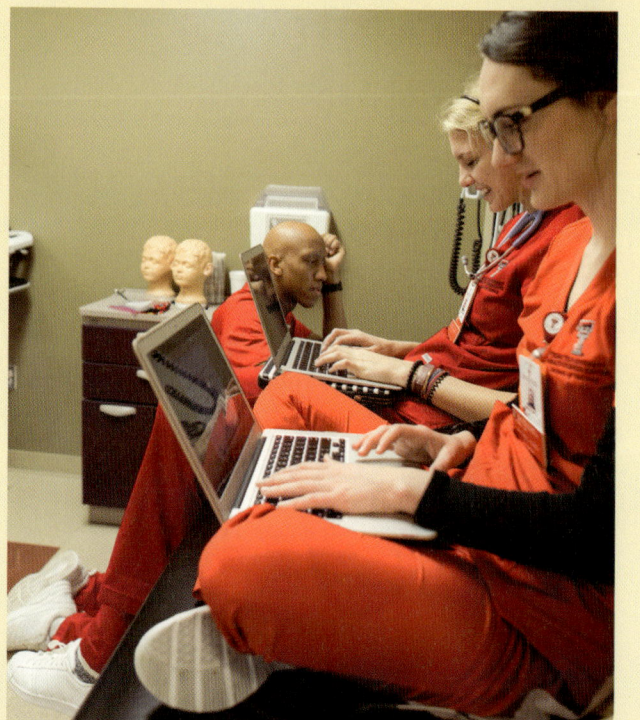

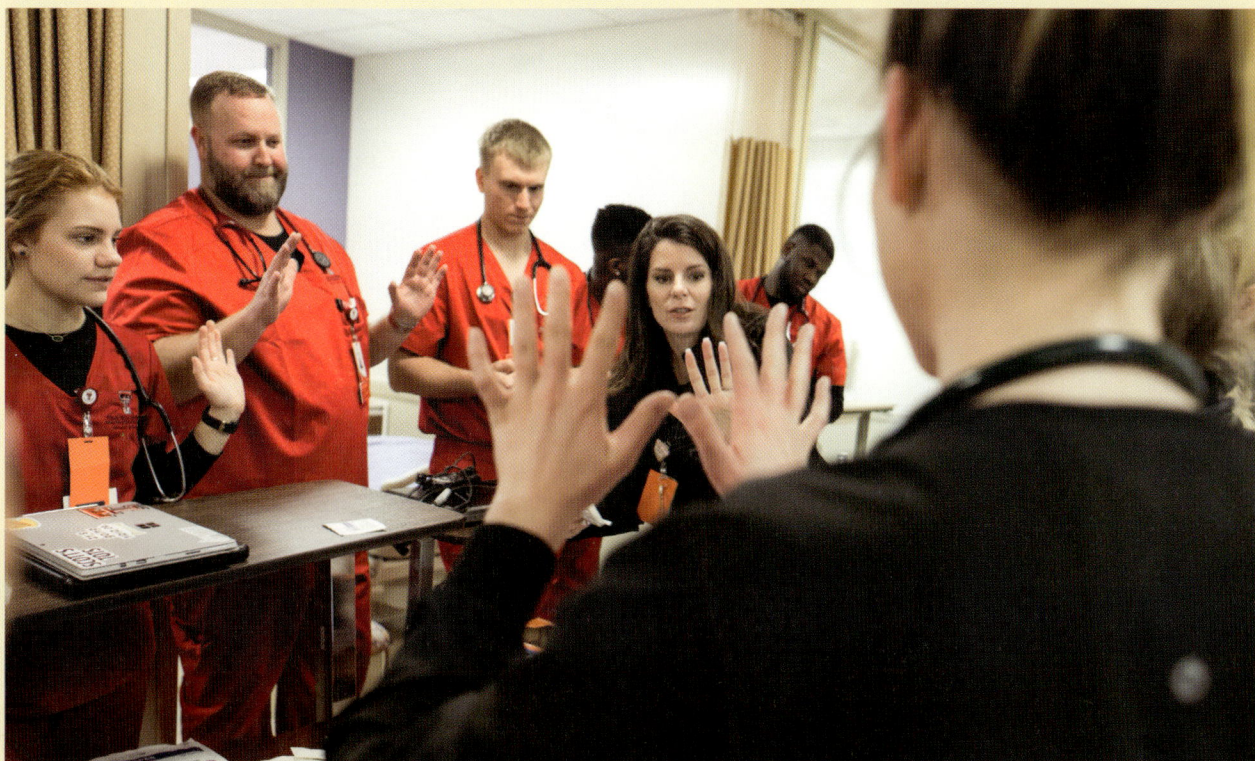

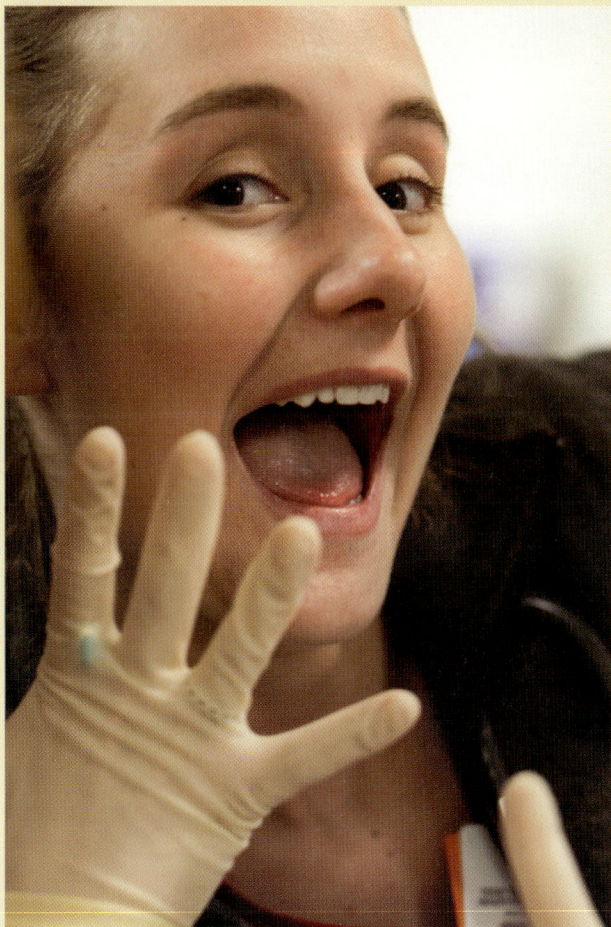

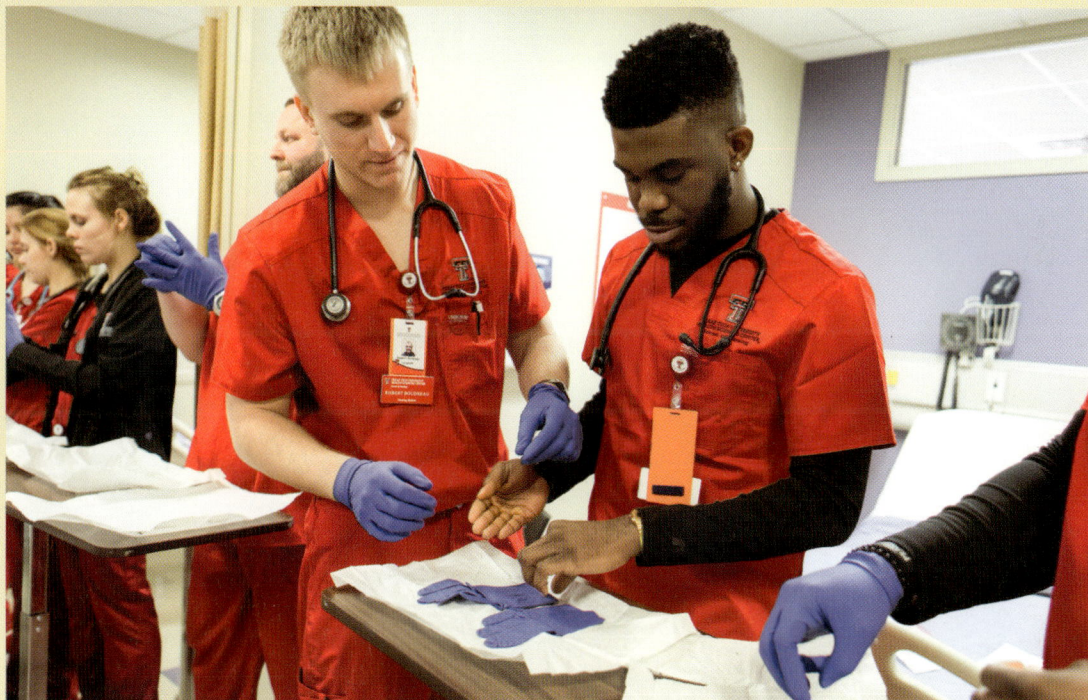

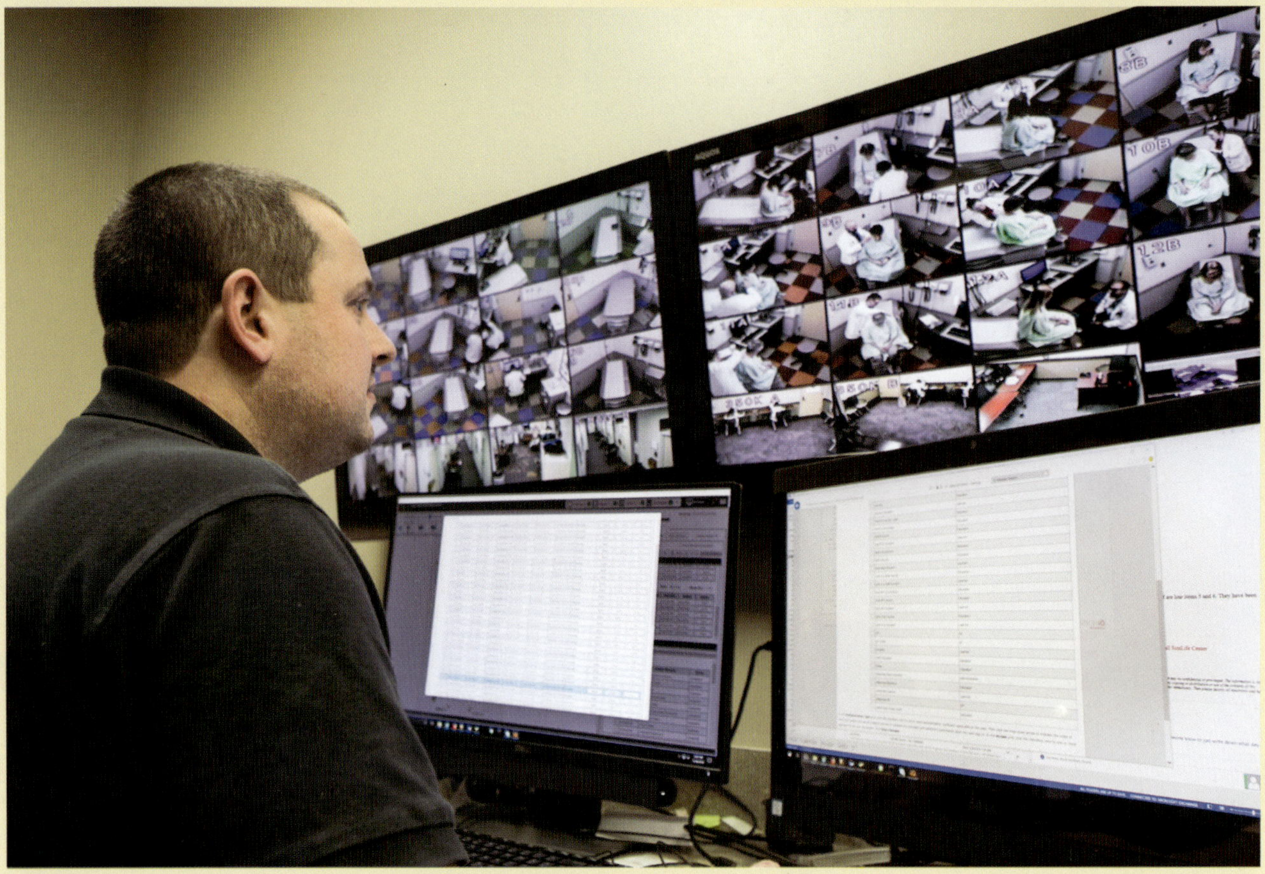

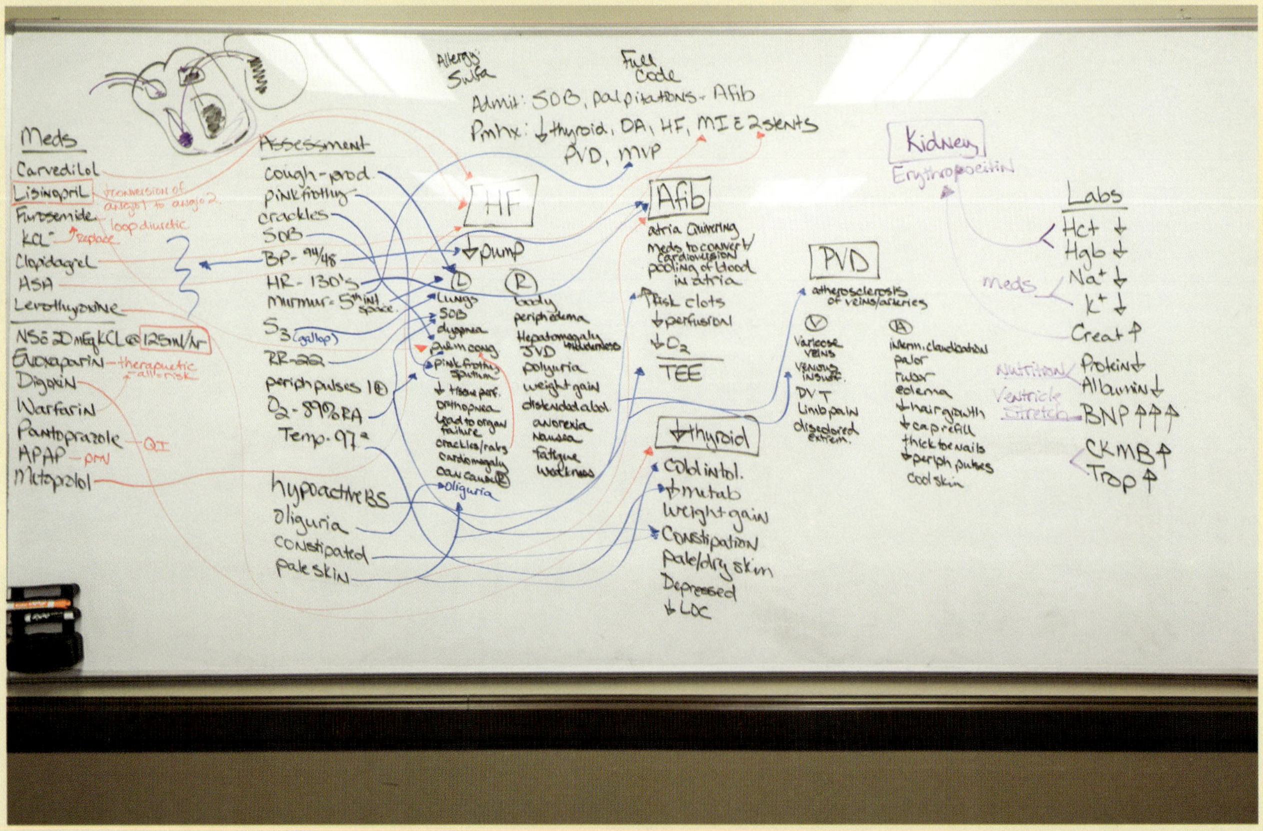
Allergy: Sulfa
Full Code
Admit: SOB, palpitations - Afib
Pmhx: ↓thyroid, DA, HF, MI c̄ 2 stents
PVD, MVP
Meds
Carvedilol
Lisinopril
Furosemide
loop diuretic
KCL
Clopidogrel
ASA
Levothyroxine
Enoxaparin
therapeutic
Digoxin
Warfarin
Pantoprazole
APAP - prn
Metoprolol
Assessment
cough-prod.
pink frothy
crackles
SOB
BP- 94/48
HR- 130's
murmur - 5th int. space
S3 (gallop)
RR-22
periph pulses
O2 - 89% RA
Temp- 97°
hypoactive BS
oliguria
constipated
pale skin
HF
↓pump
L
R
Lungs
SOB
dyspnea
pulm cong
pink frothy sputum
↓ tissue perf.
orthopnea
lead to organ failure
crackles/rales
cardiomegaly
oliguria
body
periph edema
Hepatomegaly
JVD
polyuria
weight gain
distended abd
anorexia
Nausea
fatigue
weakness
Afib
atria quivering
meds to convert/ cardioversion
pooling of blood in atria
↑risk clots
↓perfusion
↓O2
TEE
↓thyroid
Cold intol.
↓metab
weight gain
Constipation
Pale/dry skin
Depressed
↓LOC
PVD
atherosclerosis of veins/arteries
V
Varicose veins
venous insuff.
DVT
Limb pain
discolored extrem.
A
interm. claudication
palor
rubor
edema
↓hair growth
↓cap refill
thick toenails
↓periph pulses
cool skin
Kidney
Erythropoeitin
Labs
Hct ↓
Hgb ↓
Na+ ↓
K+ ↓
Creat ↑
Protein ↓
Albumin ↓
BNP ↑↑↑
CKMB ↑
Trop ↑
meds
Nutrition
Ventricle Stretch

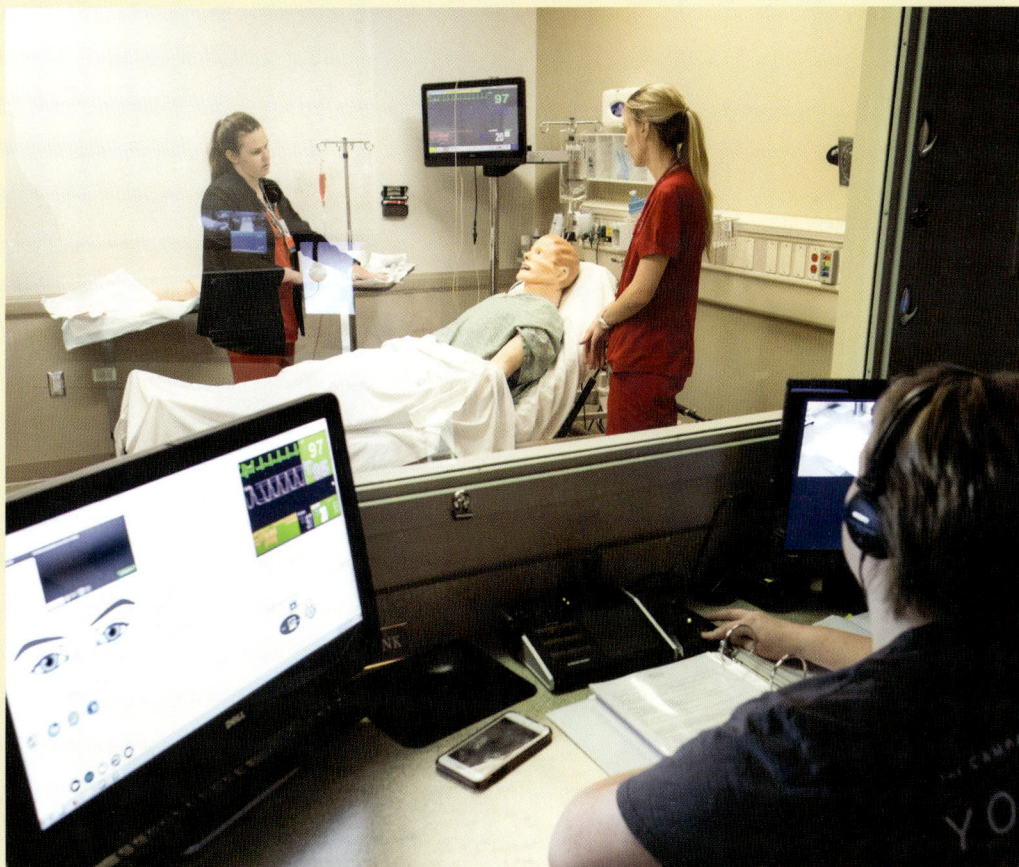

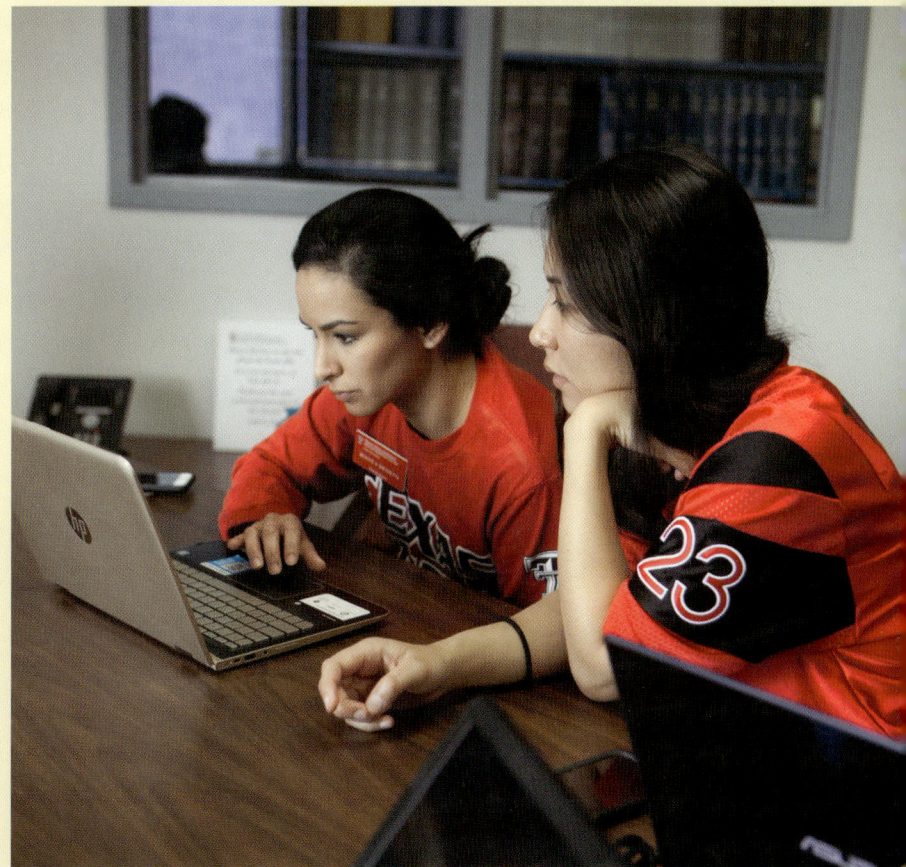

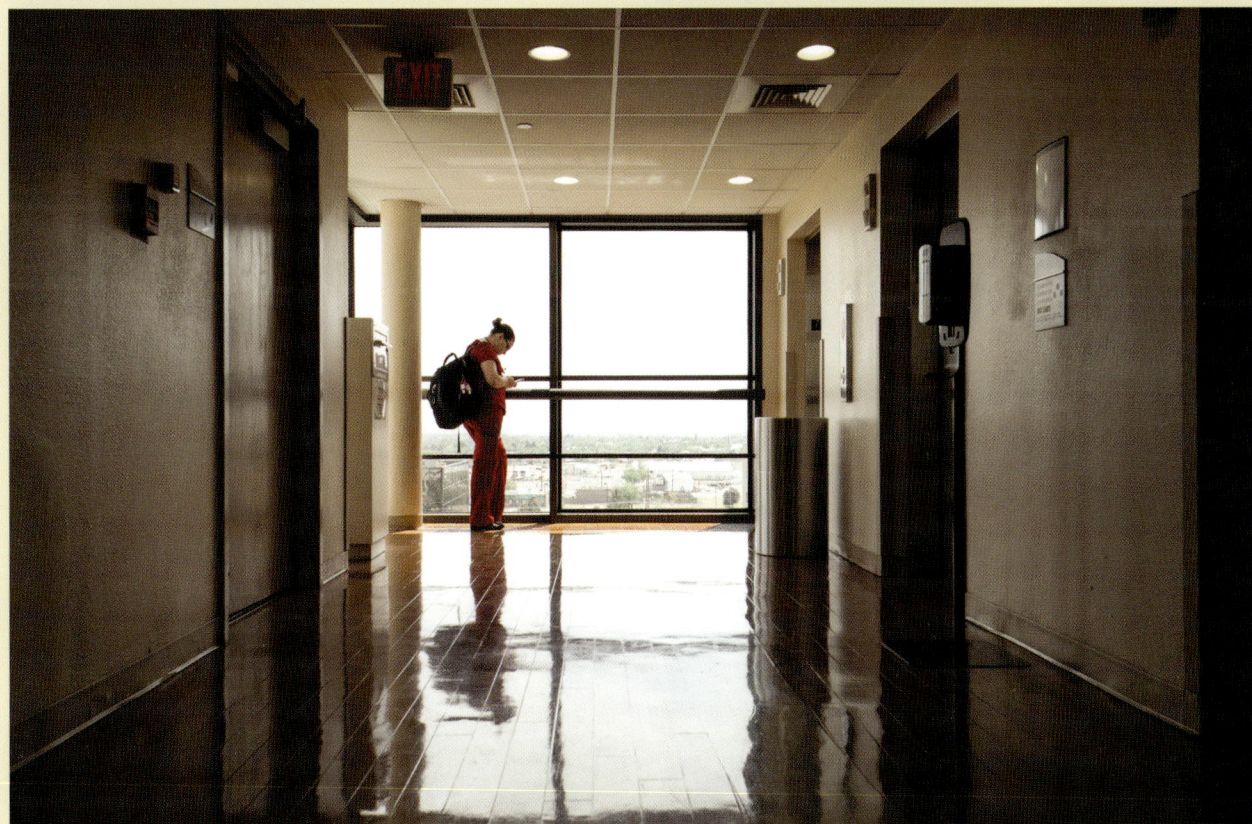

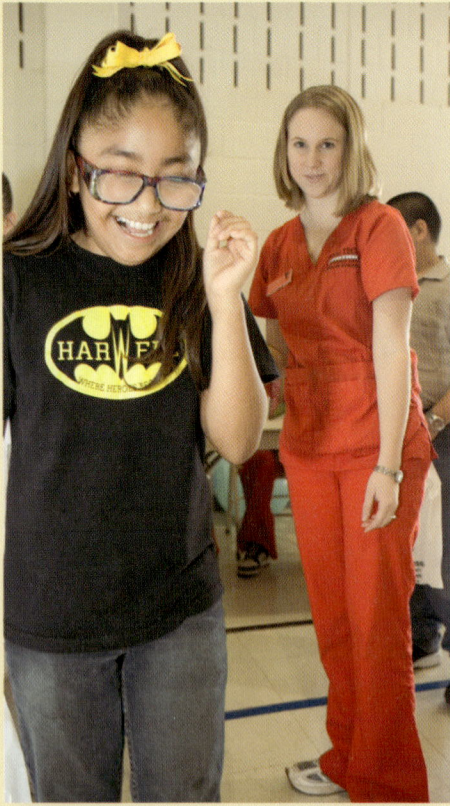
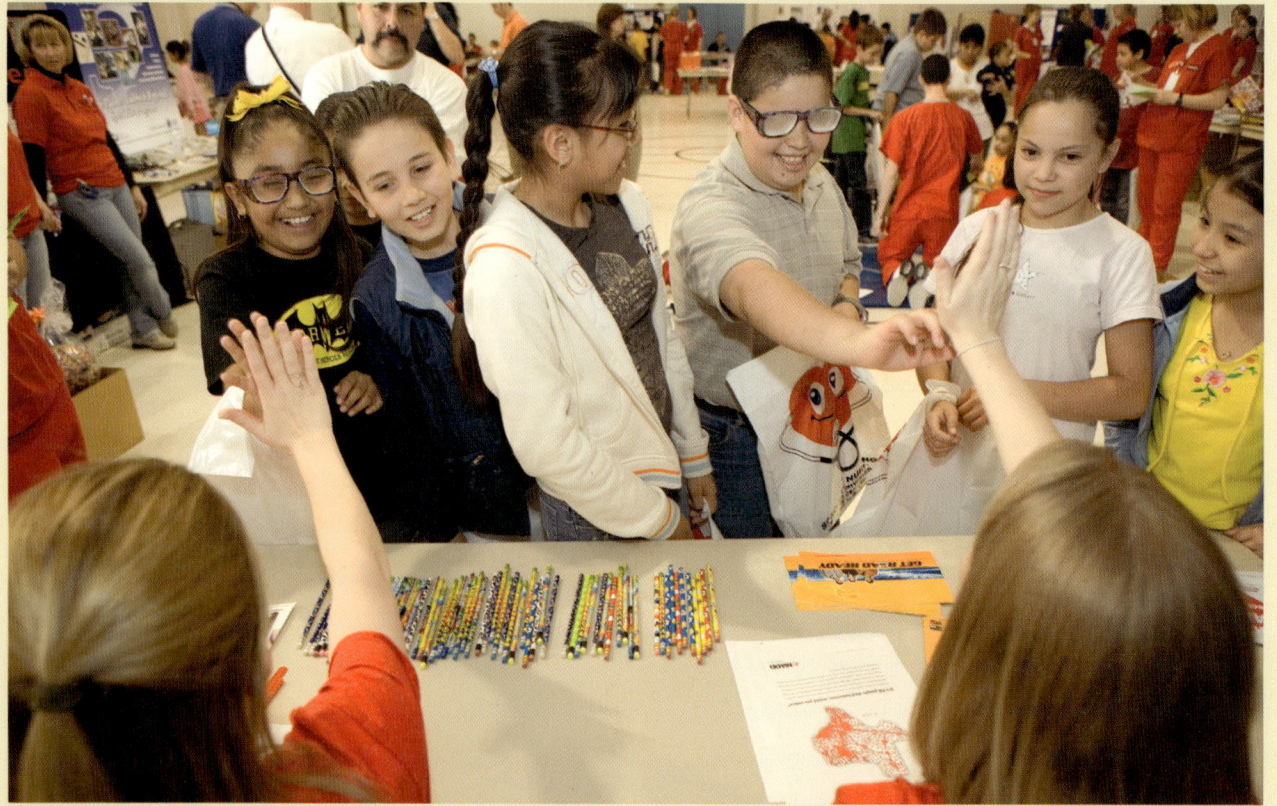
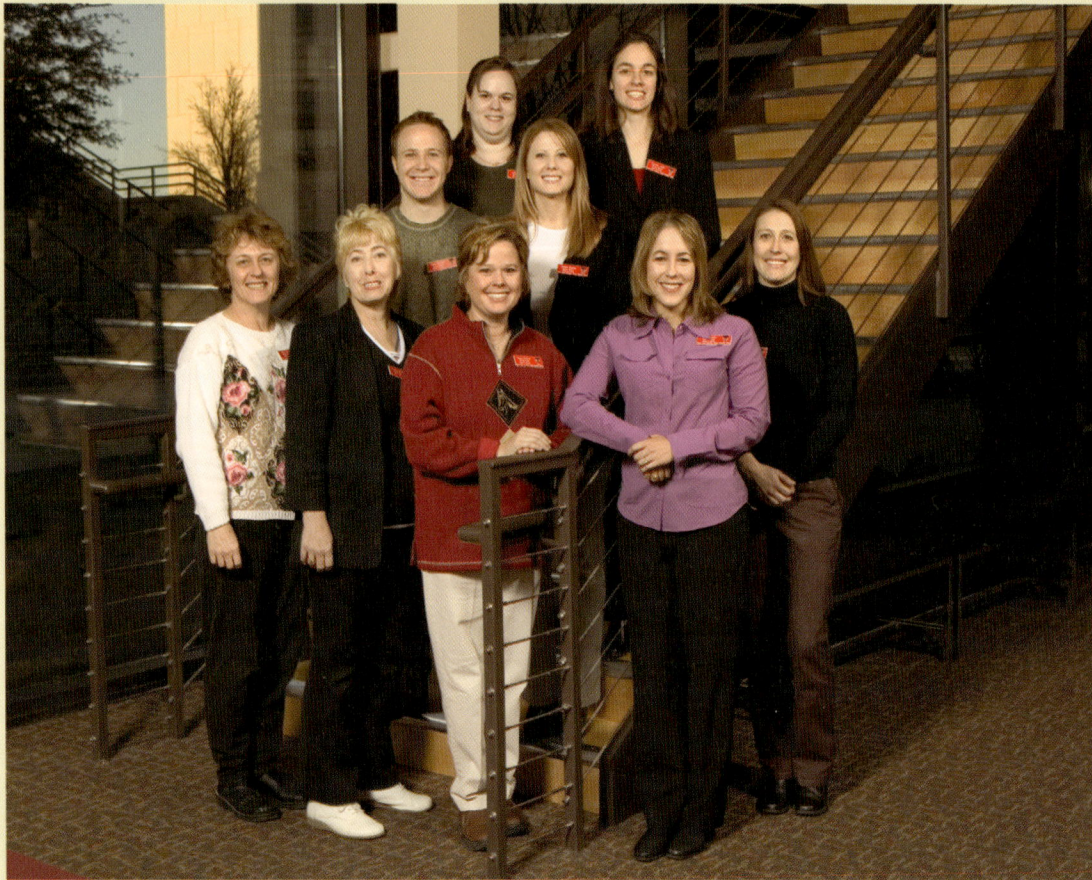
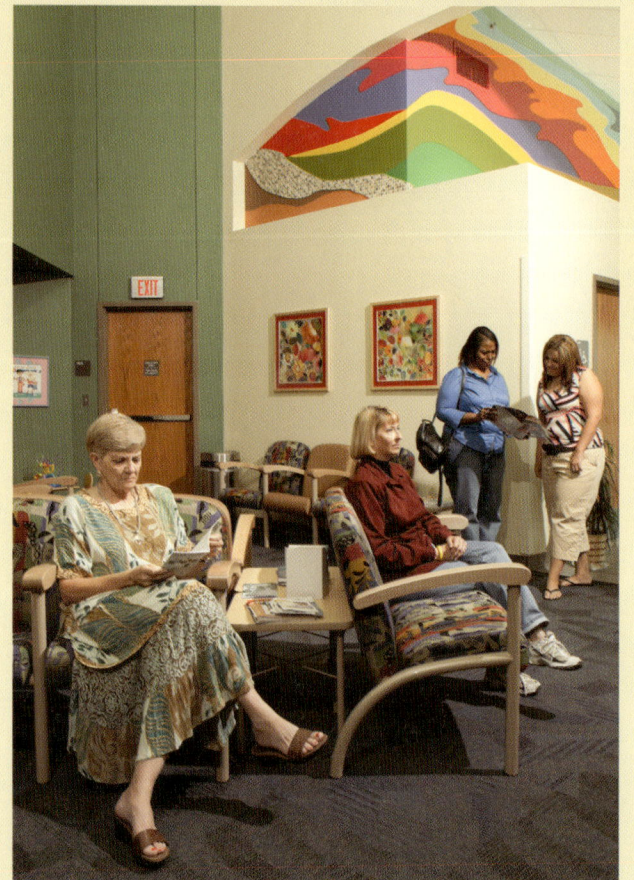

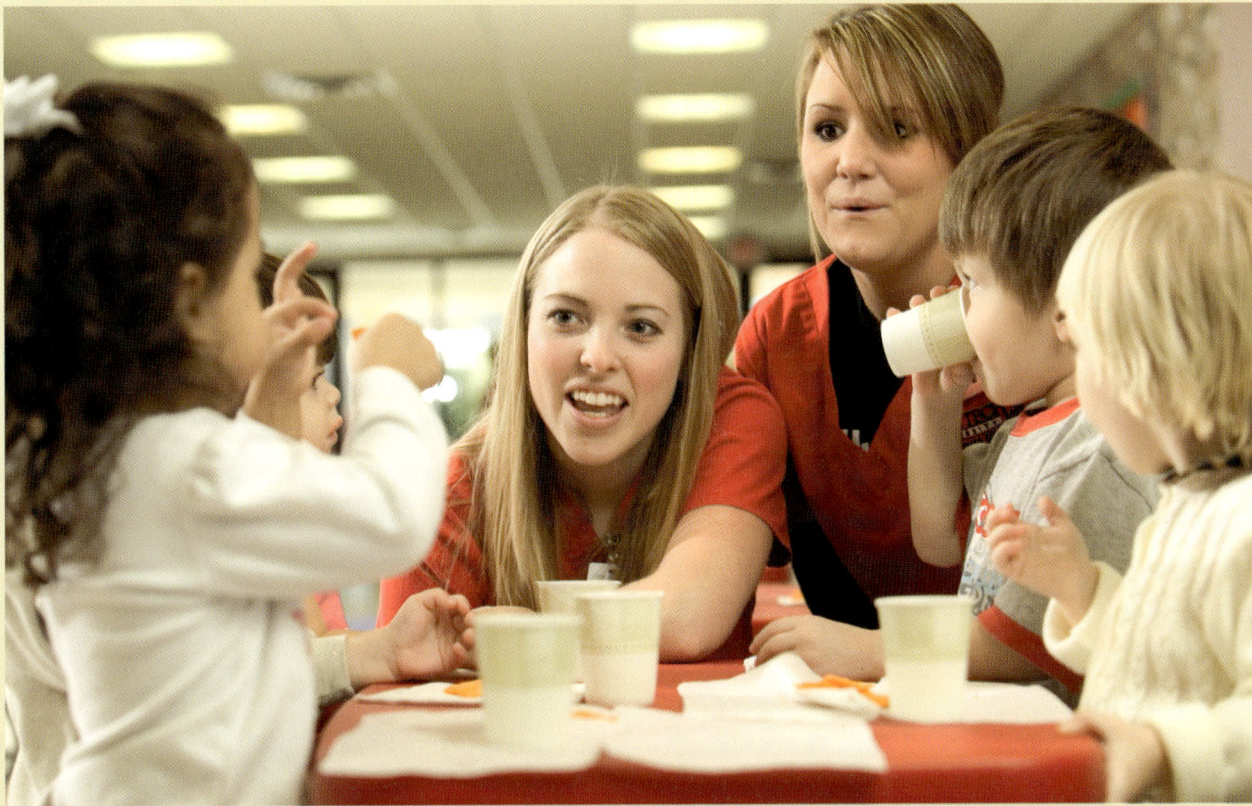
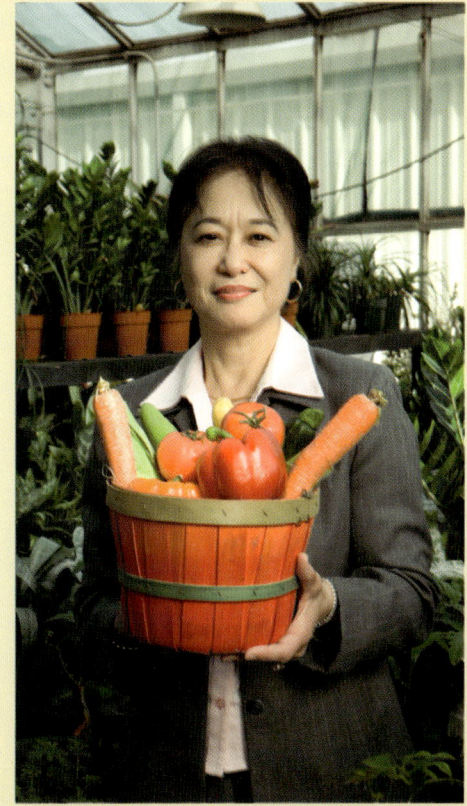
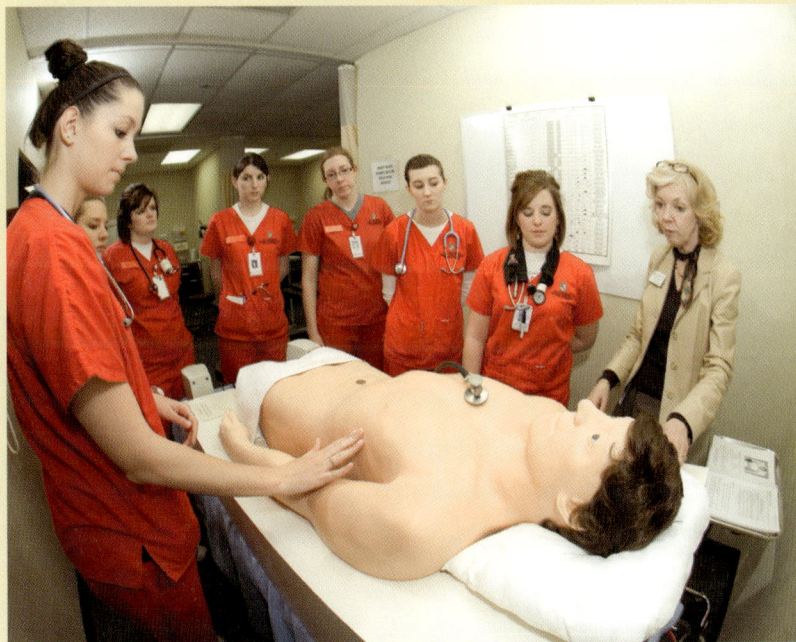
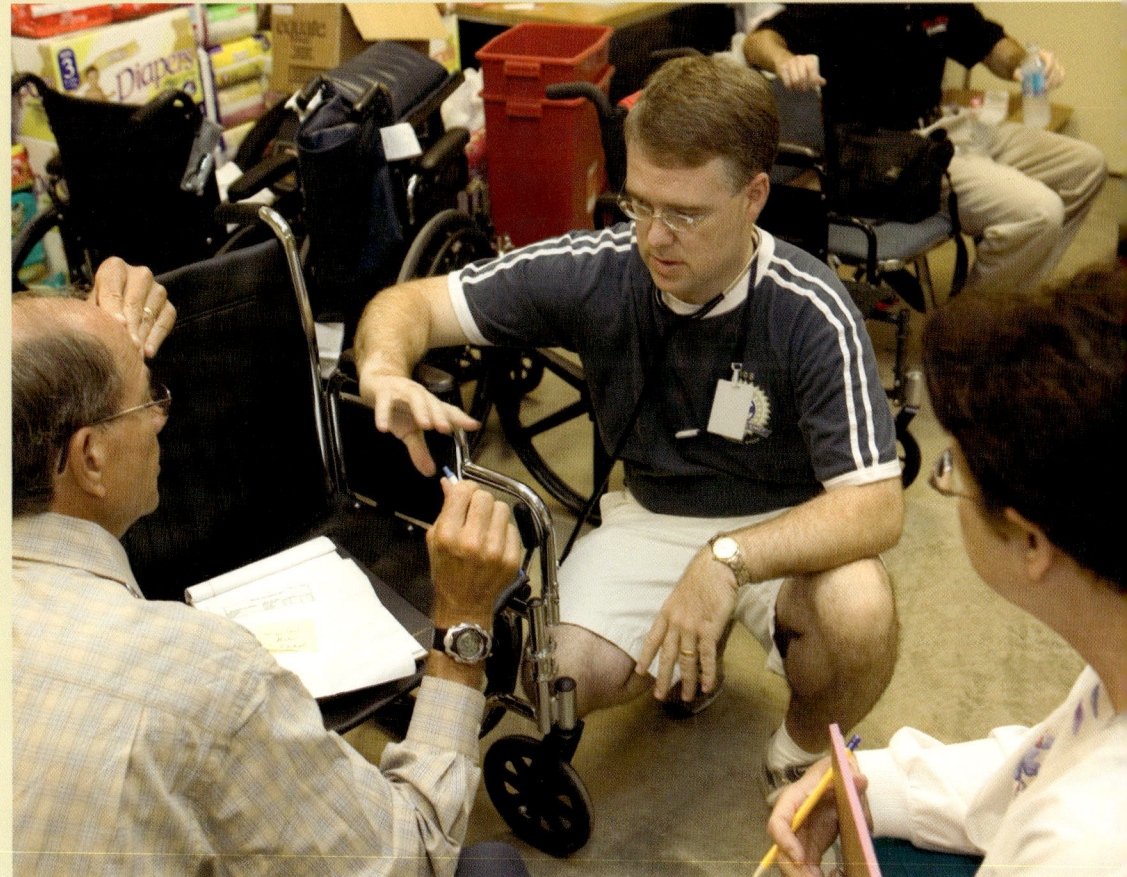

School of Nursing–Dean Michael Evans | 77

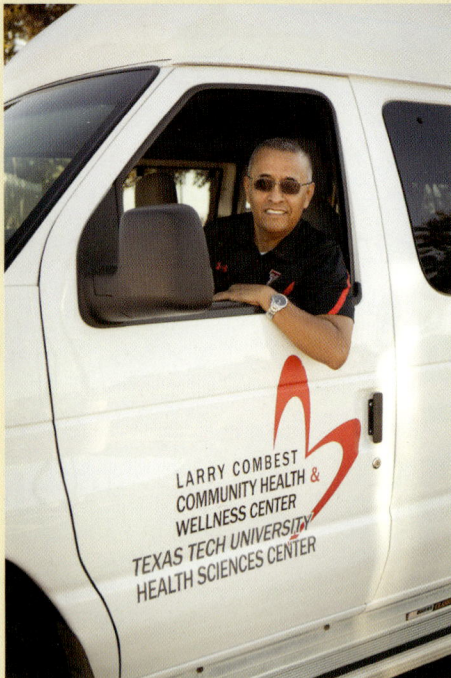

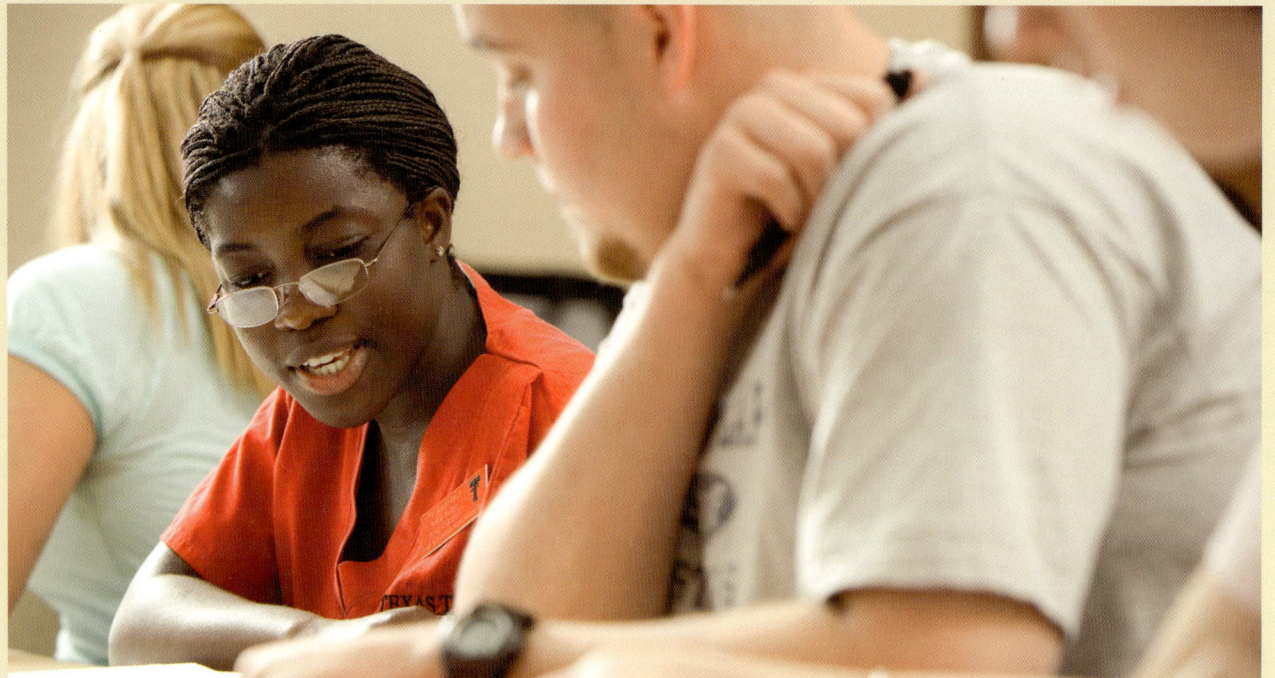

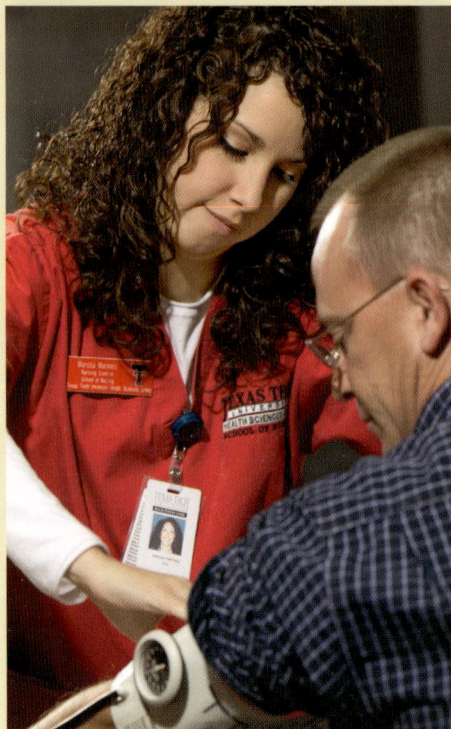

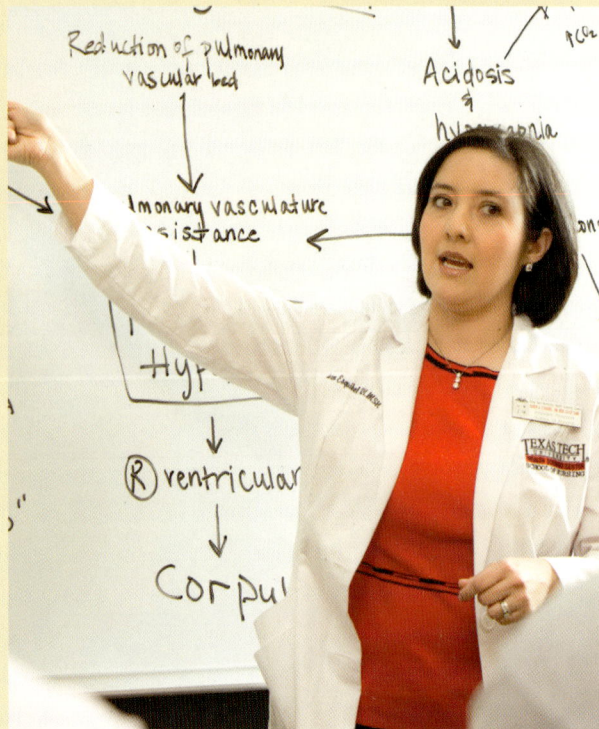

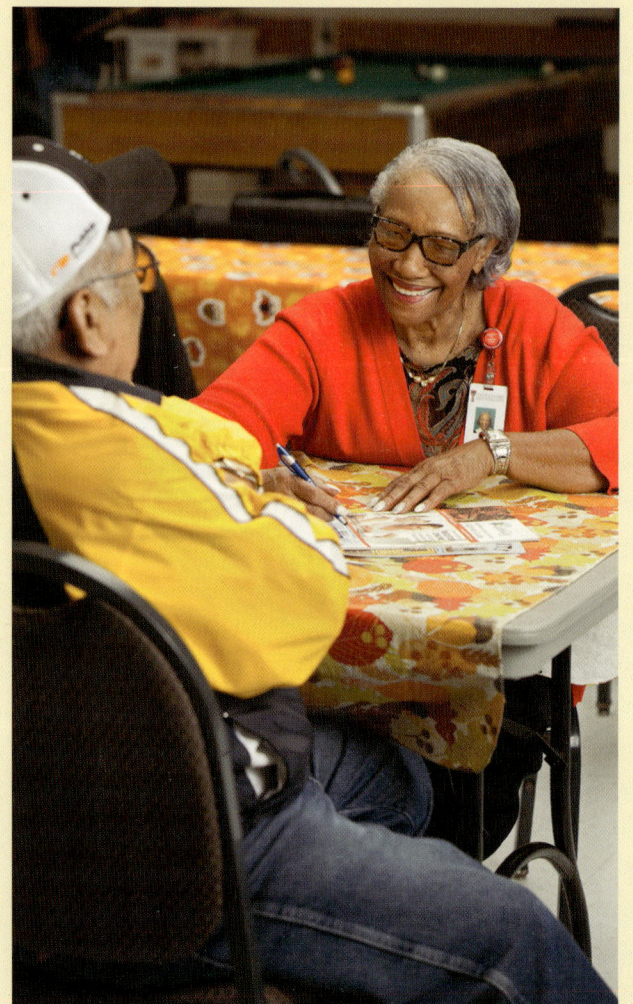

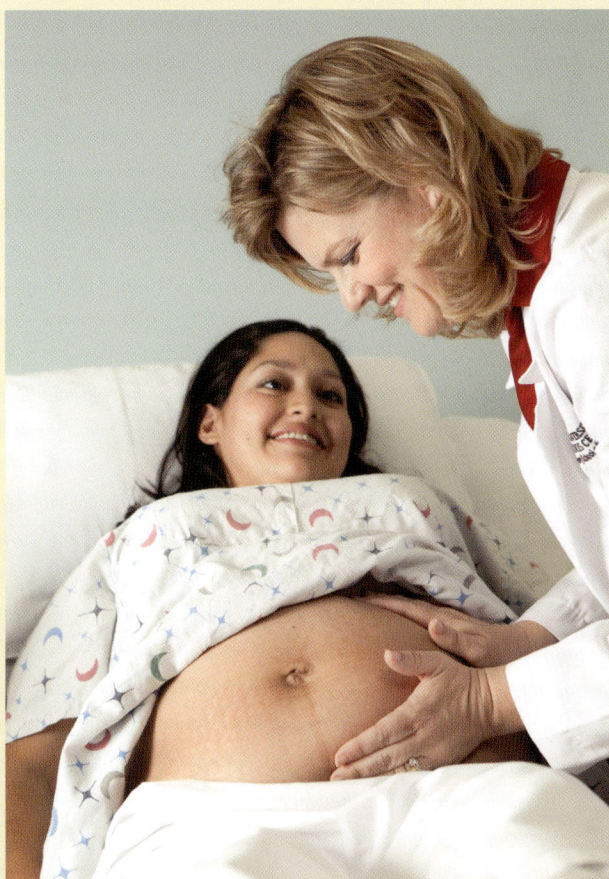
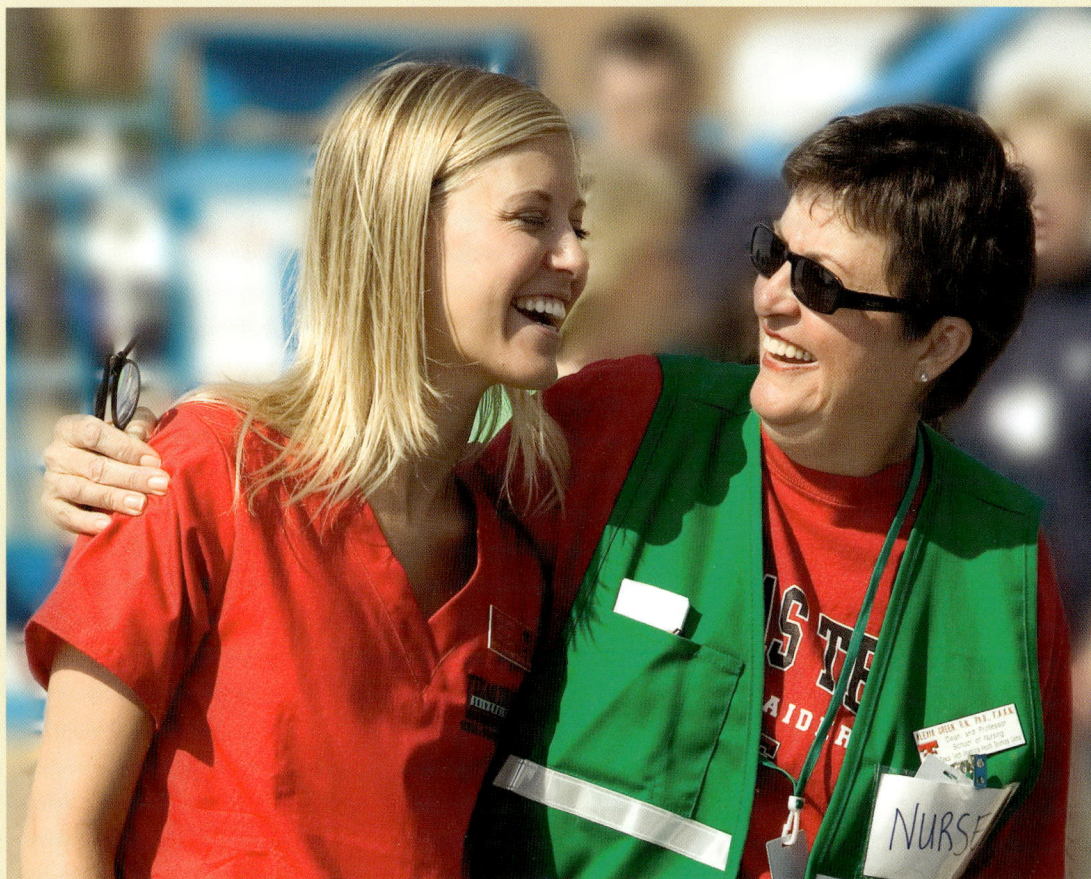
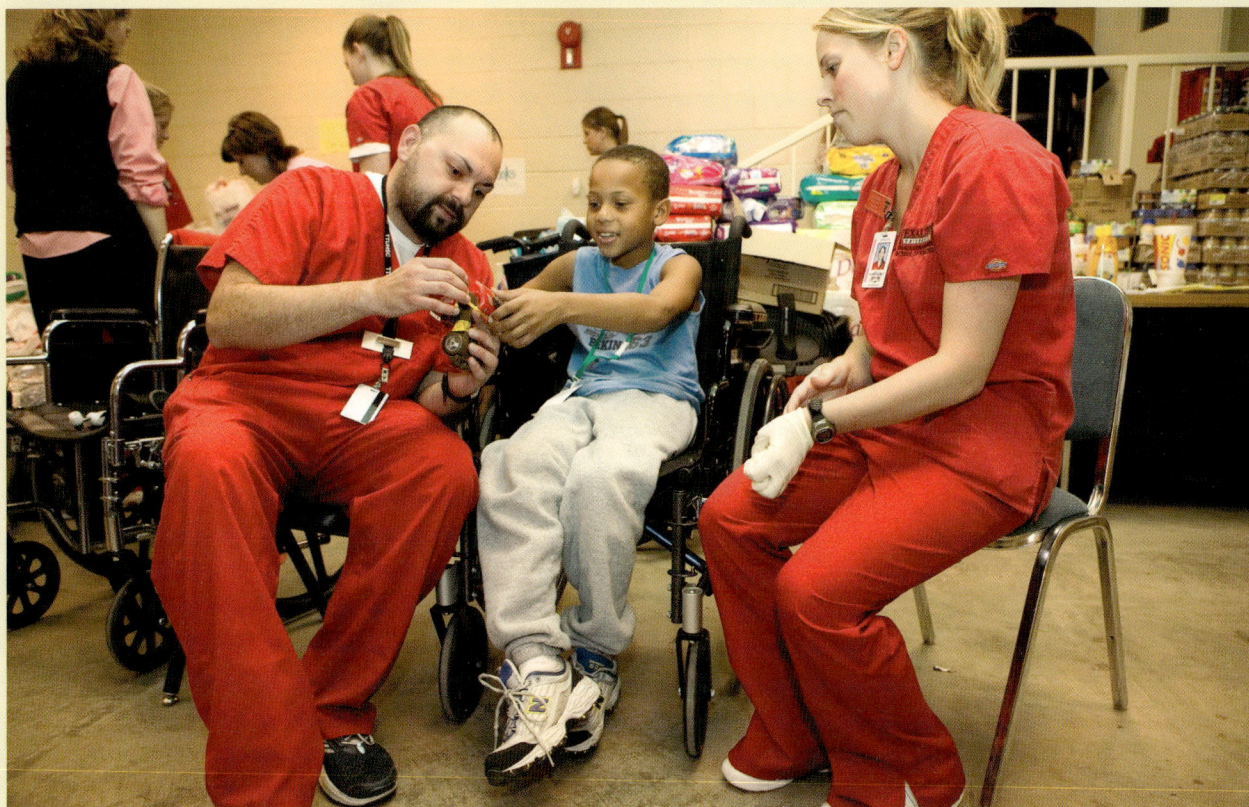
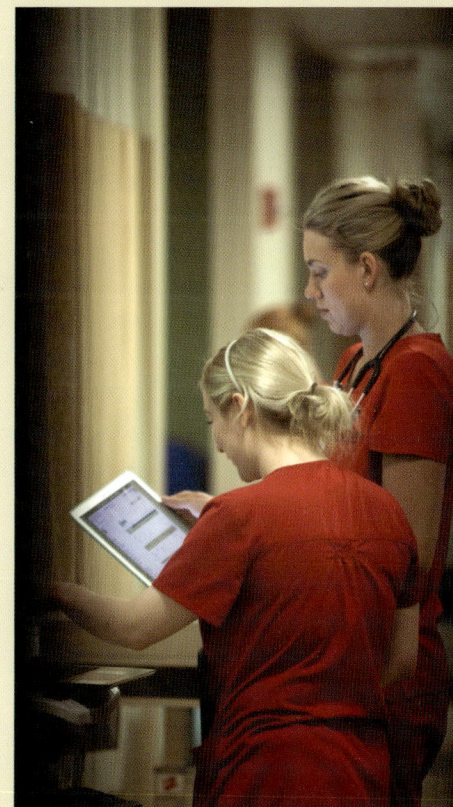

CHAPTER FOUR

SCHOOL OF HEALTH PROFESSIONS

Lori Rice-Spearman, PhD, Dean

The shortage throughout West Texas of healthcare professionals was a major reason the Texas Tech School of Medicine was created in 1969 by the Texas Legislature. The intent was to provide quality education and to develop programs that met the needs of 2.8 million Texans in the 108 counties that comprise West Texas.

It also was the reason its charter was expanded in 1979 to create the School of Nursing, the Graduate School of Biomedical Sciences, and the School of Health Professions (then known as the School of Allied Health Sciences). There was a dearth of healthcare providers needed for patient care, associated treatments, and services. In 1981, the legislature provided funding for the School of Allied Health Sciences and specified which programs should extend to Amarillo and the Permian Basin to deliver local access to health care. It was also charged with recruiting students from those underserved areas of West Texas who would be more likely to stay in the area. Today the school has five departments offering a total of 20 degree programs, enrolling 1,446 students and encompassing four campuses in Lubbock, Amarillo, Odessa, and Midland.

It started with 18 students in 1983 and offered only one degree program: a bachelor's of science in physical therapy. The school's first dean, Robert Cornesky, ScD, microbiology, arrived to take the helm after appointments at Carnegie-Mellon University, California State College,

Bakersfield, and Governor's State University in Illinois. H. H. Merrifield, PhD, PT, chaired the Physical Therapy program. The Occupational Therapy program was chaired by Lawrence Peake, OTR, and the Medical Technology program was chaired by Shirley McManigal, PhD, MT (ASCP). All three programs received accreditation in 1985. Classes during this period were held in the basement of the Health Sciences Center building, with some classrooms and labs actually located across the hall from the morgue.

Peake became the interim dean in 1985 when Cornesky took the position of director of telenetworking at the Health Sciences Center.

In 1987, Dr. McManigal, who had come to TTUHSC from the University of Southern Mississippi as chair of the Medical Technology Department, was appointed dean. Under her leadership, which lasted more than 10 years, the Physical Therapy and Occupational Therapy programs expanded to the Amarillo and Odessa campuses with increases in student enrollment and faculty hires. The school expanded by adding two new programs in emergency medical services in 1991 and a master's level degree in physical therapy.

In 1993 the Communication Disorders Department at Texas Tech University was transferred to the School of Allied Health and relocated to the TTUHSC campus in 2000. The department, now called Speech, Language

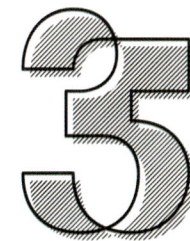

School of Health Professions 35th Anniversary Logo

and Hearing Sciences, had been a part of Texas Tech University since 1928. Both the department and its associated Center for Speech, Language and Hearing Research recently celebrated their ninetieth anniversary of service to West Texas. When McManigal retired in 1998, the School of Allied Health had five degree programs and 450 students.

In the fall of 1998, TTUHSC president David R. Smith challenged the TTUHSC schools to plan, develop, and produce strategies to grow enrollment. The president specifically challenged the School of Allied Health to become the "enrollment growth engine" of the university. The challenge coincided with the arrival of a new dean and professor, Dr. Paul P. Brooke, Jr., PhD, a retired U.S. Army colonel, who came to TTUHSC from Our Lady of the Lake University and who previously served as the first dean for the Odessa campus of the School of Allied Health. Brooke earned his master's degree in health administration at Baylor University and his PhD in health administration management at the University of Iowa.

Brooke led the School of Allied Health from 1998 to 2012, during a critical time that shaped its growth and academic reputation. The number of academic programs rose from five to 18. Today the school has 20 degree programs. Its physical presence increased to four campuses when it added facilities in Midland. Enrollment increased from 450 to 1,300 students under Brooke's leadership.

The school created an active faculty development program to encourage and provide financial support for faculty who participate in doctoral studies. With critical, national shortages of qualified faculty in the school's disciplines, this "grow-your-own" approach continued to strengthen the knowledge, skills, and abilities of the faculty. During Brooke's tenure, 37 candidates earned their terminal degree and he counted that among his most significant achievements, according to an interview published in *PULSE*, a TTUHSC publication for alumni and friends. The school was breaking new ground. It offered the first doctorate of audiology program west of the Mississippi and the first master of science in molecular pathology in the country.

The School of Health Professions research infrastructure has been improved to support SHP faculty scholarship and external funding during the previous decade. Last year it produced a more than 50 percent increase in faculty poster and platform presentations, a more than 50 percent increase in peer-reviewed publications, and a more than 175 percent increase in internal and external grant awards compared to the annual averages across the previous five years. The SHP is presently collaborating with more than 15 different departments at Texas Tech University and TTUHSC and more than 20 different Texas, national, and international universities.

Two SHP research centers support the work in allied health research: the Center for Brain Mapping and Cortical Studies within the Department of Speech, Language and Hearing Sciences; and the Center for Clinical Rehabilitation Assessment within the Department of Rehabilitation Sciences.

There was a flurry of construction, renovation, and expansion of school facilities between 1999 and 2002, reflecting the growing number of degree programs. A $2.2 million renovated home was created for the Department of Speech, Languages and Hearing Sciences on the TTUHSC campus. One year later it received approval for a Center for Brain Mapping and Cortical Studies, which would offer important research facilities for the new PhD in audiology.

About the same time, the school moved its programs on the Odessa campus into a permanent facility after it underwent a $1.2 million renovation. In 2001, the Physician Assistants program moved from its home in portable buildings into a permanent $3.3 million facility on the Midland College campus, establishing a third campus. In 2002, the school's programs in Amarillo also moved into a multi-million-dollar permanent facility.

Graduate health degree programs became more accessible to professionals by creating weekend and online courses. They helped increase enrollment and allowed more healthcare professionals to practice in West Texas communities while they pursued more advanced degrees. One example would be the Transitional DPT (doctor of physical therapy) program, which is an online program designed to provide practicing physical therapists who already have a master's degree (MPT) or bachelor's degree (BSPT) the opportunity to earn a clinical doctorate. The Transitional DPT allows MPT and BSPT clinicians to advance their knowledge to a level consistent with the current professional DPT standards by continuing their full-time employment while enrolled in the online program. Their clinical setting at work provides the ideal environment to apply newly learned information.

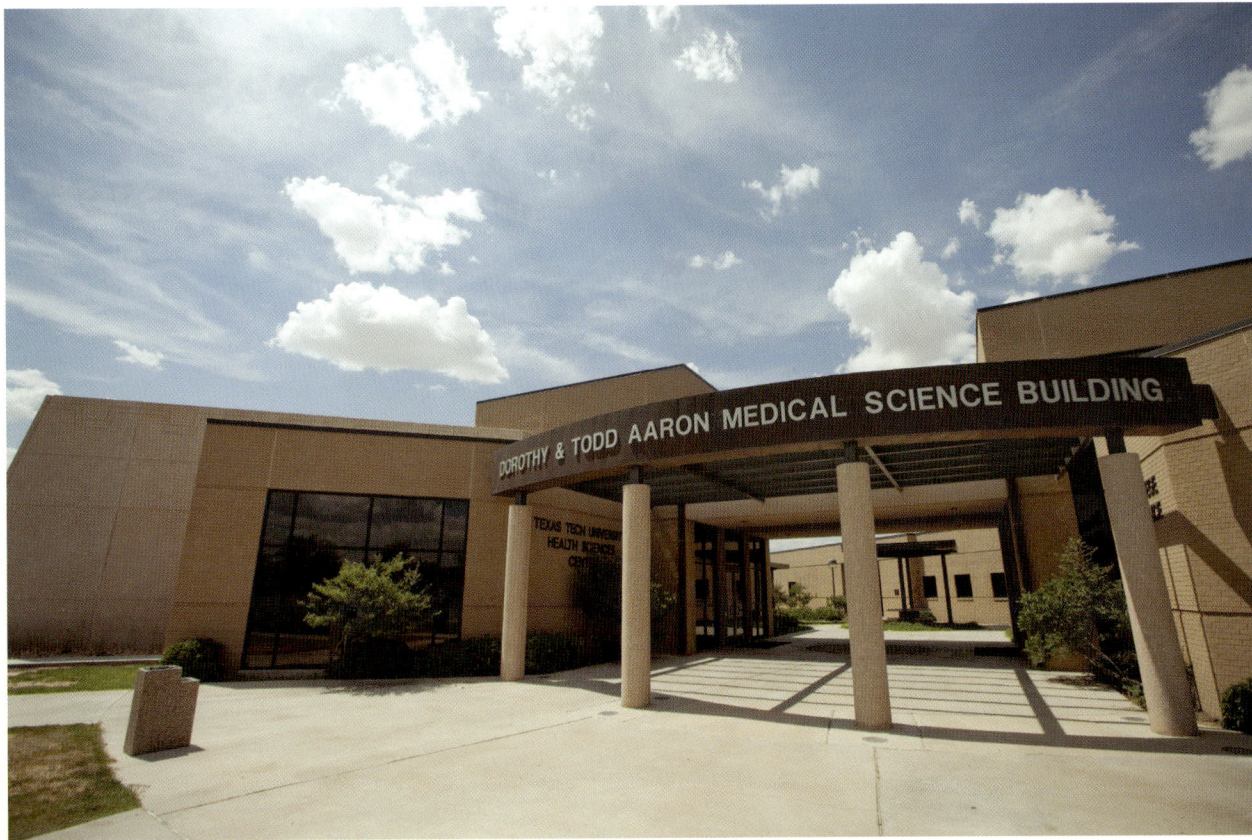

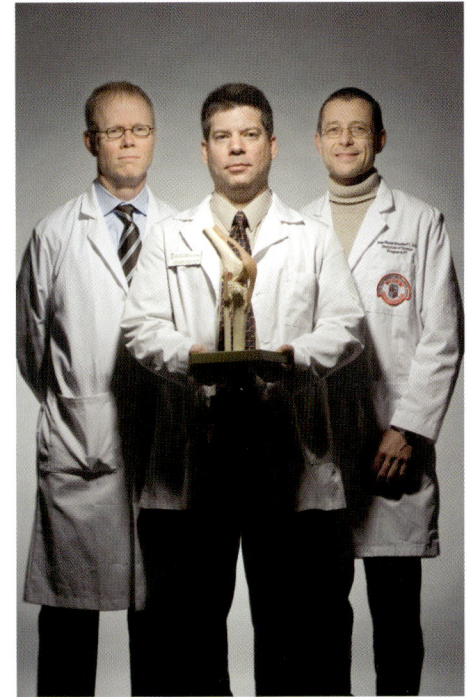

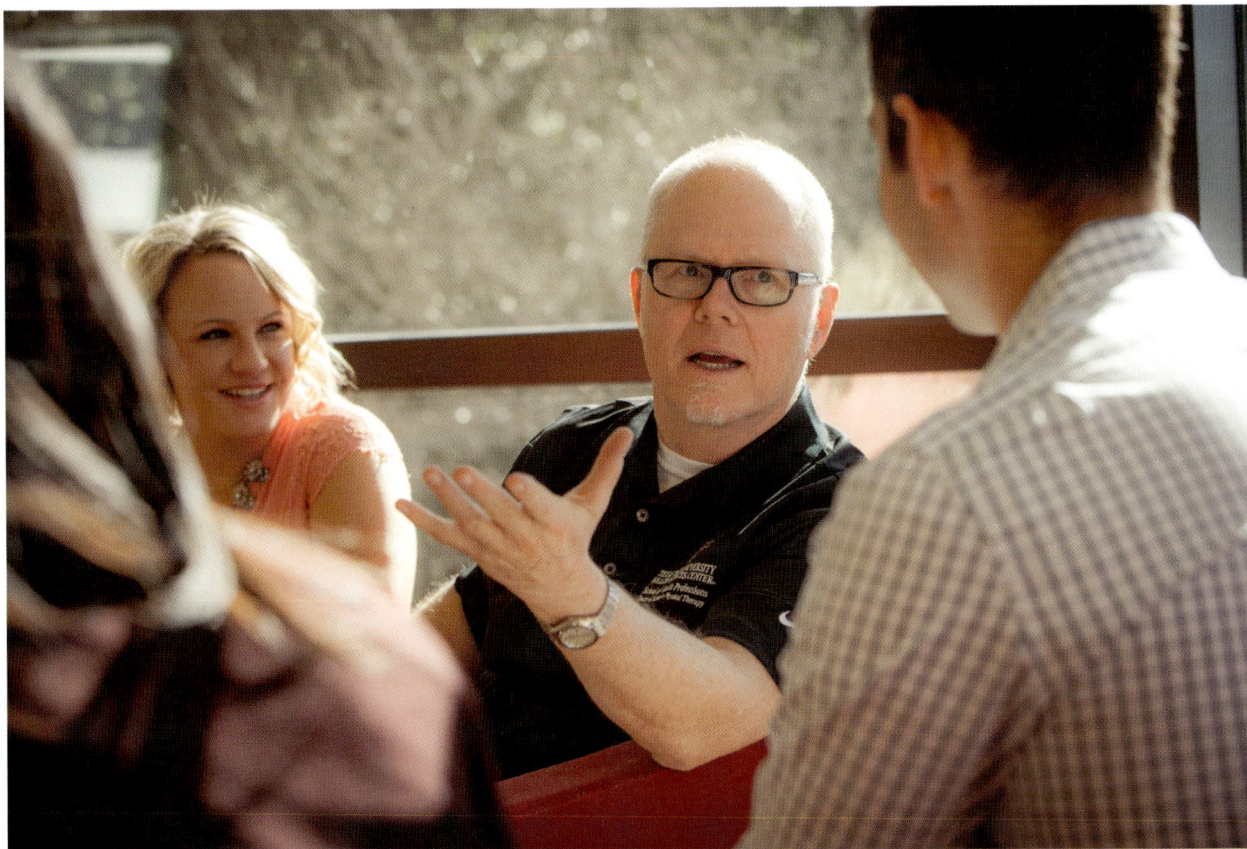

(ABOVE LEFT) SCH Physician Assistant Program—Dorothy and Todd Aaron Medical Science Building, Midland, Texas

(ABOVE RIGHT) SHP Professors: Phillip S. Sizer, Jr., PhD, PT, O CS, MOMT, FAAOMPT; C. Roger James, PhD, FACSM; and Jean-Michel Brismee, ScD, PT, OCS, FAAOMPT

(LEFT) Phil Sizer interacting with students
Artie Limmer, Photographer, Associate Director, Institutional Advancement

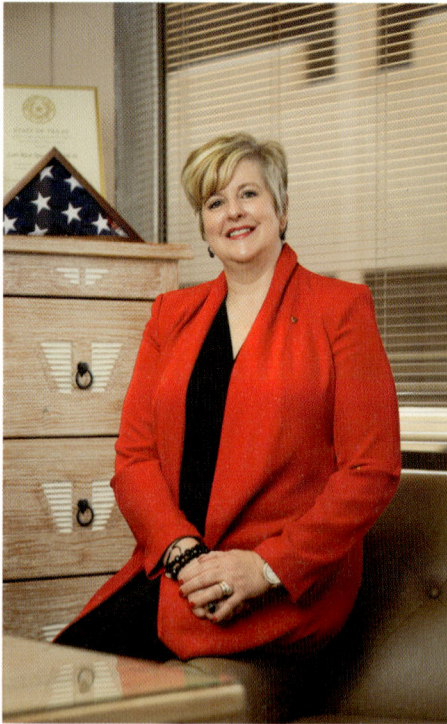

Lori Rice-Spearman, Dean

(RIGHT) Lori Rice-Spearman with students in lab

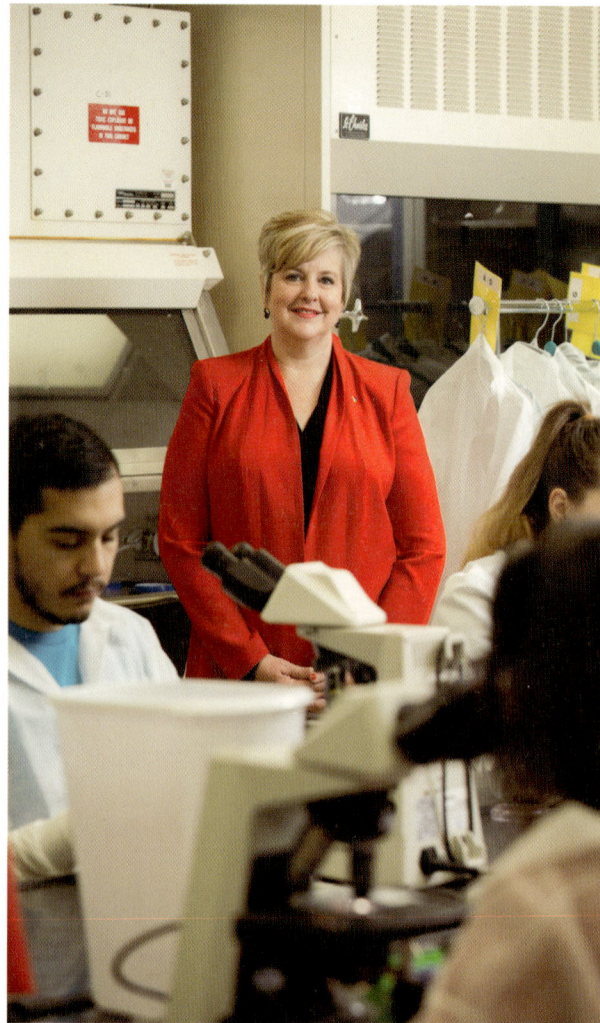

Changes like these during Brooke's time at the helm shaped a school now offering the upper tier of ranked graduate programs. It also received its first National Institutes of Health research grant before Brooke retired in 2012. "I'll say my contribution to this whole thing was creating the climate and creating a demand for creativity and then allowing folks to take reasonable risks," Brooke said in an interview for *PULSE*.

Upon Brooke's retirement, Robin Satterwhite, MBA, EdD, was named the fifth dean of the School of Allied Health Sciences. He previously served the school as associate dean for Learning Outcomes and Technologies and as professor and founding chair of the departments of Clinic Administration and Rehabilitation Counseling. Satterwhite is a Texas Tech alumnus and joined

TTUHSC in 1999 as dean of the Odessa campus. Prior to his academic positions, Satterwhite served as CEO and administrator of two separate hospitals and clinics.

In 2015, the school changed its name from Allied Health Sciences to the School of Health Professions, reflecting a growing trend among similar schools. It also marked the end of Satterwhite's leadership at TTUHSC when he left TTUHSC in July to become vice president of academic affairs at South Plains College. The following spring, he was appointed president of that college.

Hal Larsen, PhD, MT(ASCP), executive associate dean, served as interim dean in 2016 until the sixth and current dean, Lori Rice-Spearman, PhD, MT(ASCP), was selected. Dean Rice-Spearman was one of the first faculty members in the SHP's Medical Technology program in 1987, serving as lab manager. She has taken on the task of promoting research opportunities for the school as well as being involved in an extensive HSC expansion project that will add research and educational facilities for the SHP faculty and students.

The School of Health Professions had 1,446 students enrolled in fall 2017 and 20 graduate and undergraduate degree programs in five departments. All the programs lead directly to careers in critical segments of health care. The following is a list of the programs offered through the School of Health Professions:

SCHOOL OF HEALTH PROFESSIONS DEGREE PROGRAMS

Laboratory Sciences and Primary Care
Clinical Laboratory Science (postbaccalaureate certificate)—online
Clinical Laboratory Science (BS)
Clinical Laboratory Science (second degree BS)—online
Molecular Pathology (MS)
Physician Assistant (MPAS)

REHABILITATION SCIENCES

Athletic Training (MAT)
Occupational Therapy (MOT)
Physical Therapy (DPT)
Physical Therapy (ScD)—online
Transitional Doctor of Physical Therapy (tDPT)—online
Rehabilitation Science (PhD)

SPEECH, LANGUAGE AND HEARING SCIENCES

Audiology (AuD)

Speech, Language and Hearing Sciences (BS)

Speech, Language and Hearing Sciences (second degree BS)

Speech-Language Pathology (MS)

HEALTHCARE MANAGEMENT AND LEADERSHIP

Healthcare Administration (MS)—online

Healthcare Management (BS)—online

CLINICAL COUNSELING AND MENTAL HEALTH

Addiction Counseling (MS)—online

Clinical Mental Health Counseling (MS)—online

Clinical Rehabilitation Counseling (MS)—online

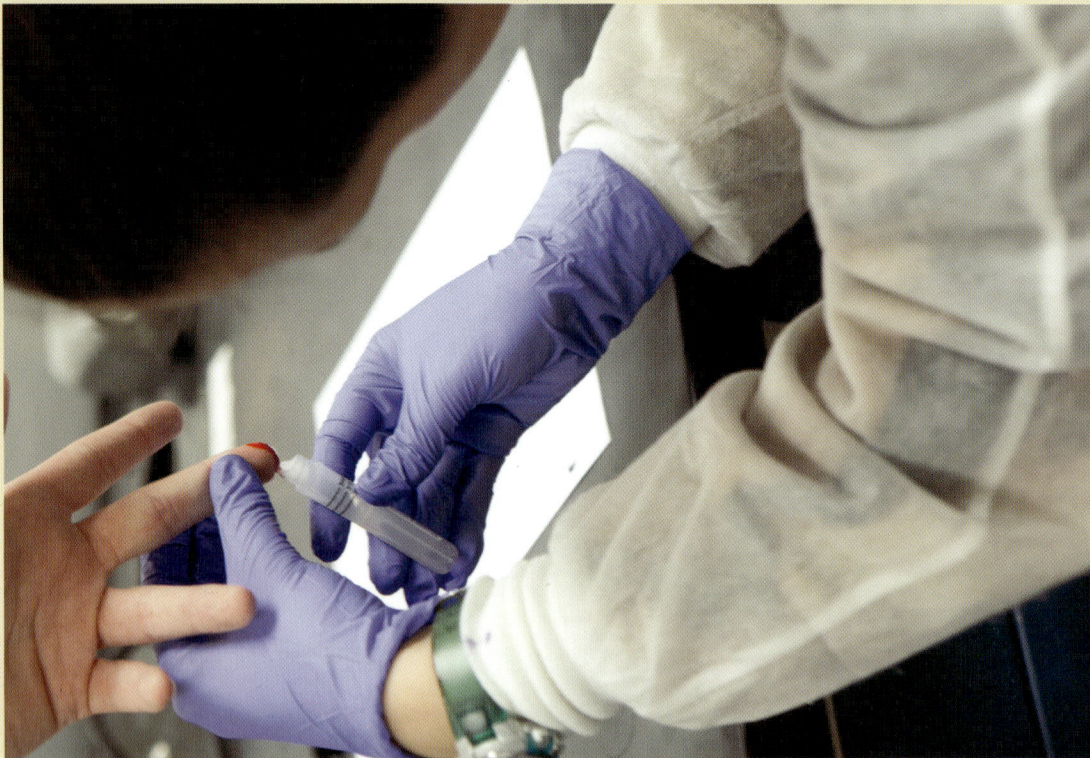
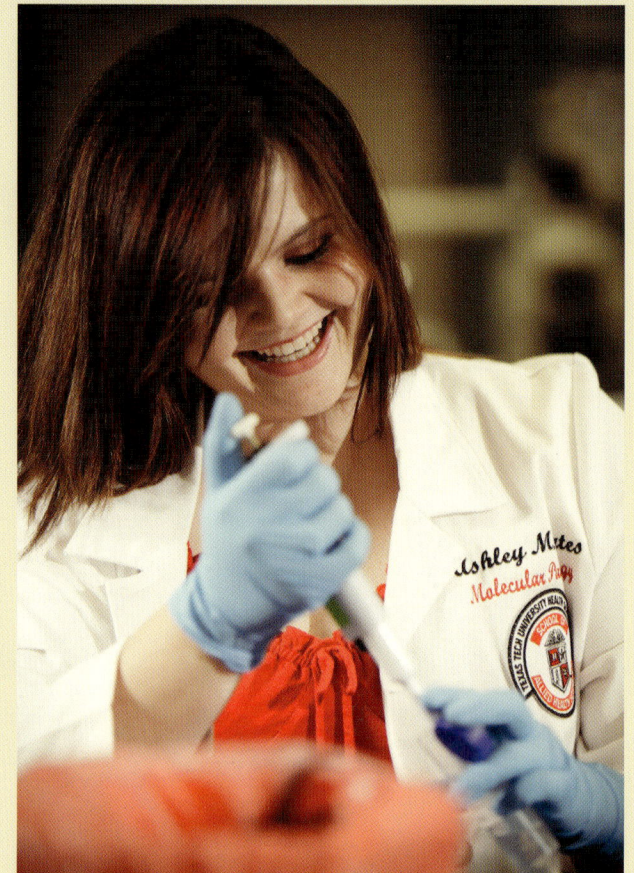
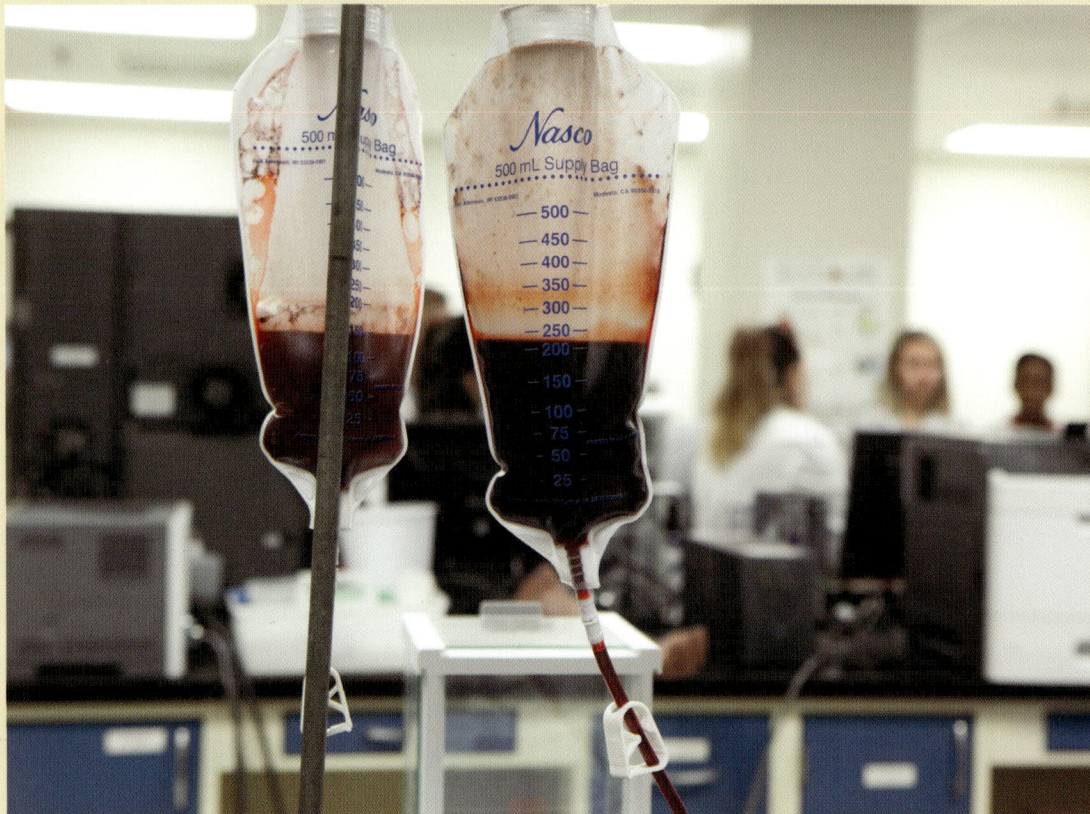
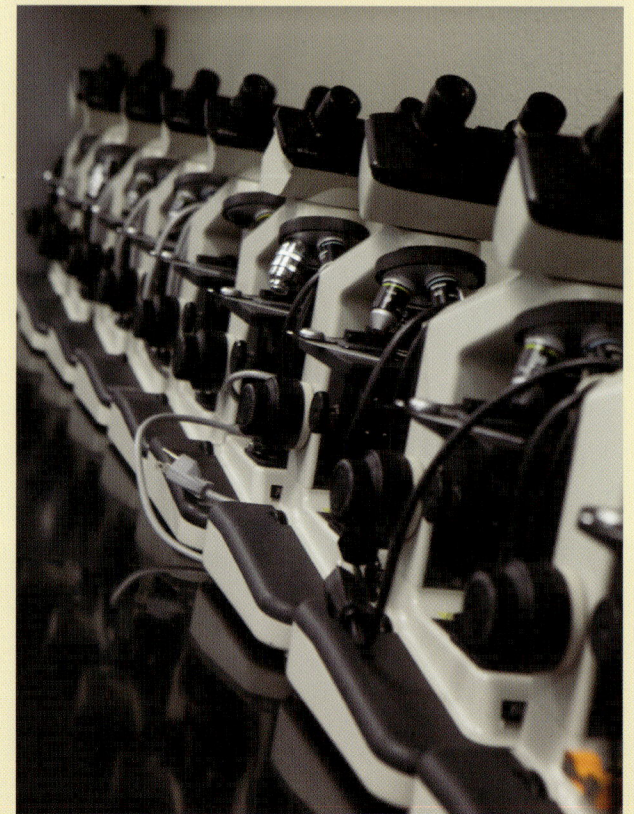

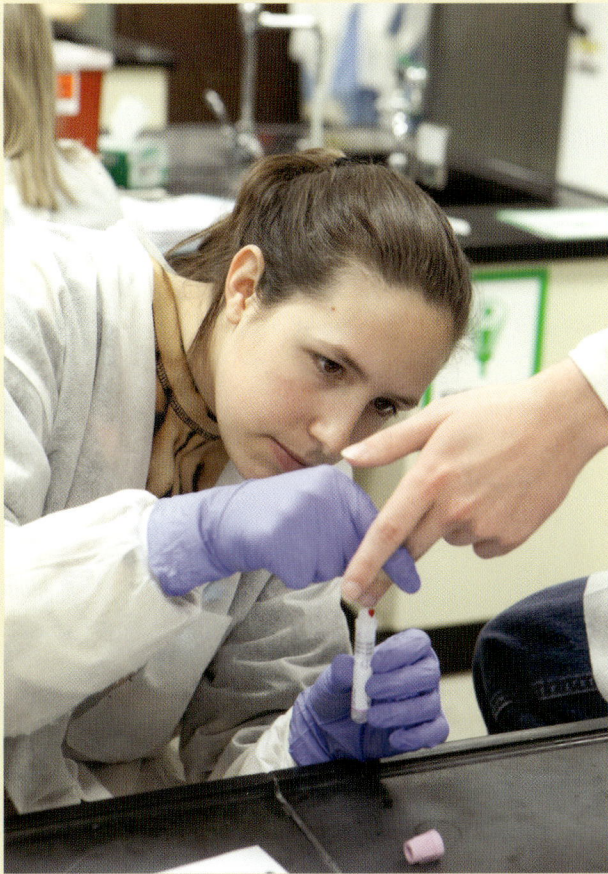
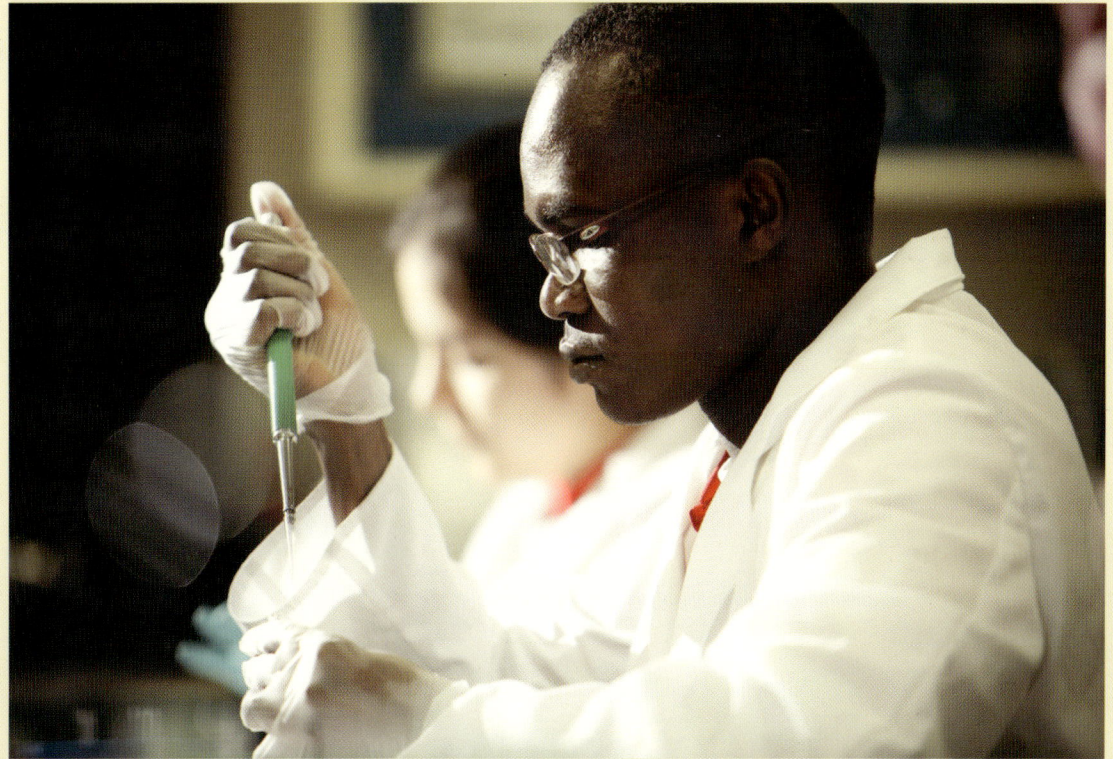
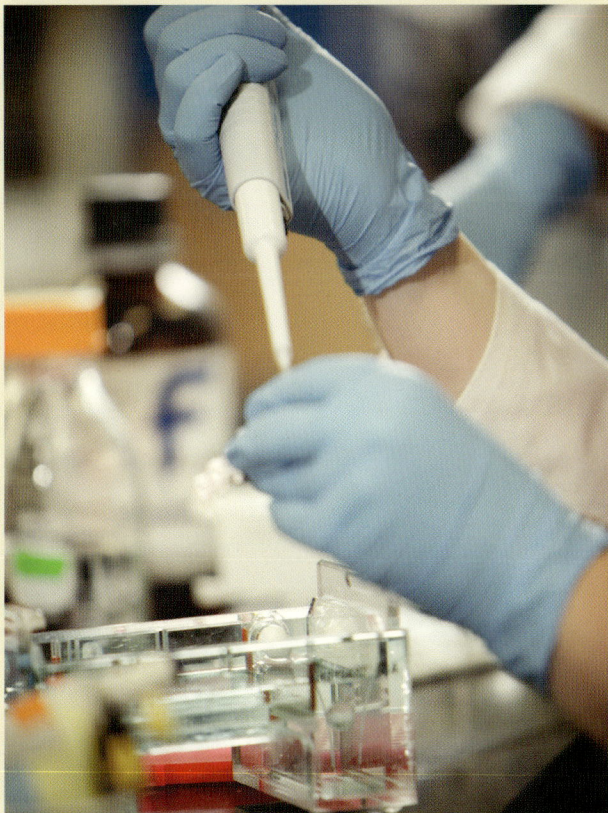
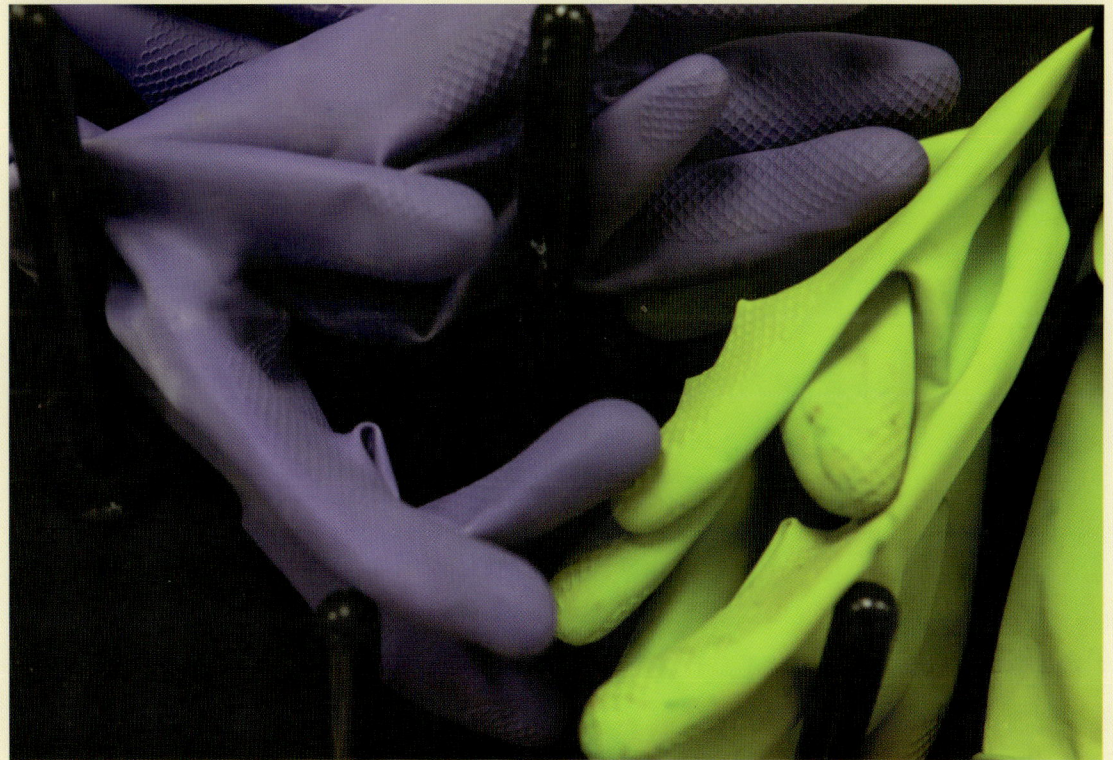

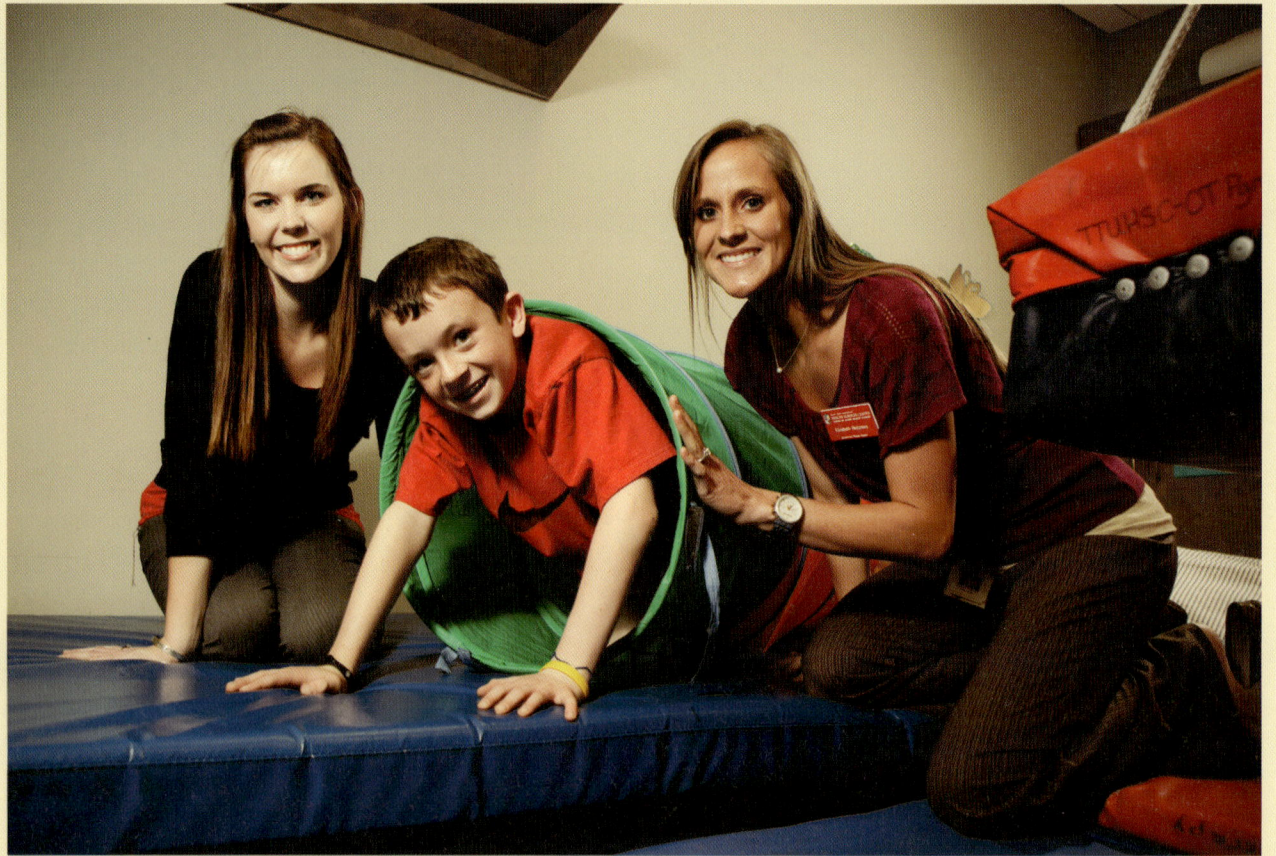

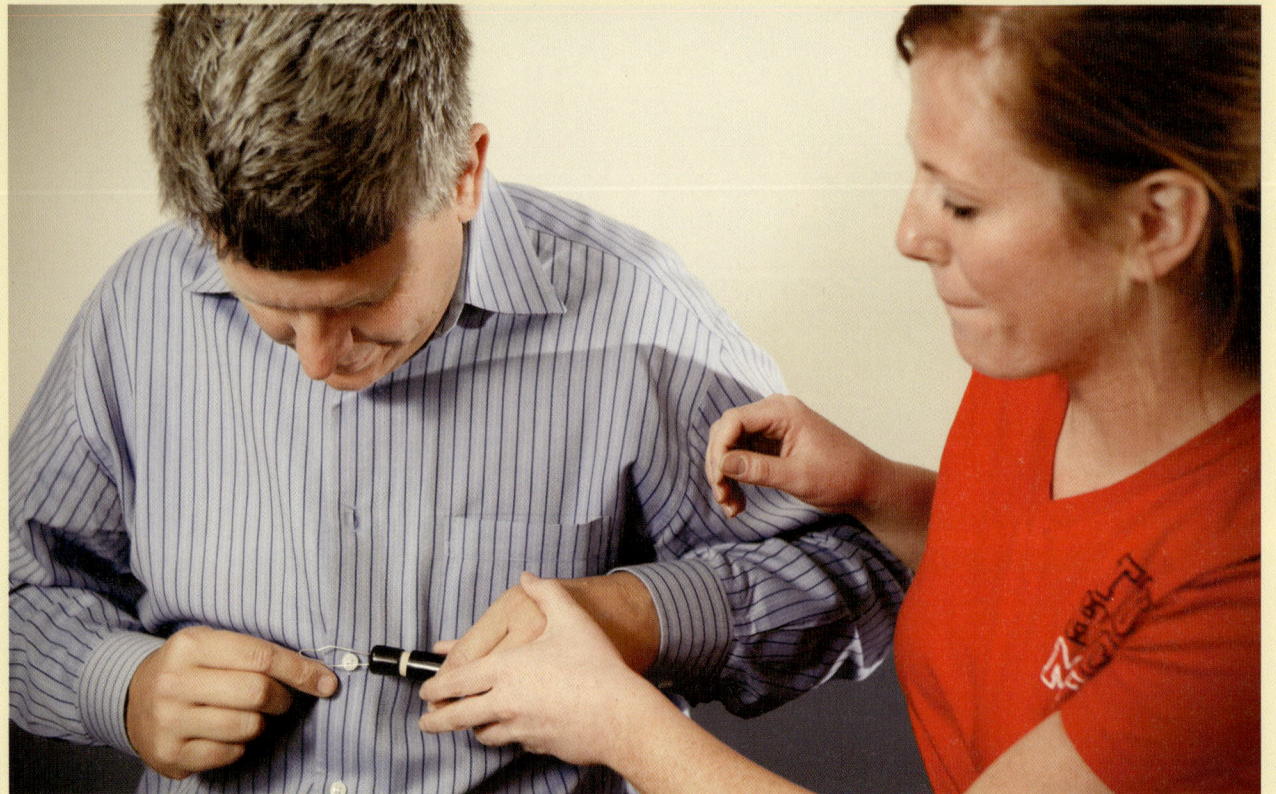

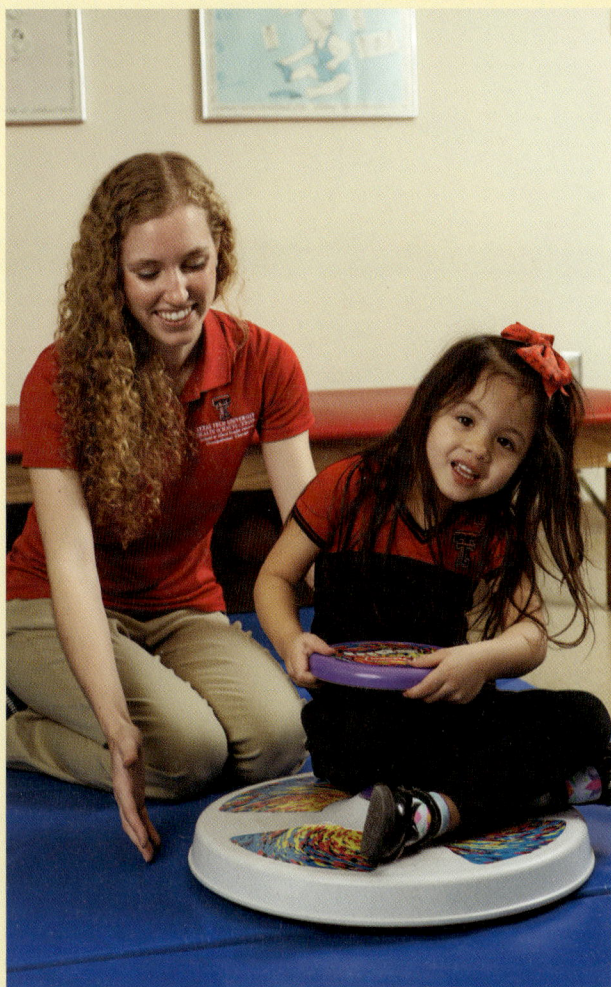
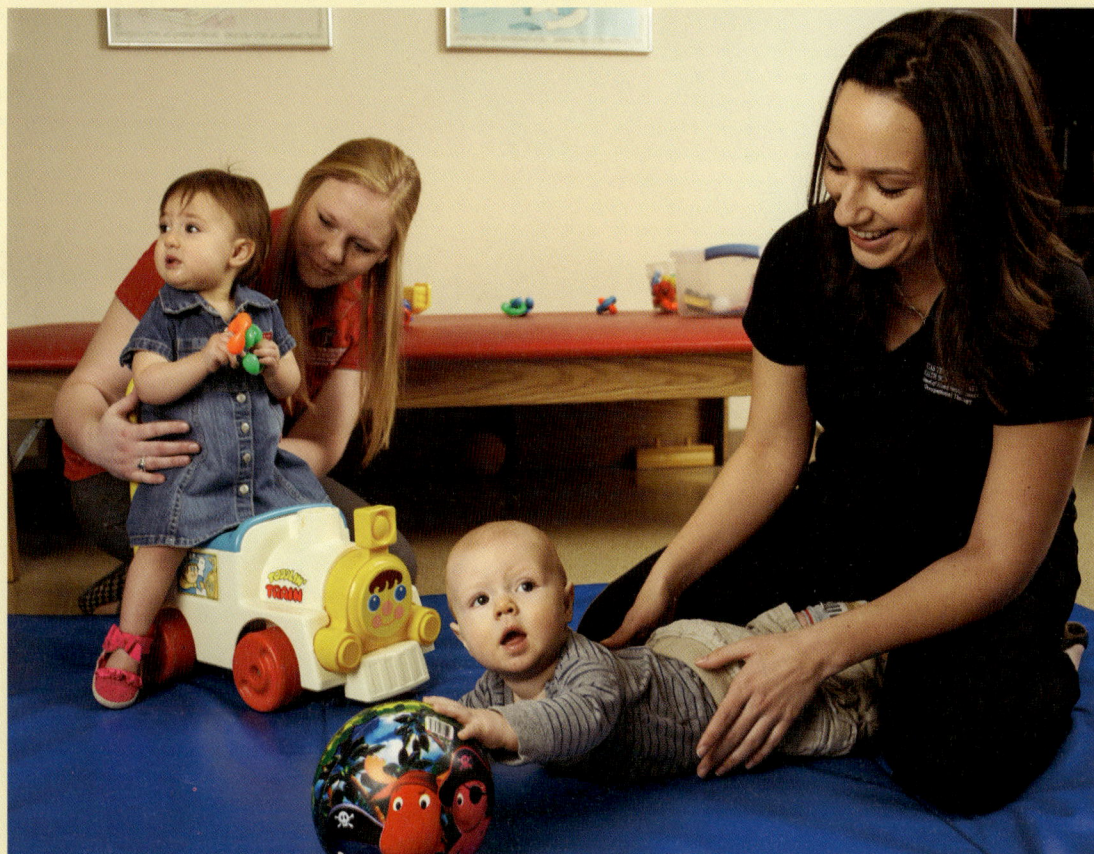
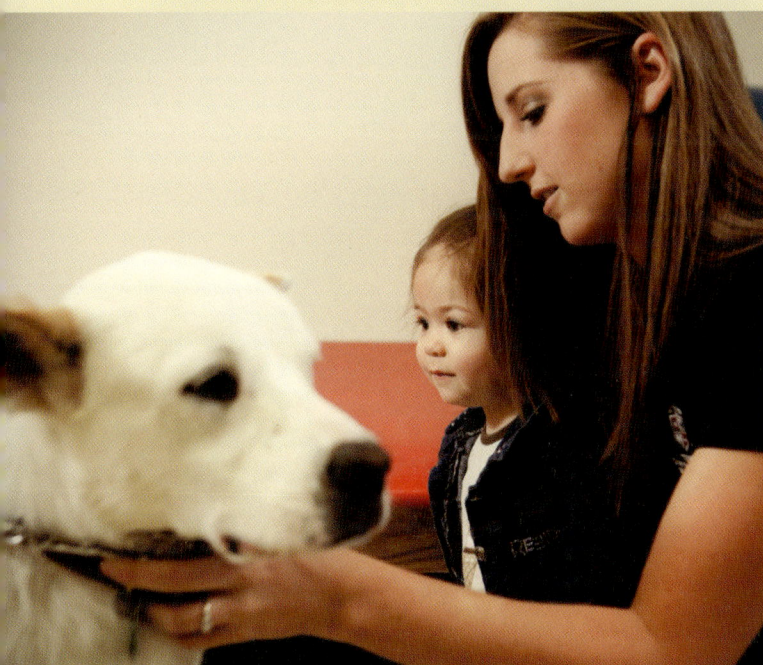
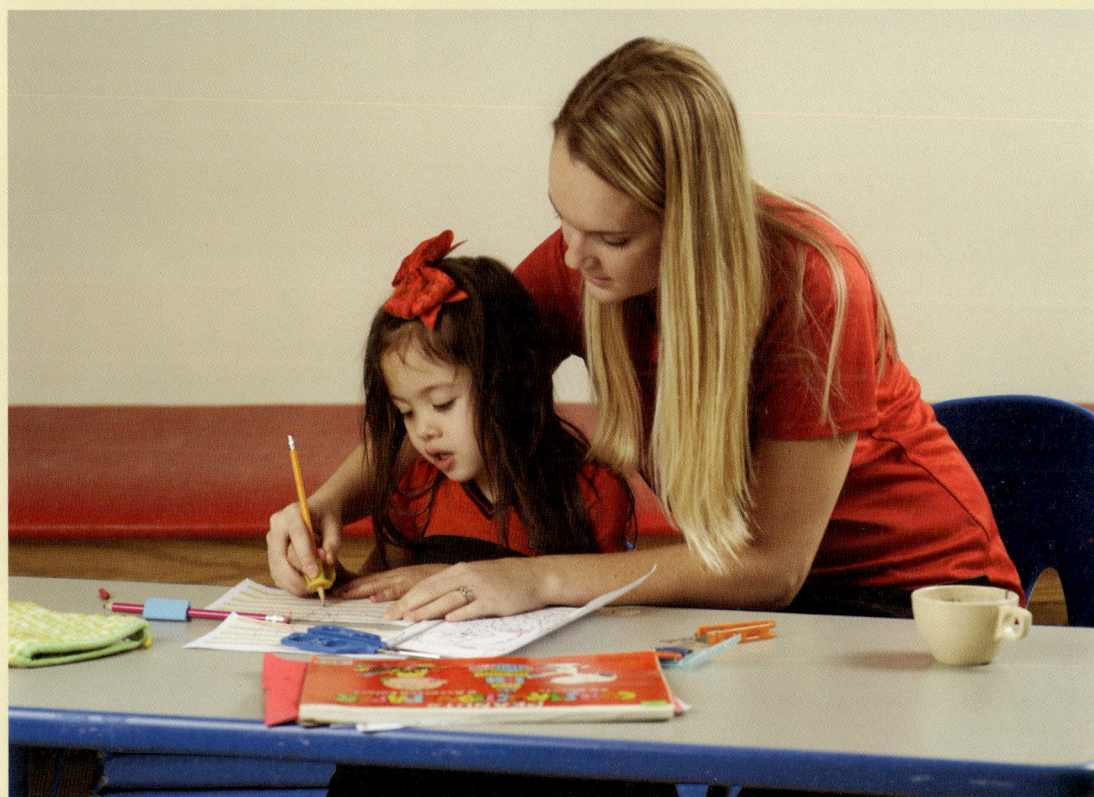

School of Health Professions—Dean Lori Rice-Spearman | 89

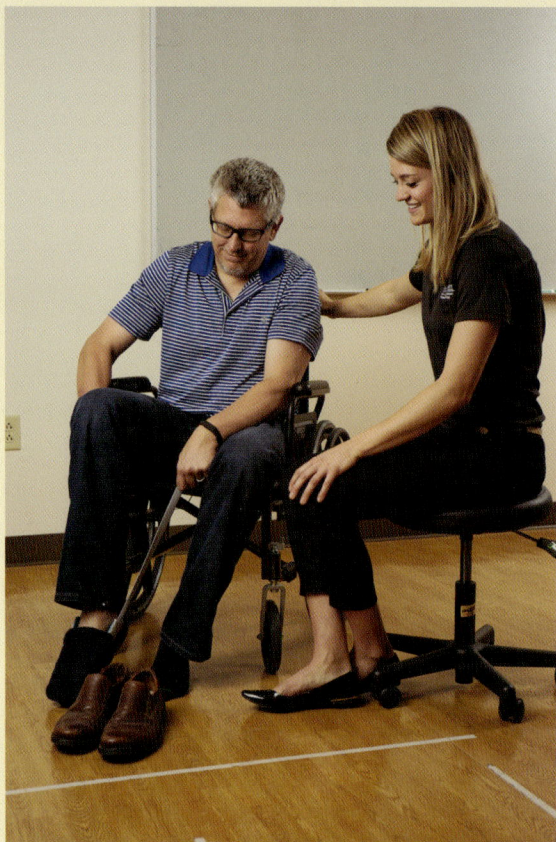
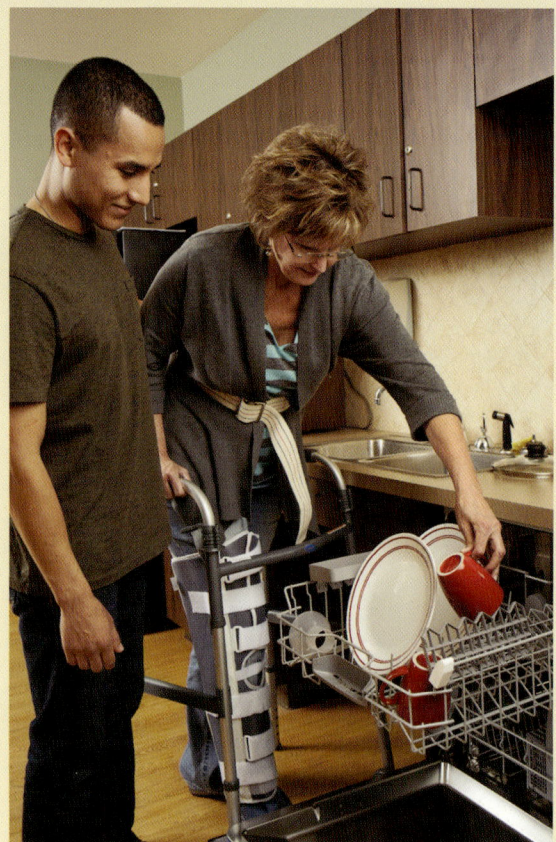
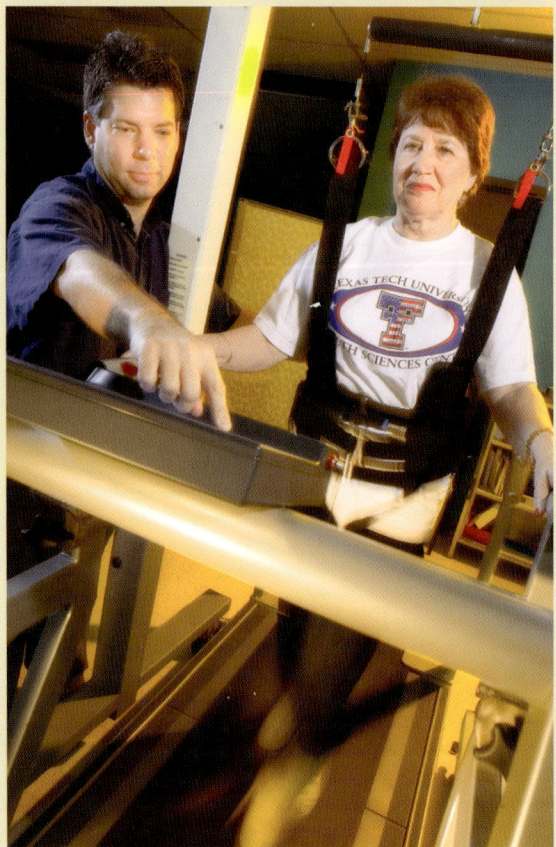
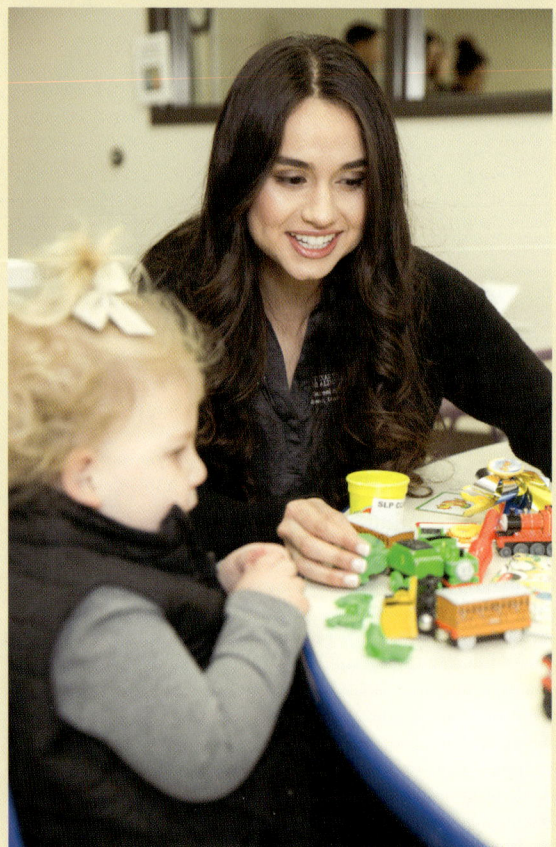

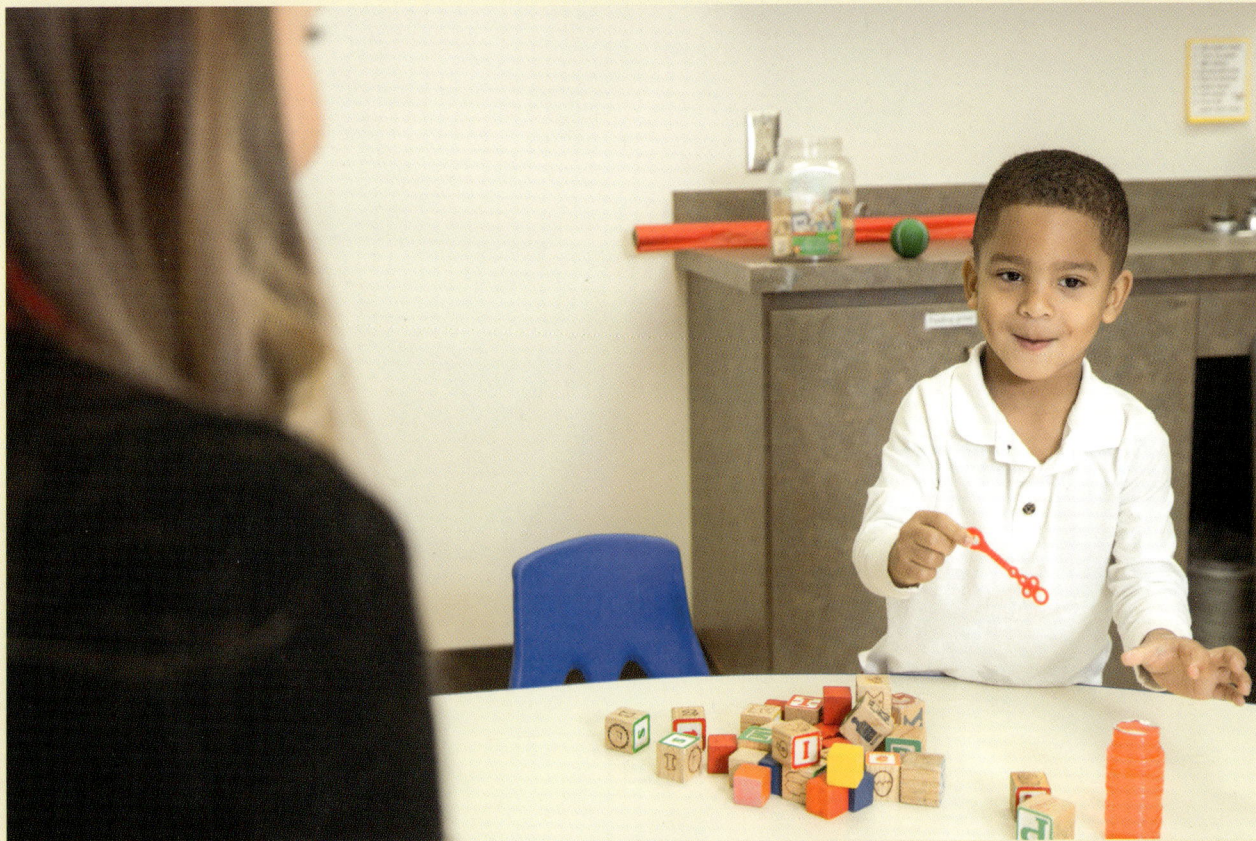

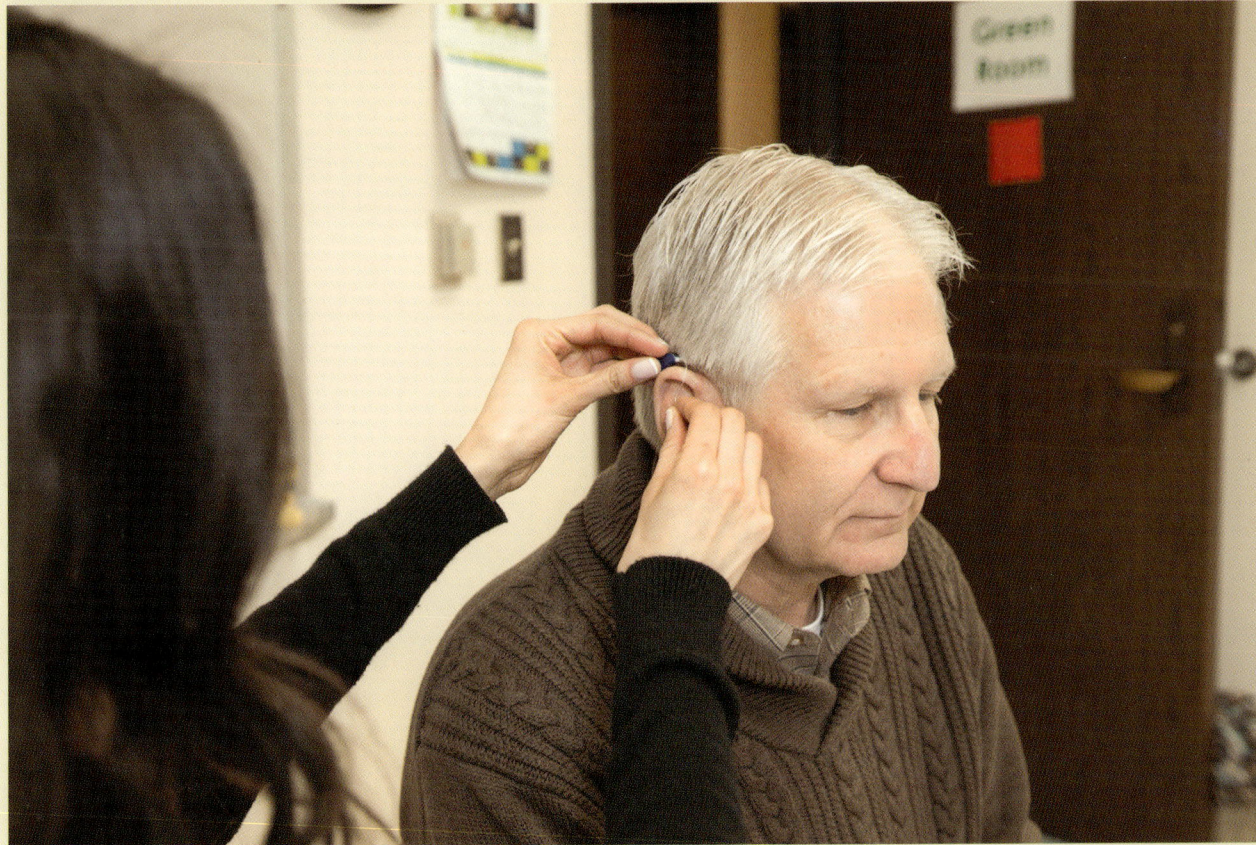

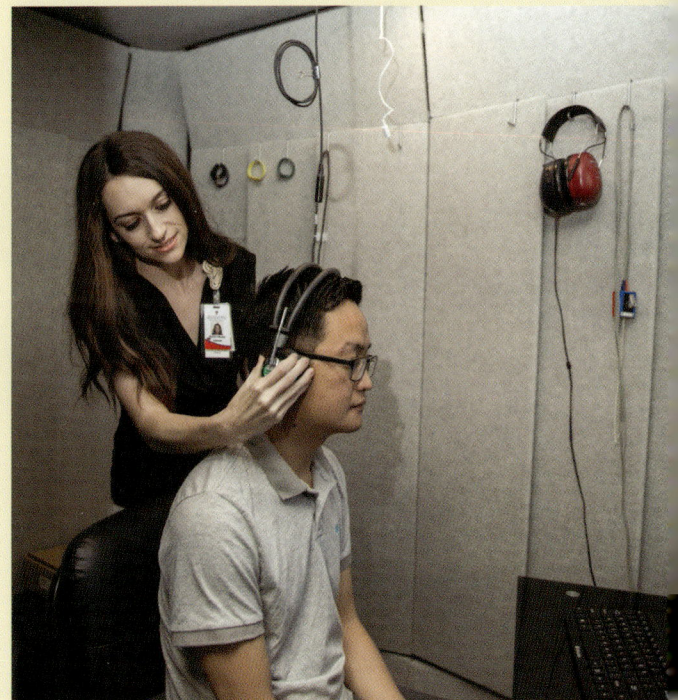

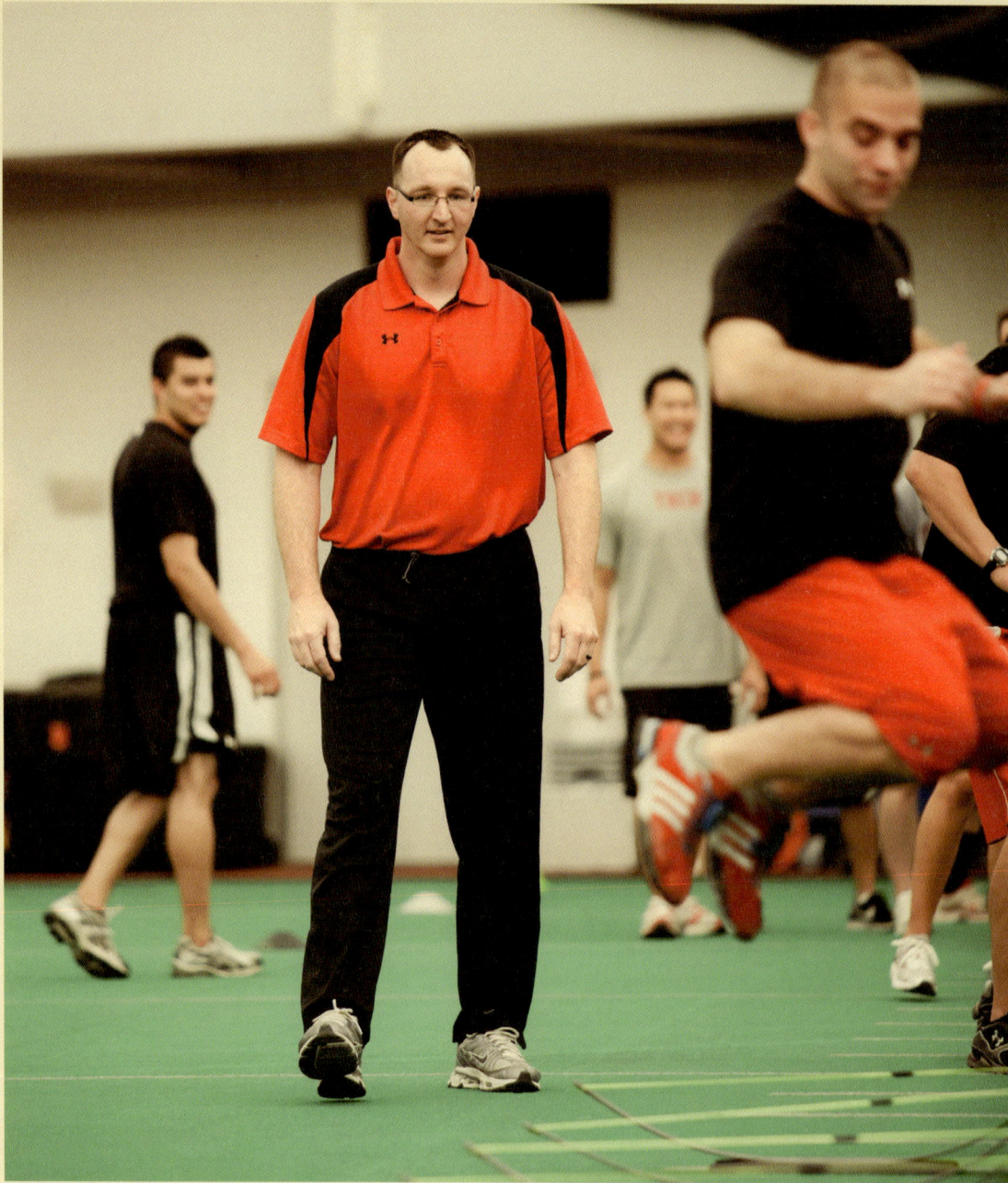
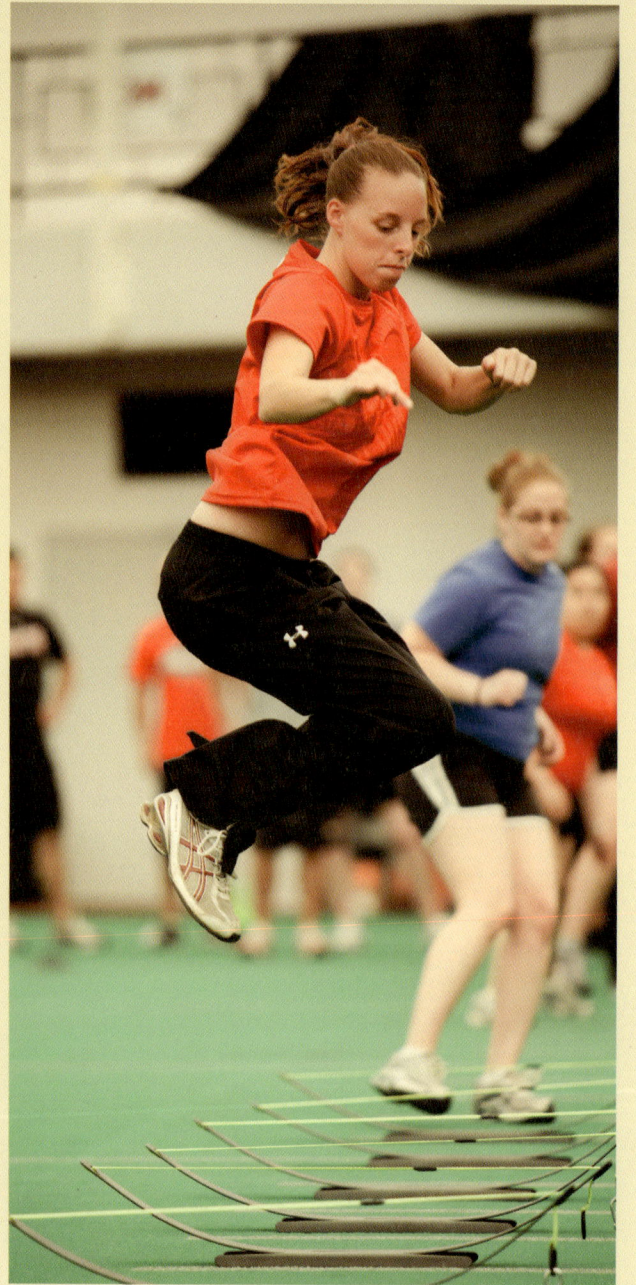

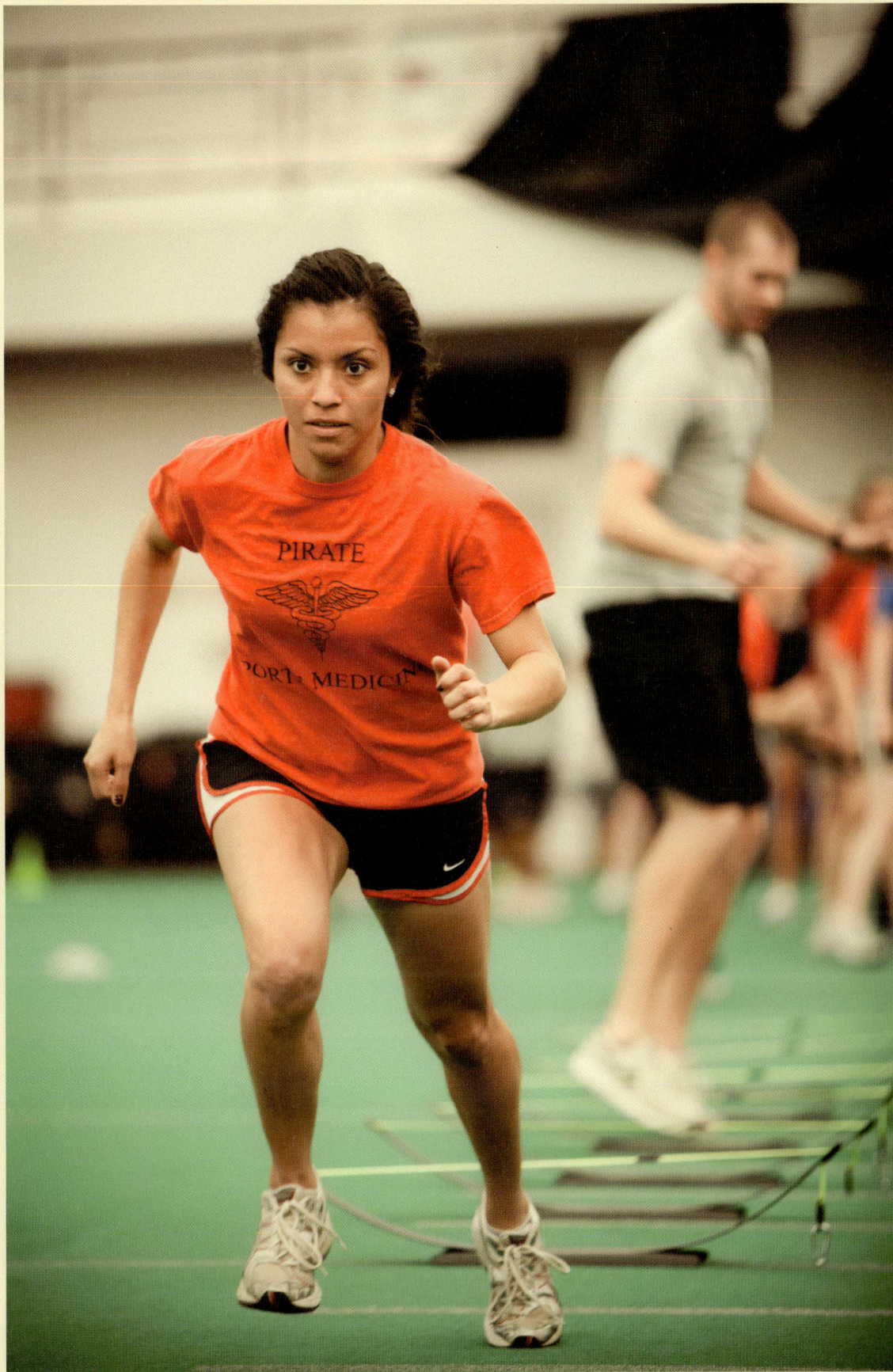

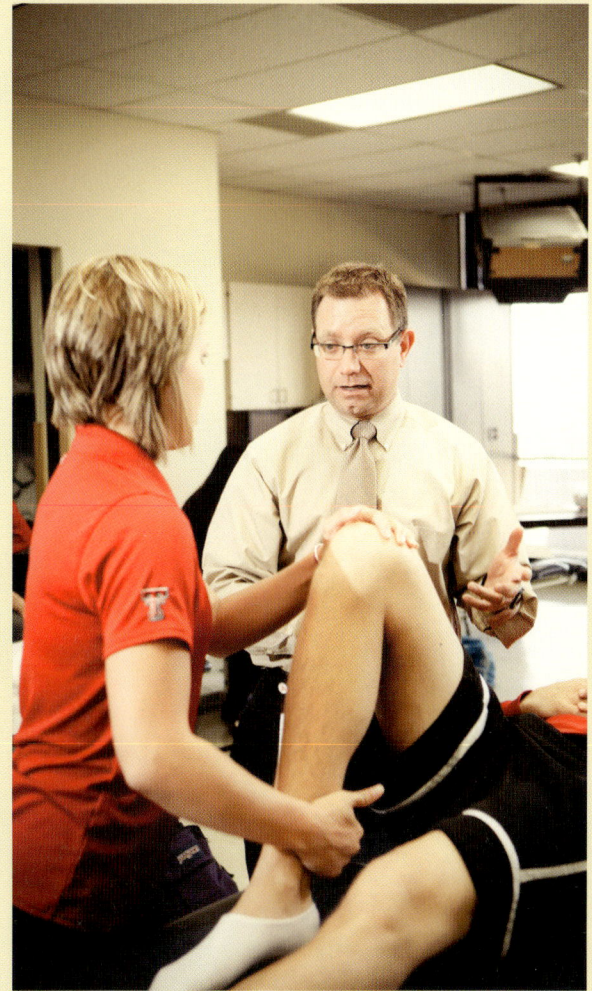

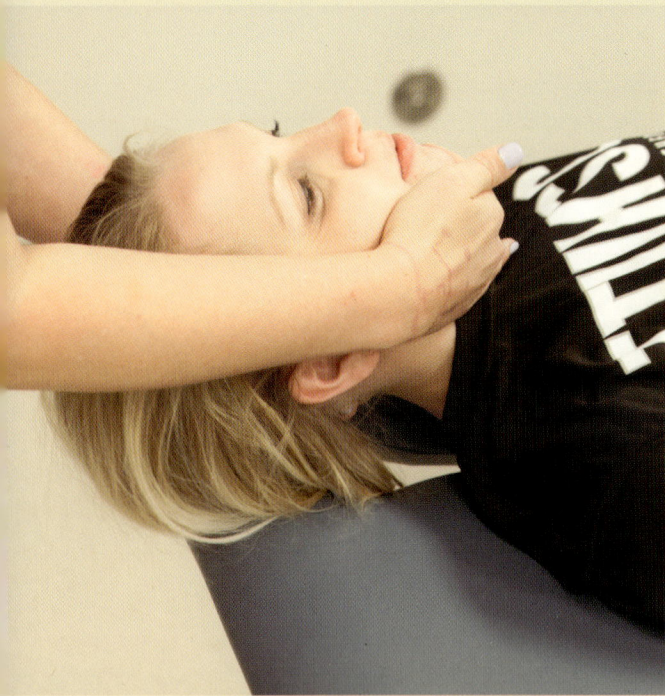
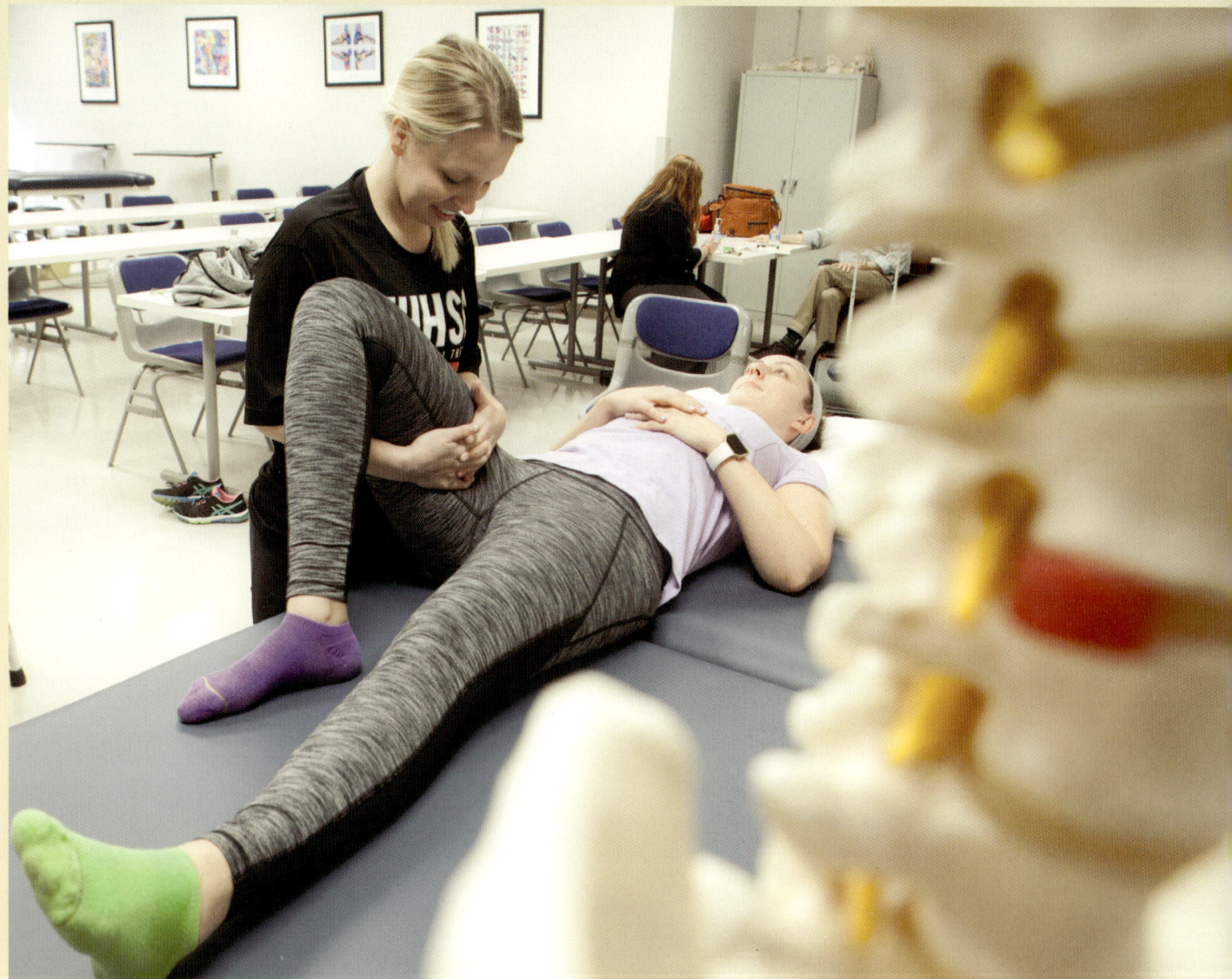

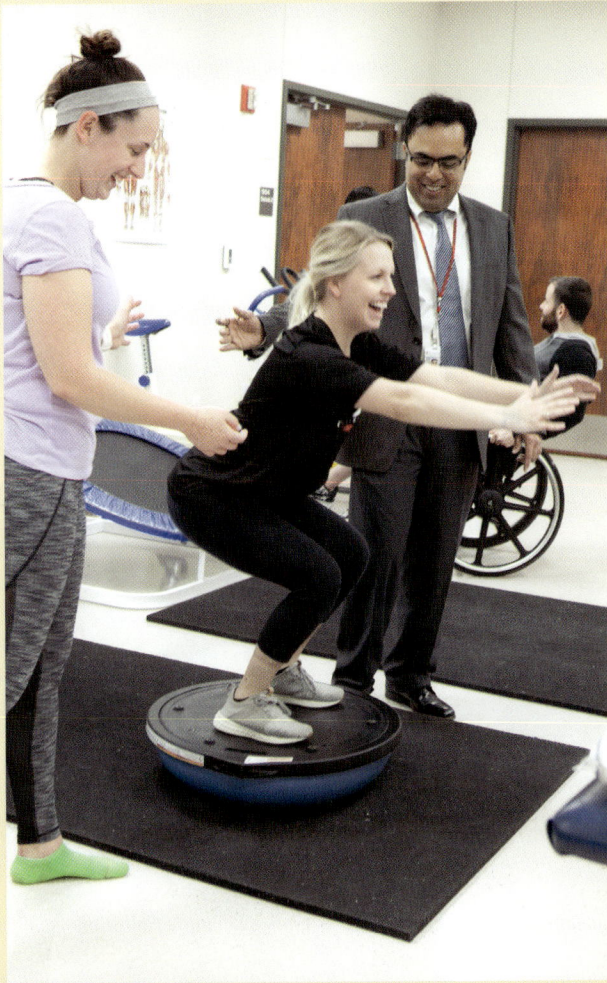

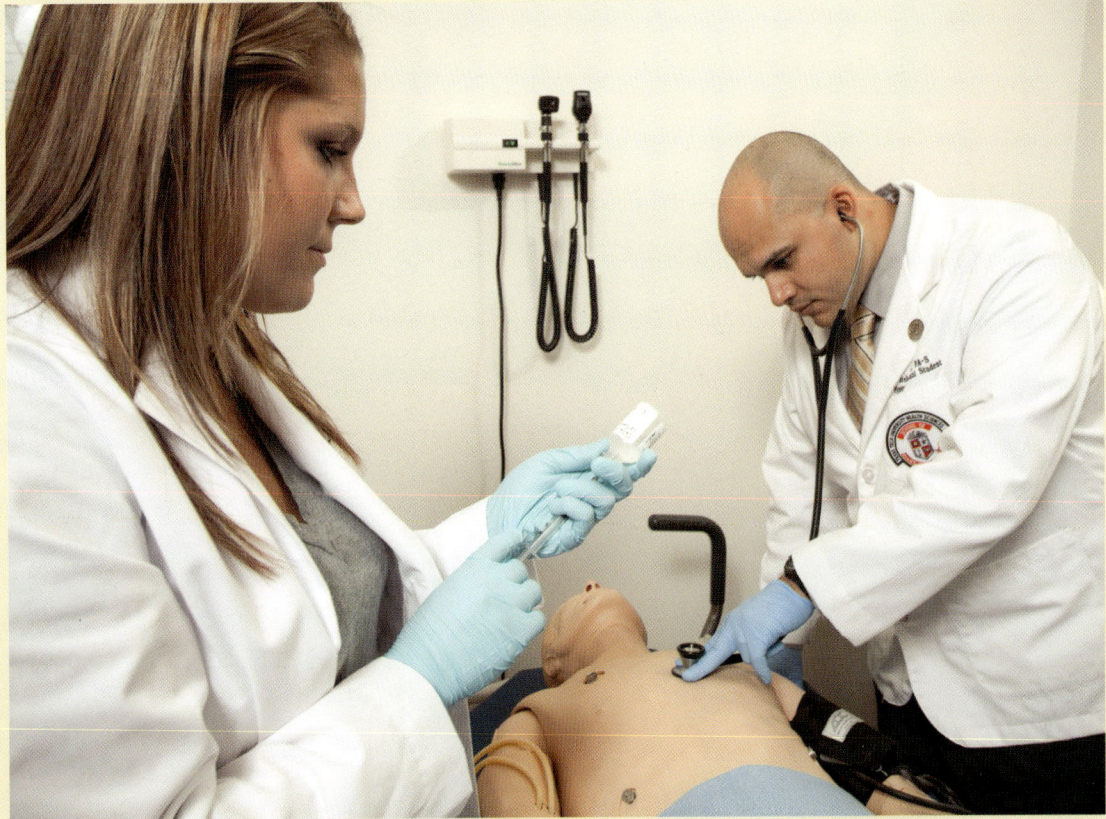

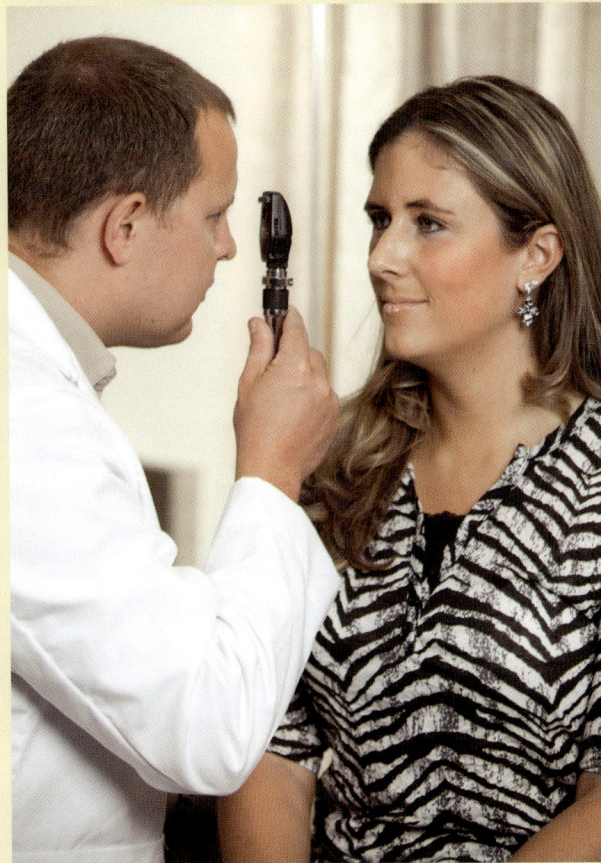

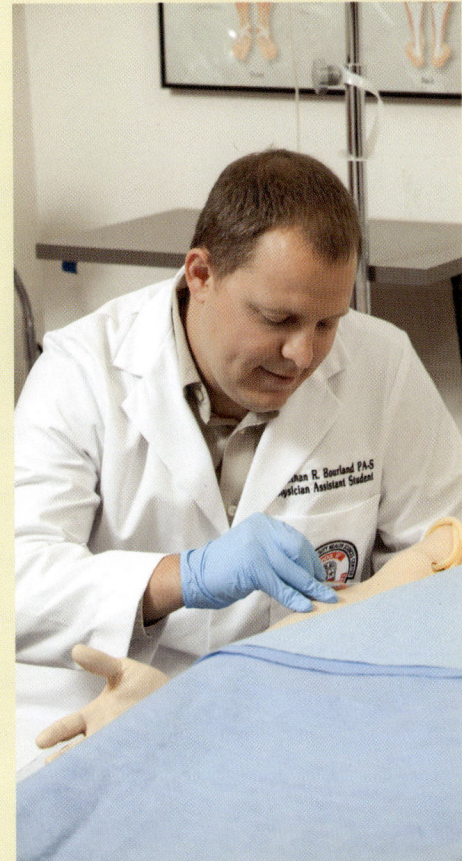

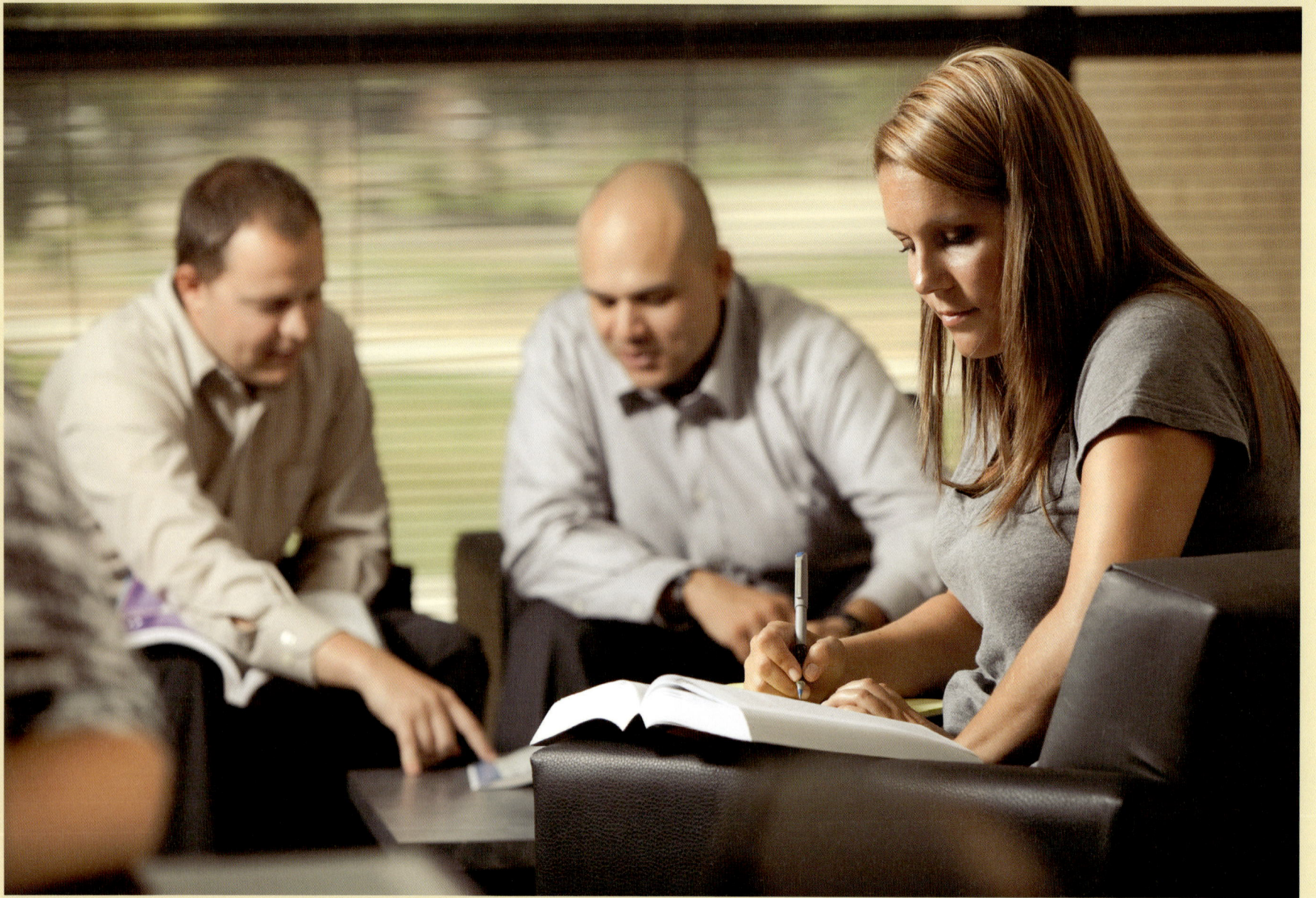

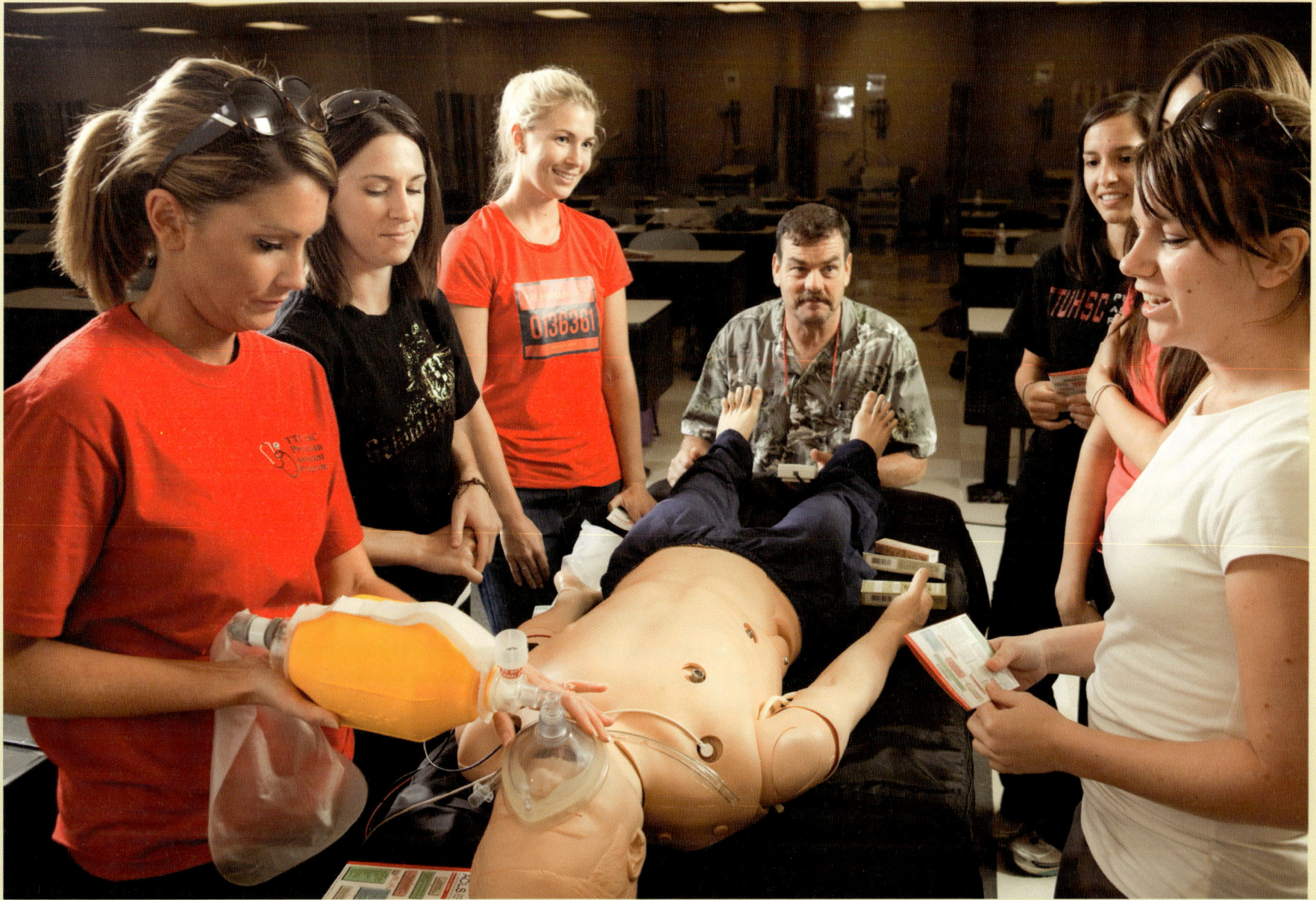

CHAPTER FIVE

SCHOOL OF PHARMACY

Quentin Smith, PhD, Dean

Although the Seventy-third Texas Legislature established the TTUHSC School of Pharmacy in Amarillo in 1993, there were hurdles to clear and skeptics who thought it would be difficult to create a first-rate school. One of them was the school's first dean, Arthur Nelson, RPh, PhD. Even after a consultant from the search committee flew in for a dinner meeting to confer, Nelson was reticent. West Texas faced a shortage of clinical practitioners required to staff the school and Nelson was told that attracting faculty to West Texas would be difficult. And, not only would the new dean need to build a school, he would need to raise the construction funds to do so.

Nelson was dean of the Idaho State University College of Pharmacy and the search committee thought he might be interested in coming to West Texas to start a new pharmacy school that also would open as a PharmD program. Though Nelson was persuaded to take a closer look, he remained skeptical of the TTUHSC situation. New pharmacy schools were all but unheard-of in the mid-1990s. There had only been two new pharmacy schools in the country since the 1950s and they were opened at private universities.

When Nelson visited Amarillo, State Senator Teel Bivins and Dr. Lee Taylor, dean for the Amarillo TTUHSC School of Medicine, met him the airport. After talking with them, Nelson's skepticism began to dis-

sipate and before he boarded his flight back to Idaho, the idea of moving to Amarillo to start a new pharmacy school had become an interesting challenge.

Nelson accepted the offer and began assembling staff and faculty for the school he envisioned. In addition to establishing an all-PharmD program, the school would add a graduate program and a residency program. It would emphasize clinical pharmacy practice for its PharmD graduates. From the moment it opened its doors, the TTUHSC School of Pharmacy required more clinical training hours than any program in the country. Once Nelson turned to hiring advanced clinical practitioners and faculty members, he found the outlook a good deal brighter than he anticipated. At the time there were only six advanced clinical practitioners in West Texas. Fortunately, five of those practitioners worked in Amarillo.

Similarly, Nelson found that the gloomy predictions about recruiting good faculty were not so accurate. Nelson was able to recruit national leaders like Chester (CAB) Bond and his wife, Cynthia Raehl, from the University of Wisconsin. The new pharmacy school also attracted young talented postdoctoral fellows from the National Institutes of Health such as David Allen and Jim and Carolyn Stoll; some of the most talented residency graduates in the country such as Glenn Anderson and Sherry Luedtke; and some very talented local practitioners, including Butch Habeger and Ranee Lenz.

A significant amount of senior faculty leadership was

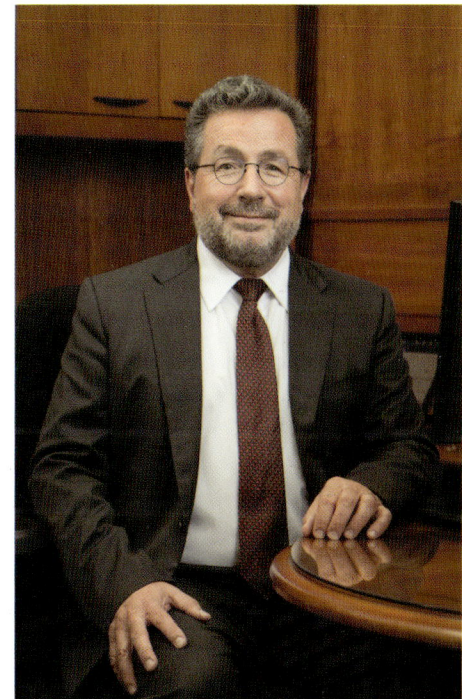

Quentin Smith, PhD, Dean

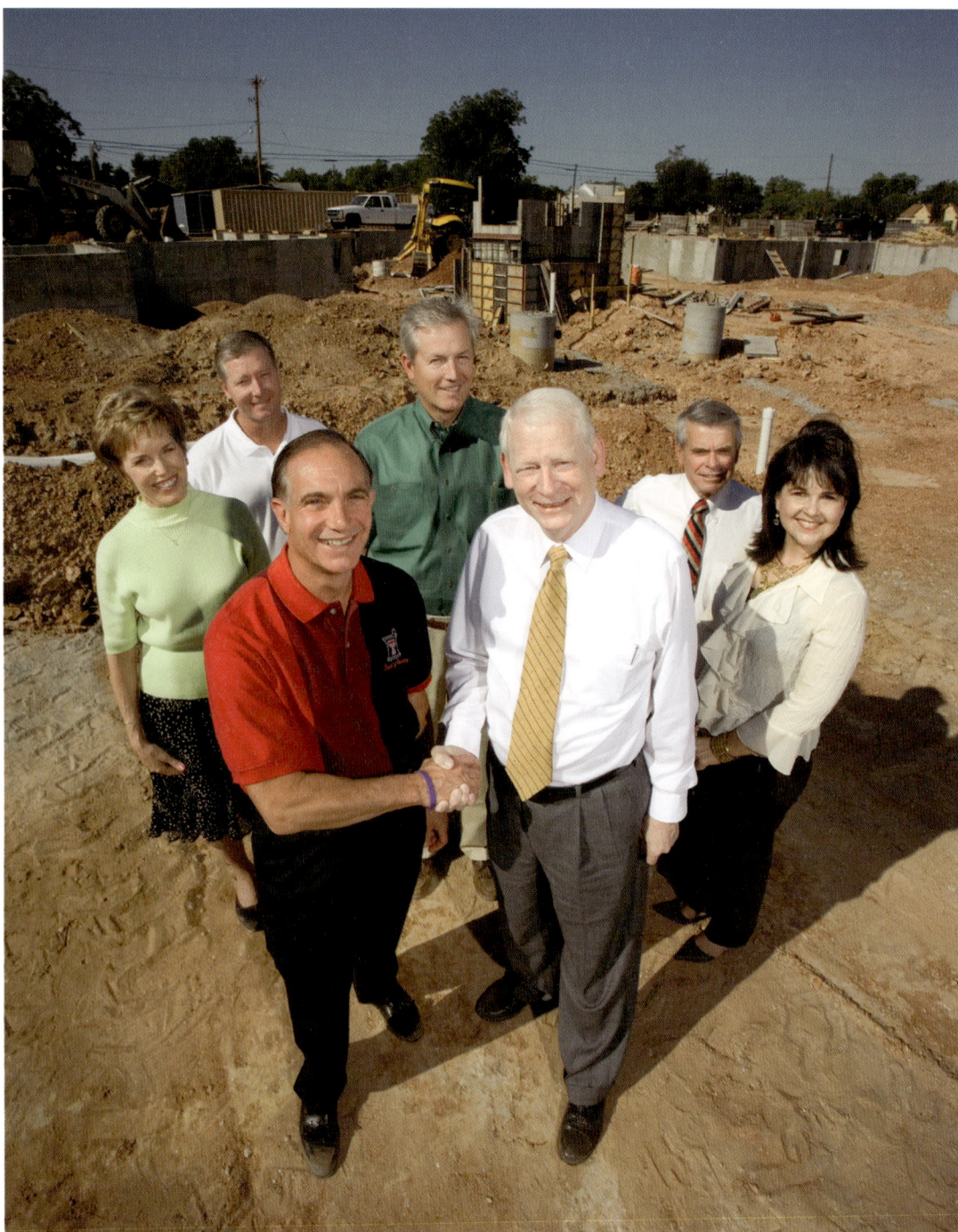
SOP construction site Abilene

put into place when Bond and Raehl agreed to sign on. In addition to their national reputations as pharmacy practice educators, their 20-year study of more than 1,000 U.S. hospitals demonstrated how clinical pharmacists are associated with reductions in mortality rates, total care and drug costs, lengths of stay, and medication errors. Their research data catalyzed fundamental change in the United Kingdom's National Health Service, which was cited in the U.S. congressional debate on Medicare reform.

Bond died in 2009. Raehl, the founding co-chair for the school's Department of Pharmacy Practice, then led in that position until she became the dean for the school's Abilene campus in 2013. She served in Abilene until she retired in 2017. During her career, Raehl served as president of the American Association of Colleges of Pharmacy and the American Society of Health-System Pharmacists. Her career honors included a TTUHSC President's Outstanding Professor Award.

Glenn Anderson left TTUHSC in 2011 to become associate dean for academic and curricular affairs and a professor of pharmacy practice for the Marshall University School of Pharmacy in West Virginia. Jim Stoll was working at the NIH when Allen, a co-worker and friend, suggested Stoll apply to TTUHSC's new pharmacy school. Eventually they both accepted positions as founding faculty members for the school. Stoll is still with the School of Pharmacy and has served as associate dean for faculty enhancement since 2009. In 2006, Allen became the founding dean for the Northeast Ohio Medical University School of Pharmacy.

Like Stoll and Allen, Quentin Smith came to TTUHSC from the NIH where he had served as the neurochemistry and brain transport section chief for the laboratory of neurosciences at the NIH–National Institute on Aging. Smith served as chair for the School of Pharmacy's Department of Pharmaceutical Sciences until 2009 when he assumed the role of senior associate dean for pharmacy sciences. TTUHSC honored Smith as a University Distinguished Professor in 2007, and in 2009 he was named the sixth recipient of the Grover E. Murray Professorship, the highest honor TTUHSC bestows upon its faculty members. In 2011, Smith was one of 13 Texas Tech University System's faculty members to receive a Chancellor's Council Distinguished Teaching and Research Award.

After Nelson retired in 2012, Smith was named the School of Pharmacy's second dean. Under Smith's leadership, school faculty voted in 2016 to adopt a curricular renewal process to keep the school on the cutting edge of pharmacy education.

Just as Nelson put to rest any doubts about attracting top-notch faculty and staff, by 1995 he had worked with TTUHSC to secure $13 million in donations to build a 102,000-square-foot, state-of-the-art facility for training future pharmacists. He had wide support from TTUHSC, Amarillo organizations, corporations, and private donors.

Construction began in March 1995 on land donated by the Harrington Regional Medical Center and the building was officially dedicated on August 14, 1996. The founding class included 65 students supported by 26 faculty and 10 staff. There were two departments: Pharmacy Practice and Pharmaceutical Sciences. Only a year later, the School of Pharmacy would begin creating a constellation of campuses beginning in Dallas–Fort Worth with a handful of clinical placements. The school also started its residency program that same year. In 1998, the Lubbock campus of the School of Pharmacy opened at the main TTUHSC building under the direction of Charles Seifert, PharmD, who still serves as the Lubbock dean. Also in 1998, the school began a small program in El Paso under the direction of Maumi Villarreal, PharmD, and started its graduate program in Pharmaceutical Sciences.

The Dallas/Fort Worth campus officially opened in 1999 using space leased from Baylor University Medical Center. Now PharmD students, completing their first two years at the main campus in Amarillo, had the option of remaining in Amarillo or transferring to either Lubbock or Dallas/Fort Worth to complete their final two years. In 2002, Richard Leff, PharmD, was named Dallas/Fort Worth dean and the campus was relocated to a renovated 4,800-square-foot building on the grounds of the North Texas Veterans Affairs Hospital. This building was expanded to approximately 8,000 square feet in 2003, and in August 2008, the Dallas/Fort Worth campus expanded to a second location within the Dallas Medical District.

In 2013, Leff became senior associate dean for clinical and translational research for the School of Pharmacy and Roland Patry, DrPH, another of the school's founding faculty members, moved from the Amarillo campus to the Dallas/Fort Worth campus to assume the dean's position. Patry, who joined Raehl as a founding co-chair for the school's Department of Pharmacy Practice, came to TTUHSC after a successful run as a senior hospital practice administrator at Baylor University Medical Center.

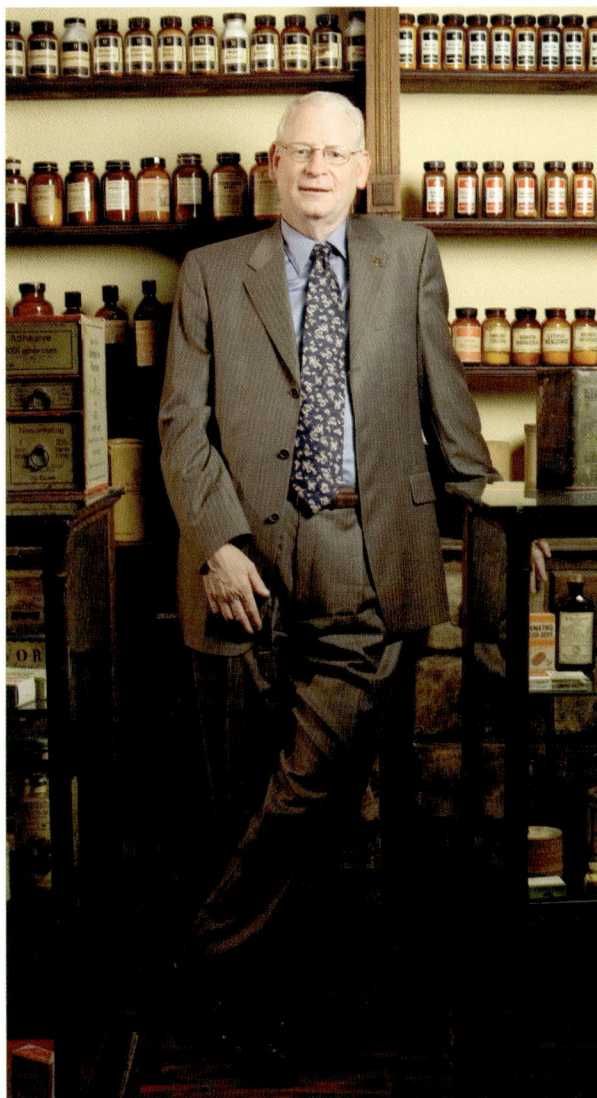

Arthur Nelson,
Retired Dean

While based in Amarillo, Patry worked with Texas Tech University's Rawls College of Business to establish the PharmD/MBA dual degree program at the School of Pharmacy, which awarded its first degree in 2010.

Leff was awarded the James A. "Buddy" Davidson Endowed Professorship in Pediatric Pharmacology in 2012, and in 2017 he received the Chancellor's Council Distinguished Faculty Award, the Texas Tech University System's highest faculty honor, before retiring. Patry was named a TTUHSC University Distinguished Professor in 2015 and he retired in 2017. Steven Pass, Pharmd, became the Dallas/Fort Worth dean, succeeding Patry.

In 2004, Abilene mayor Norm Archibald approached Nelson at a Texas Tech football game to discuss a four-year campus in Abilene. By the time the School of Pharmacy celebrated its tenth anniversary in 2006, construction was

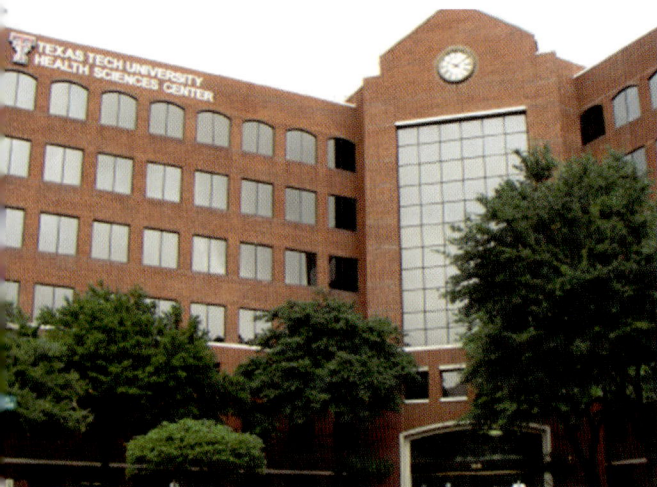

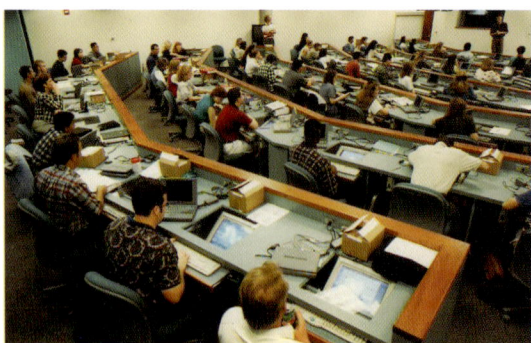

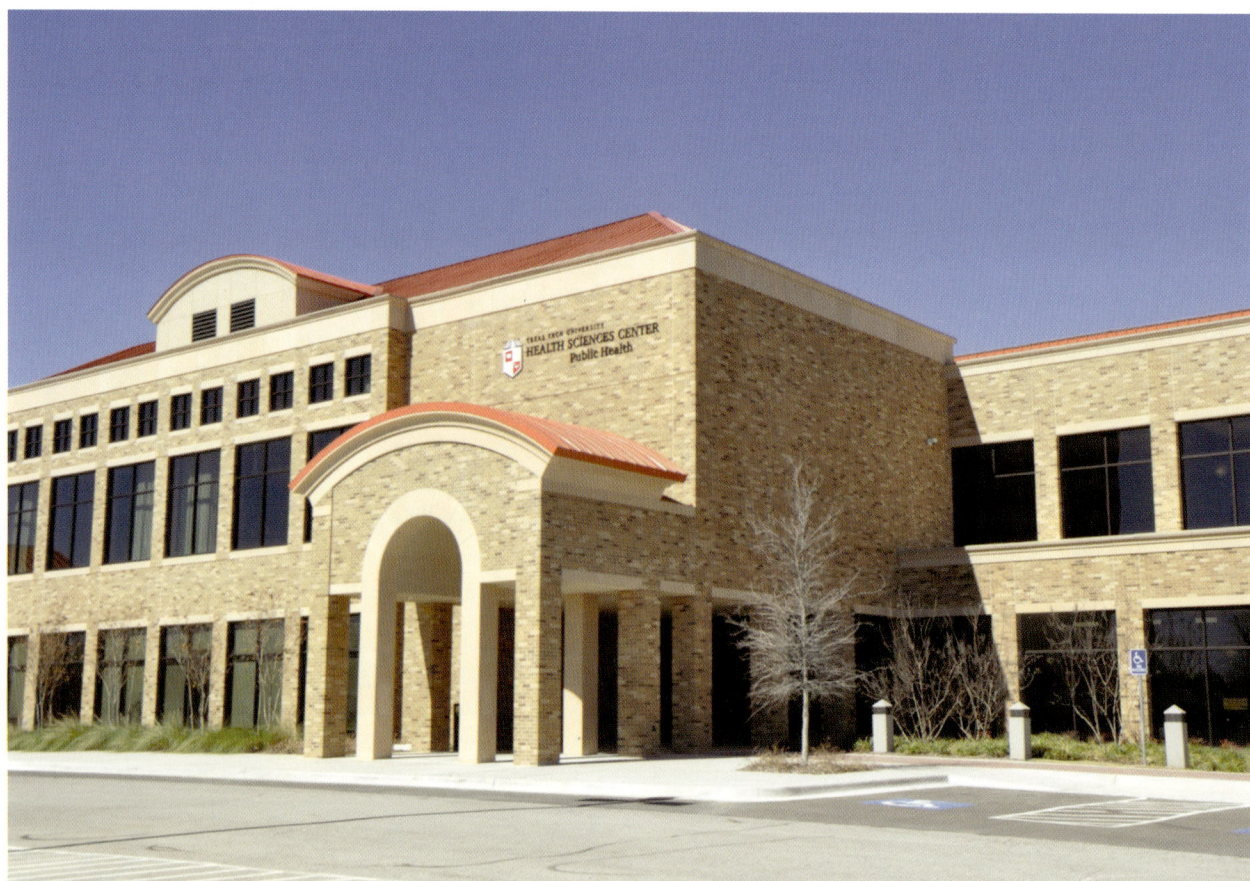

(TOP) SOP Dallas Campus Building

(BOTTOM) SOP students listening to lecture

(ABOVE RIGHT) SOP, Amarillo Building

underway in Abilene. The new campus opened in August 2007 with a 40-member founding class. Kim Powell was the founding dean and in May 2011 the first graduates crossed the stage.

In 2012, the Texas Tech University System Board of Regents approved construction of a 13,000-square-foot expansion on the Abilene campus for the School of Pharmacy's newly established Department of Immunotherapeutics and Biotechnology. Virgil Van Dusen, RPh, JD (2010–2011) also served as Abilene dean, as did Debra Notturno-Strong, RPh (2011–2013) and Cynthia Raehl, PharmD (2013–2017). Sara Brouse, PharmD, was named to the position in 2017 when Raehl retired.

Expansion came to the Amarillo campus in 2009. In March of that year, the TTUHSC Schools of Pharmacy and Medicine opened the 48,000-square-foot Amarillo Research Building to provide additional space for up to 15 School of Pharmacy laboratories and offices for researchers, graduate student researchers, and support

personnel. In November, the Amarillo campus also cut the ribbon on its 23,000-square-foot Pharmacy Academic Center. The facility includes two 120-student classrooms and a 12-room patient simulation training and assessment center.

That same year, Thomas Thekkumkara was named the first dean for the Amarillo campus and the school's annual extramural research funding topped $5 million for the first time.

Growing the Mission

The School of Pharmacy's Department of Pharmacy Practice is comprised of seven divisions: geriatrics, adult medicine, clinical sciences and research, primary care, pediatrics, community care, and practice management. The department also oversees the Office of Experiential Programs and the Graduate Pharmacy Education (Residency) program. Raehl and Patry were the department's

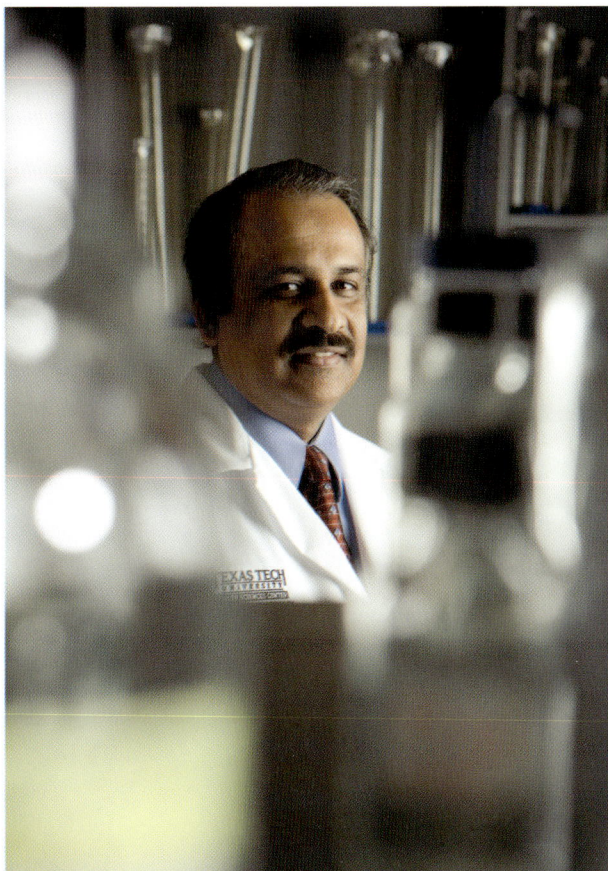

Thomas Thekkumkara, PhD, Amarillo Regional Dean

a Crystal Academic–Practice Partnerships for Learning Excellence (Crystal APPLE) Award from the American Association of Colleges of Pharmacy for fostering experiential education.

The Graduate Pharmacy Education (Residency) program was established in 1997 and has developed into one of the nation's largest school-funded, postgraduate residency programs. It supports the School of Pharmacy's mission by offering unique training opportunities through pharmacy practice.

The graduate program in Pharmaceutical Sciences (GPPS) was established in 1998 as part of TTUHSC's Graduate School of Biomedical Sciences. The program offers masters' and doctoral degrees in integrated biomedical/pharmaceutical research, and many GPPS graduates go on to fill important positions within academia, research labs, government agencies, and private companies.

The School of Pharmacy reorganized its science-based research faculty in 2009 to create two departments: the long-standing Department of Pharmaceutical Sciences and the newly formed Department of Biomedical Sciences. The Department of Immunotherapeutics and Biotechnology was opened in 2012 on the Abilene campus. These departments are comprised of more than 80 research-based faculty, postdoctoral associates, graduate students, and technicians at the Amarillo and Abilene campuses.

In 2001 the School of Pharmacy established a grant program, resulting in the development of three centers for research excellence: the Center for Cancer Biology Research, the Center for Pathophysiology and Treatment of Stroke, and the Pediatric Pharmacology Research and Development Center. A fourth research center—The Center for Immunotherapeutic Research and Development—was established in 2007 in Abilene.

In 2008, the Center for Pathophysiology and Treatment of Stroke was reorganized as the Vascular Drug Research Center to take advantage of important collaborations, which developed between several investigators.

founding co-chairs. Eric MacLaughlin, PharmD, was named department chair in 2014 after Raehl and Patry were promoted to dean positions.

The Office of Experiential Programs places TTUHSC pharmacy students in actual practice settings in Texas and has earned high marks from both students and preceptors. Craig Cox, PharmD, an associate professor on the Lubbock campus, was named the School of Pharmacy's vice chair of experiential programs in 2005.

In 2007, and again in 2008, the school and its affiliation with the North Texas VA Medical Center received

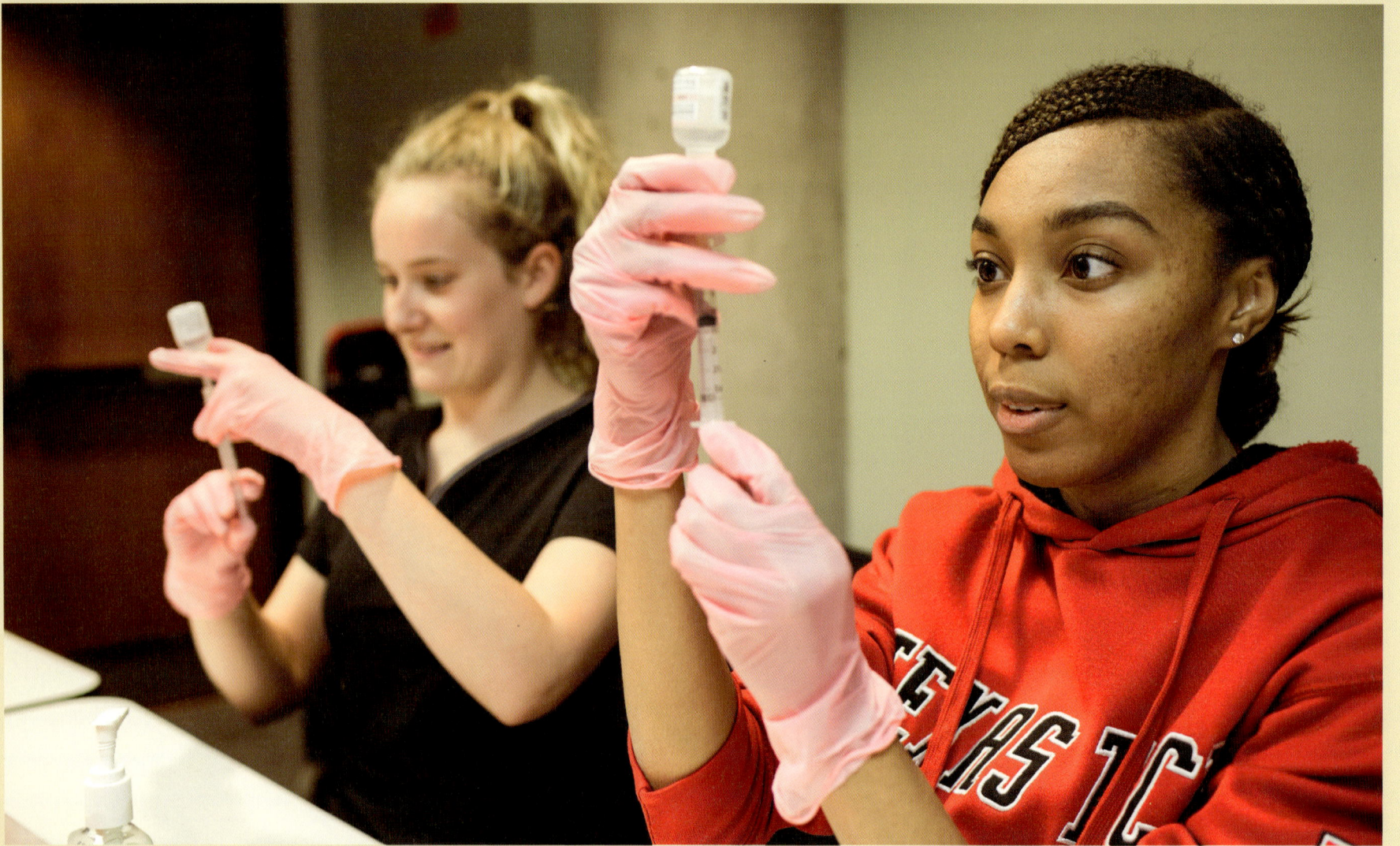
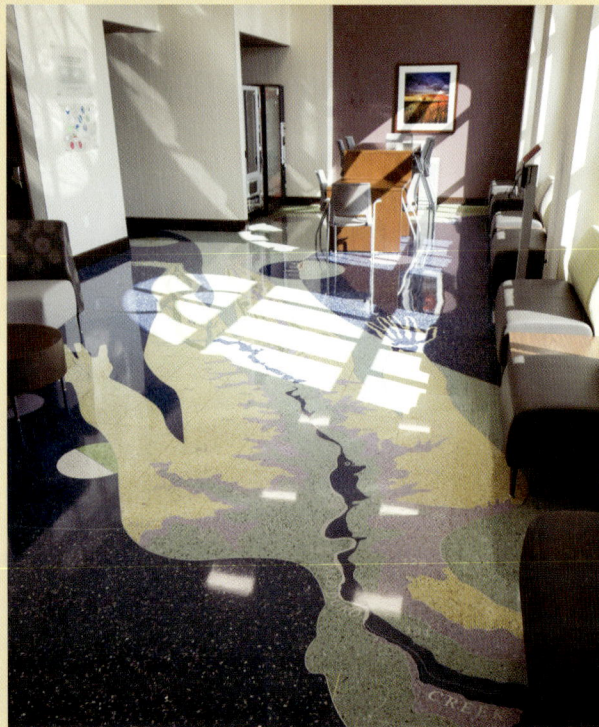
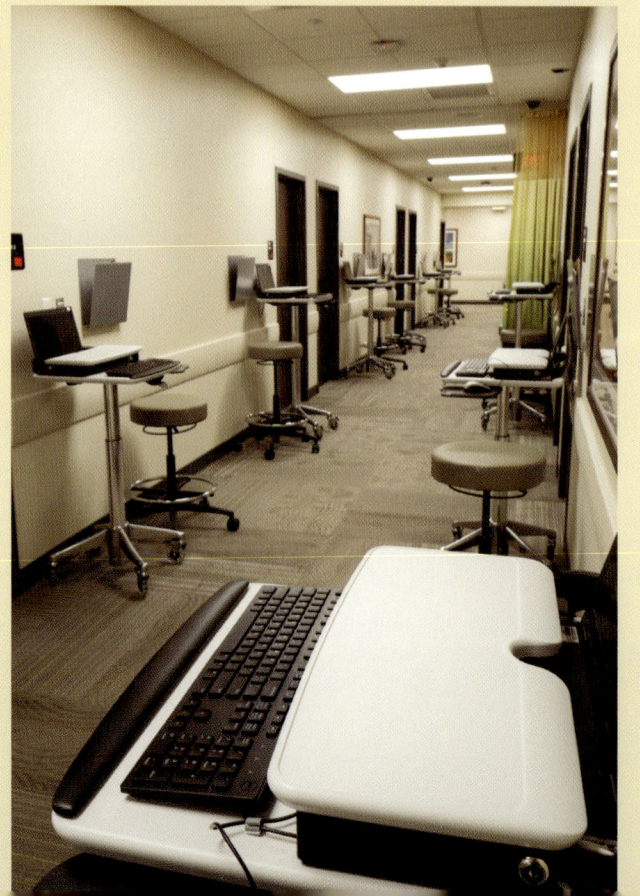

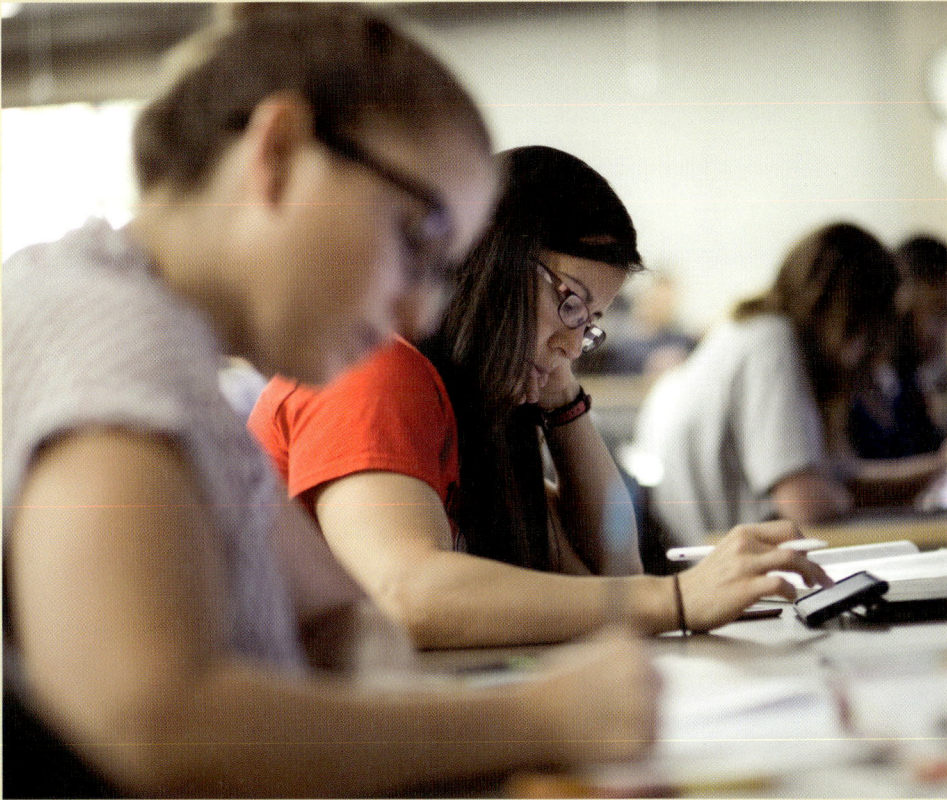
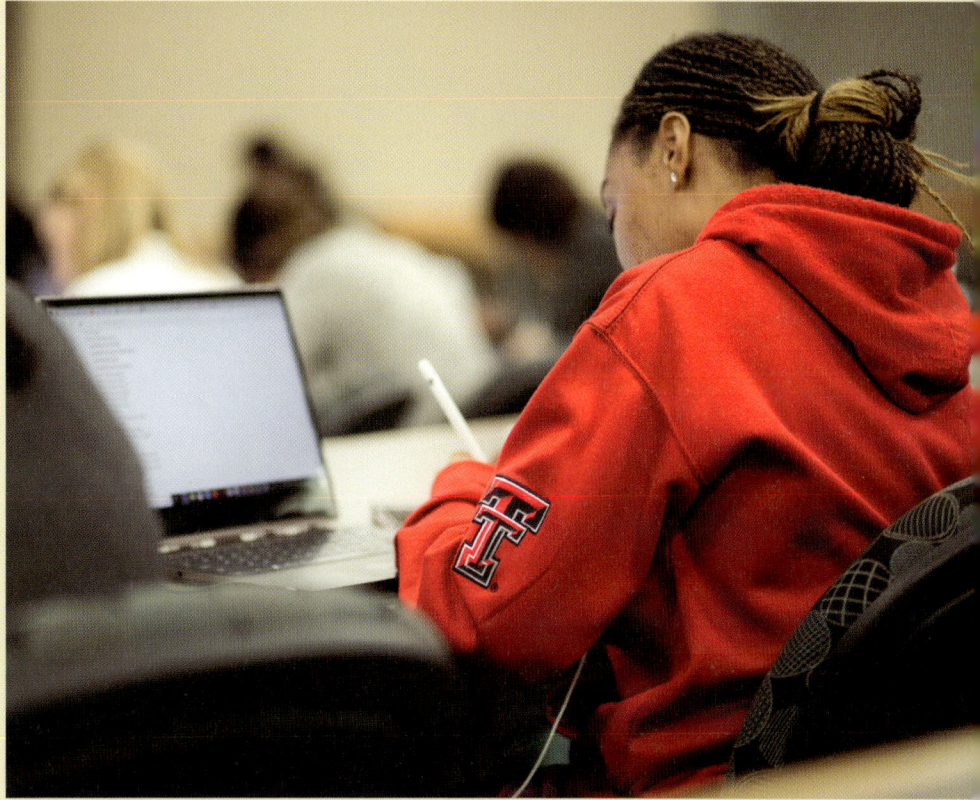
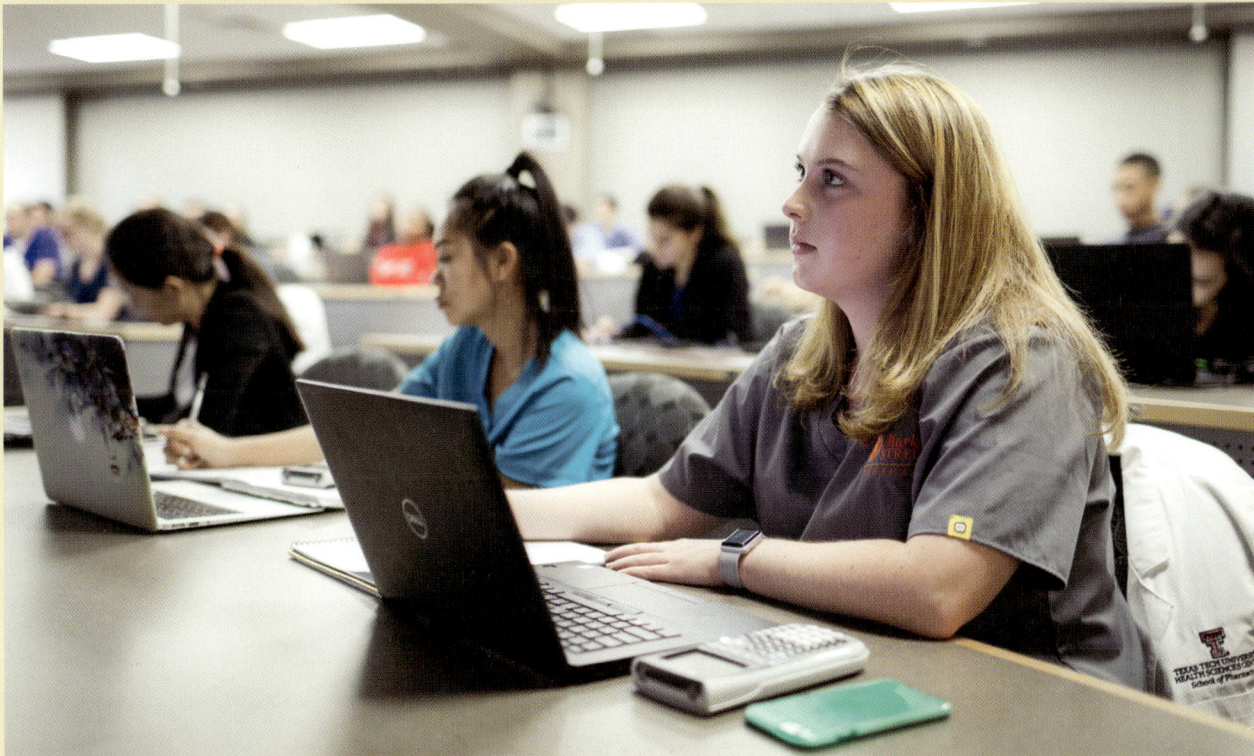
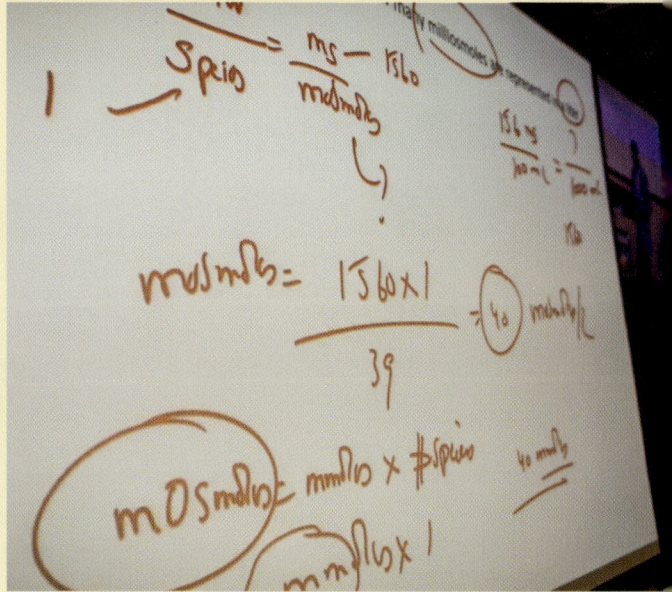

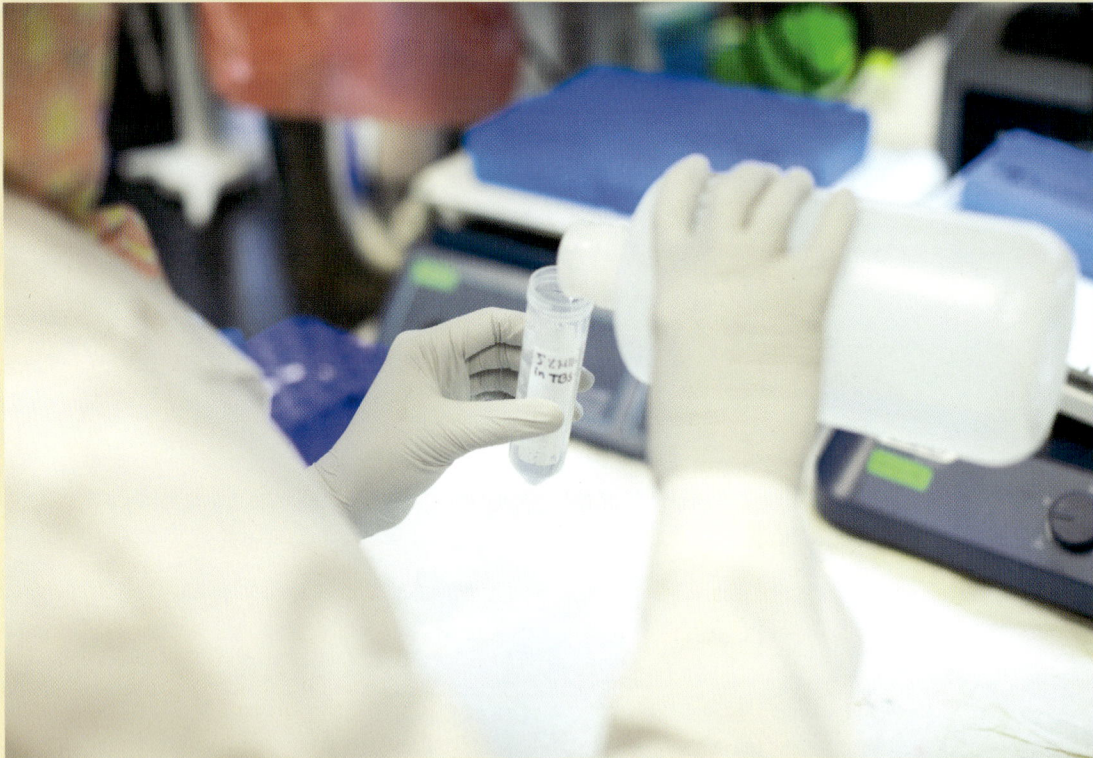
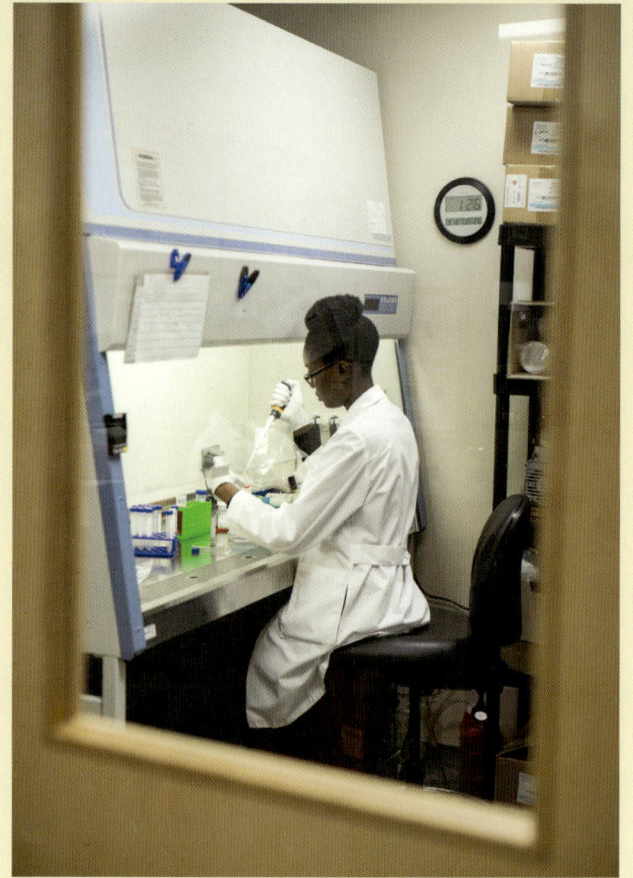
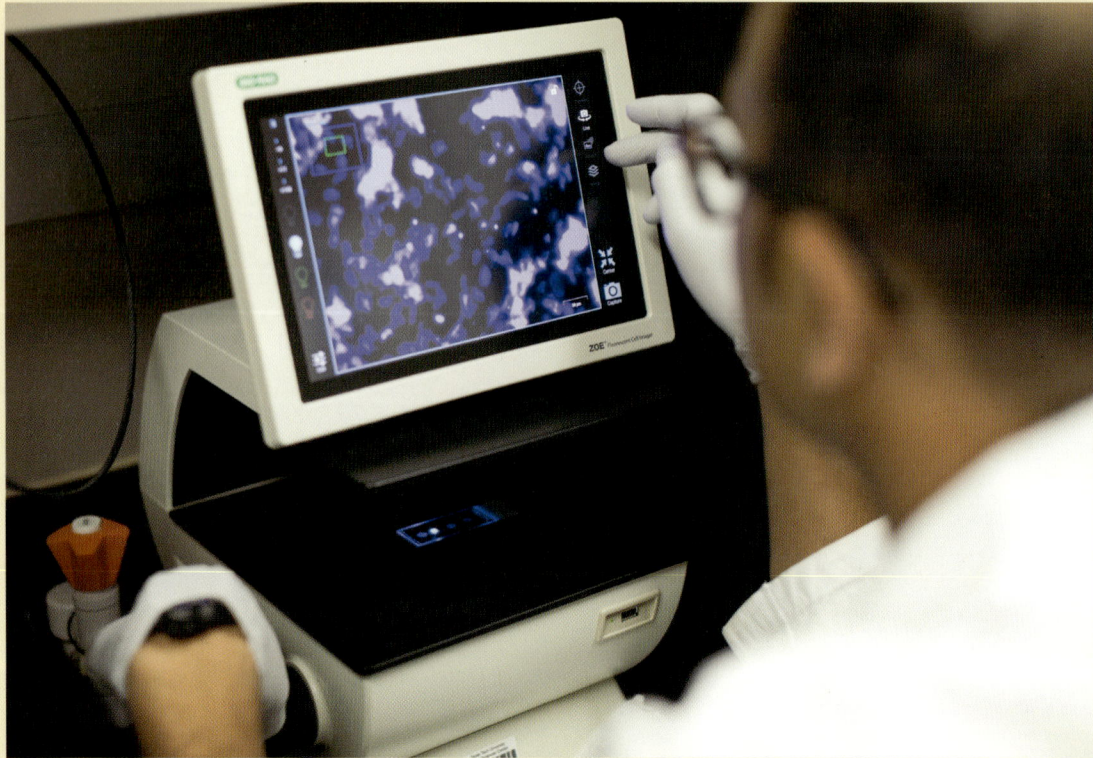
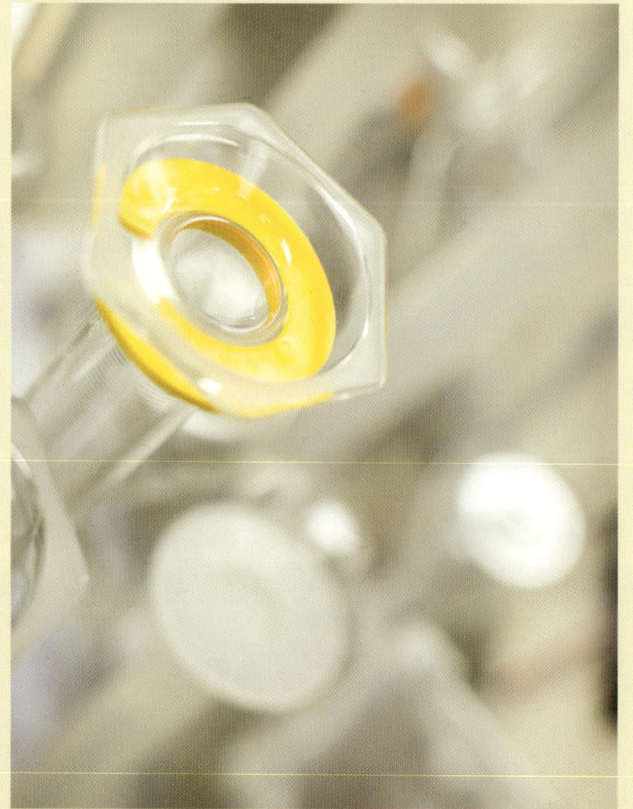

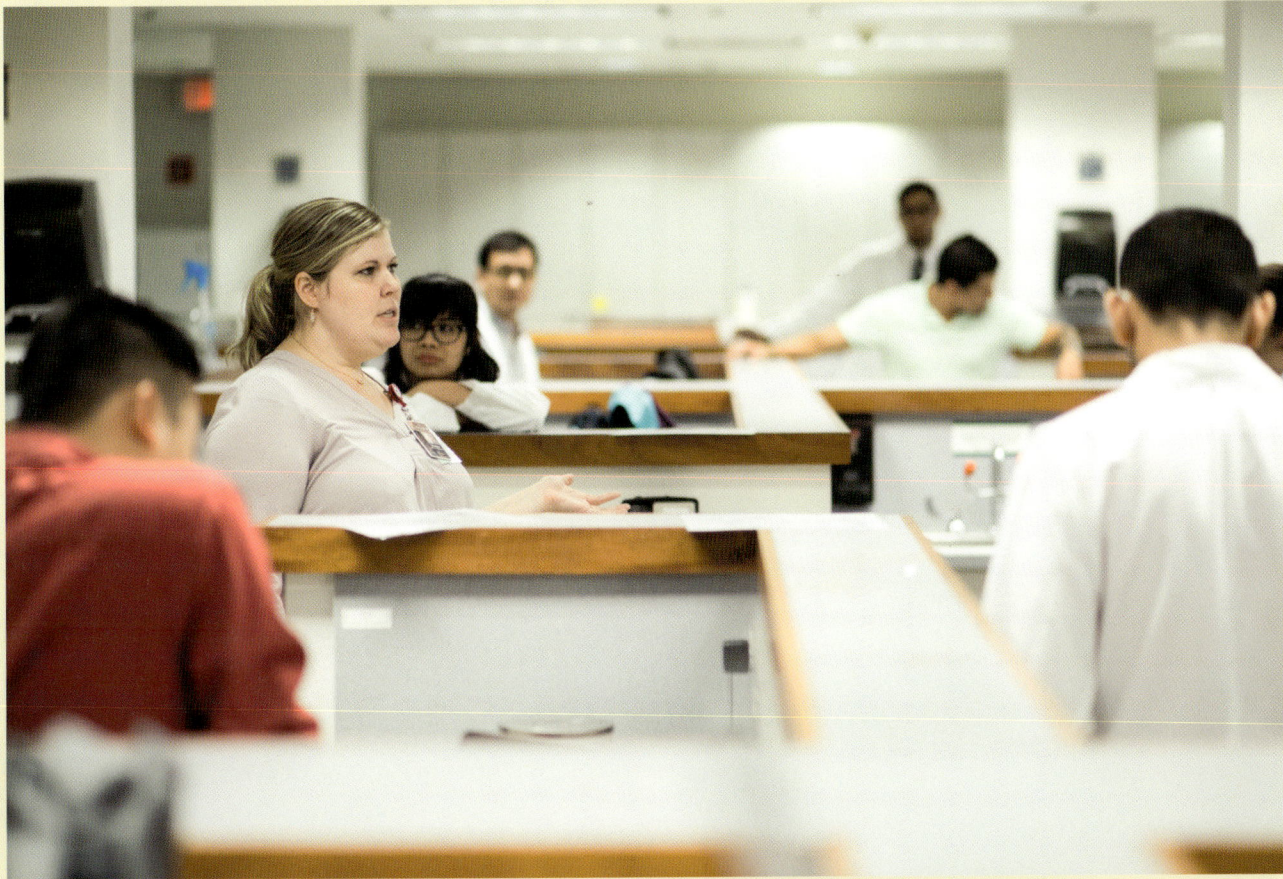

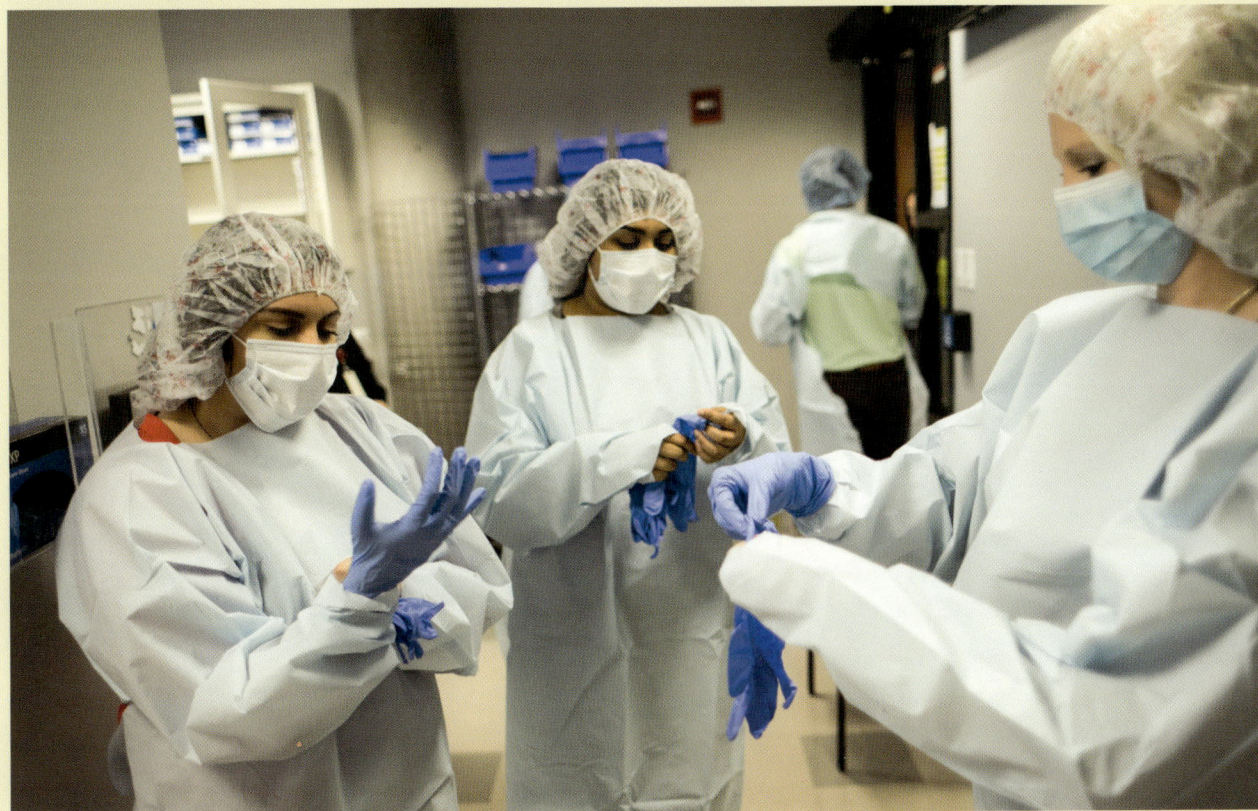

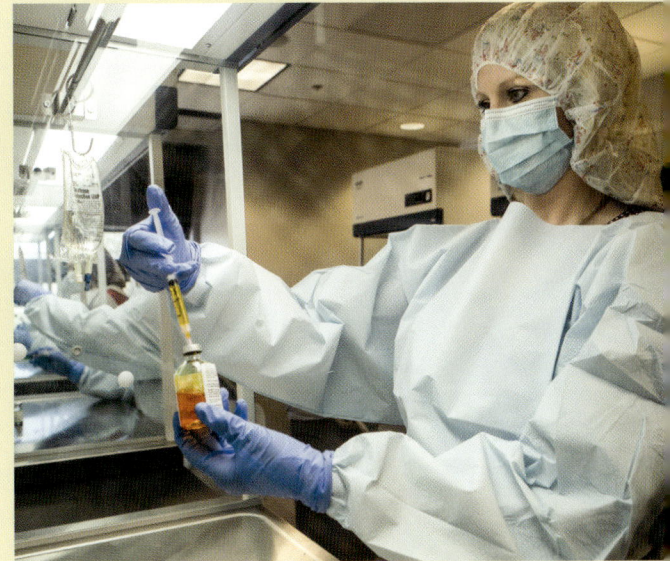

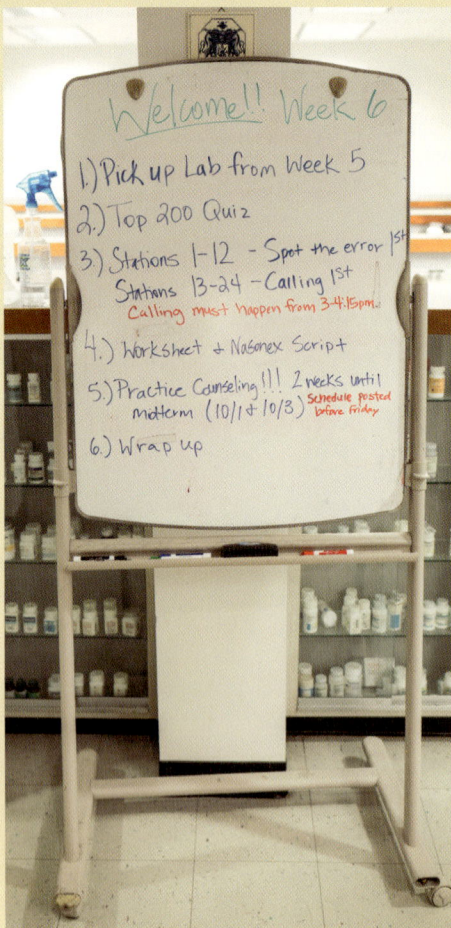

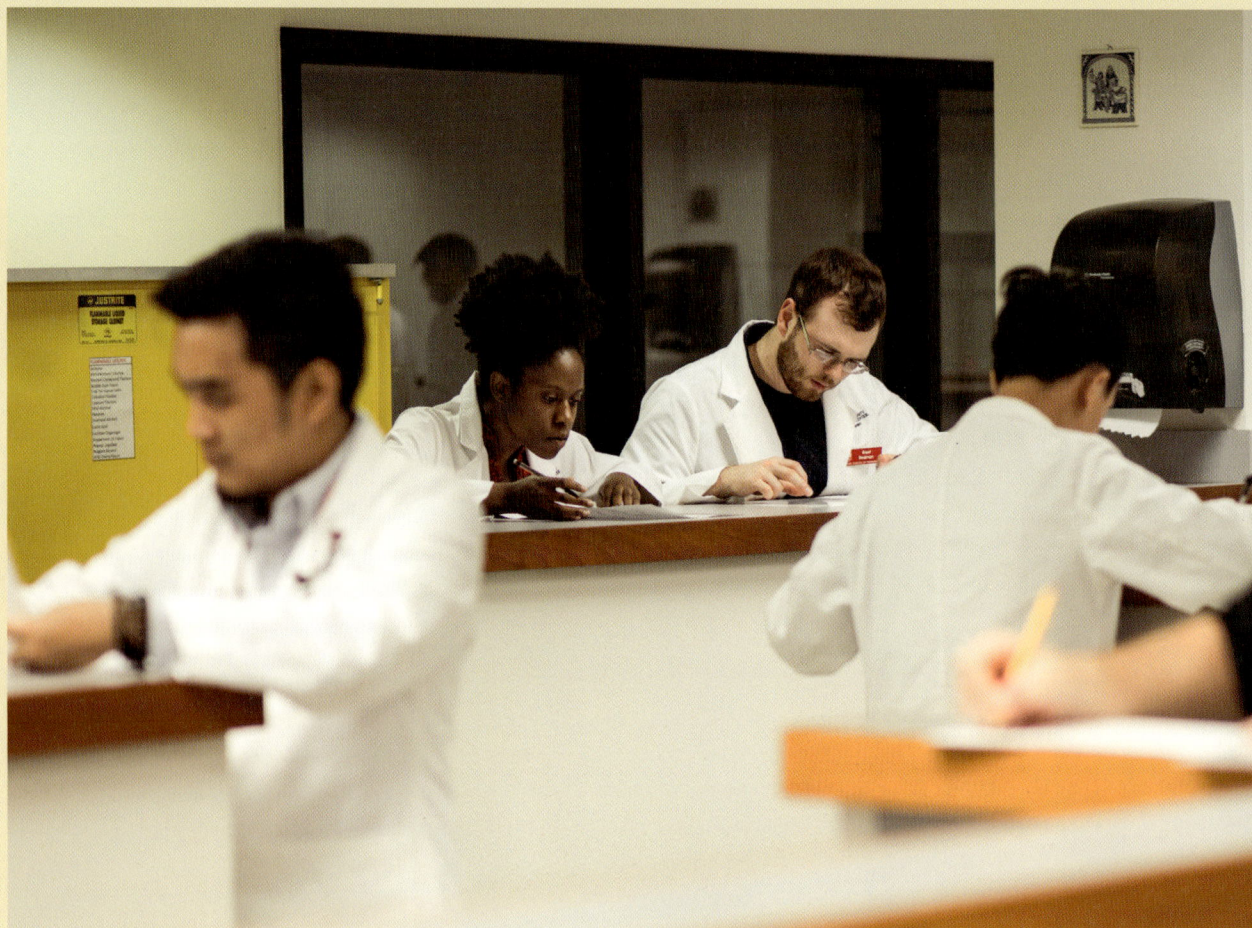

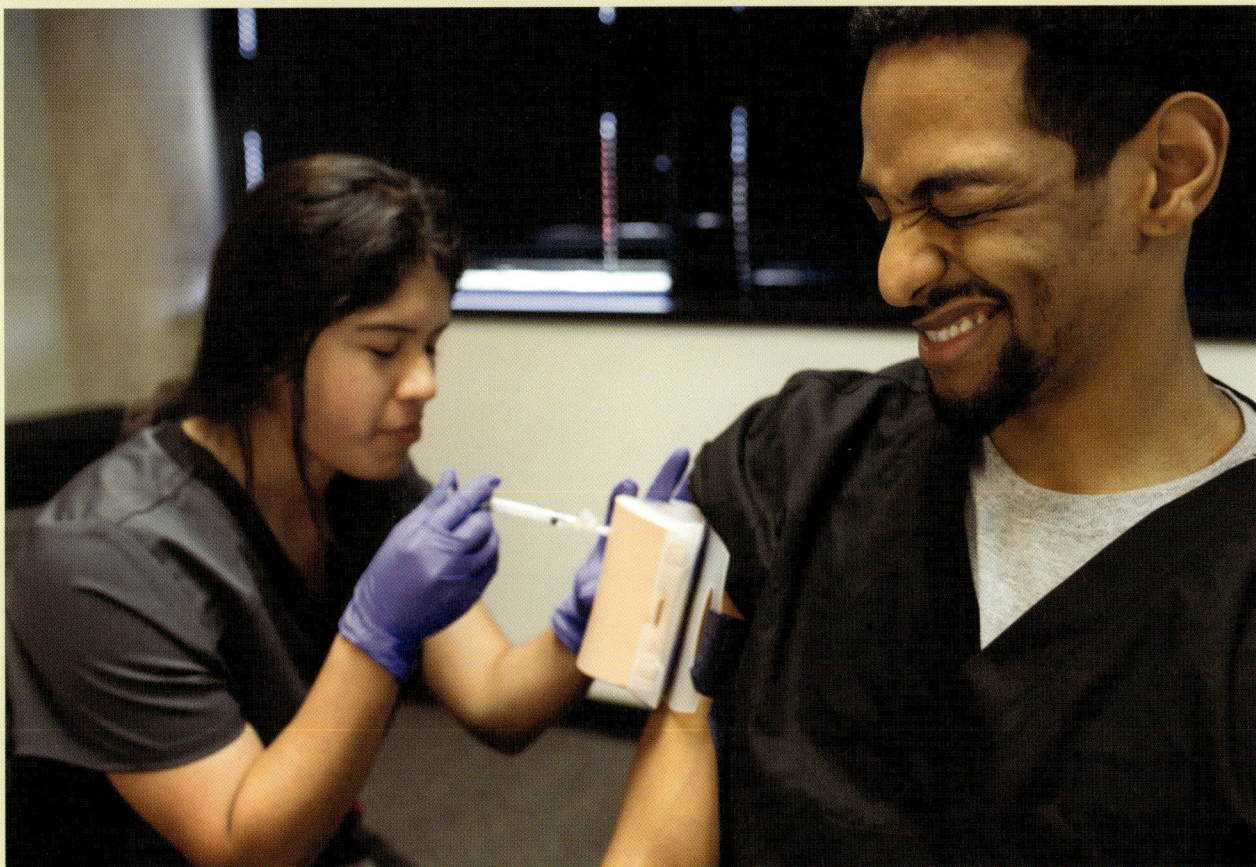

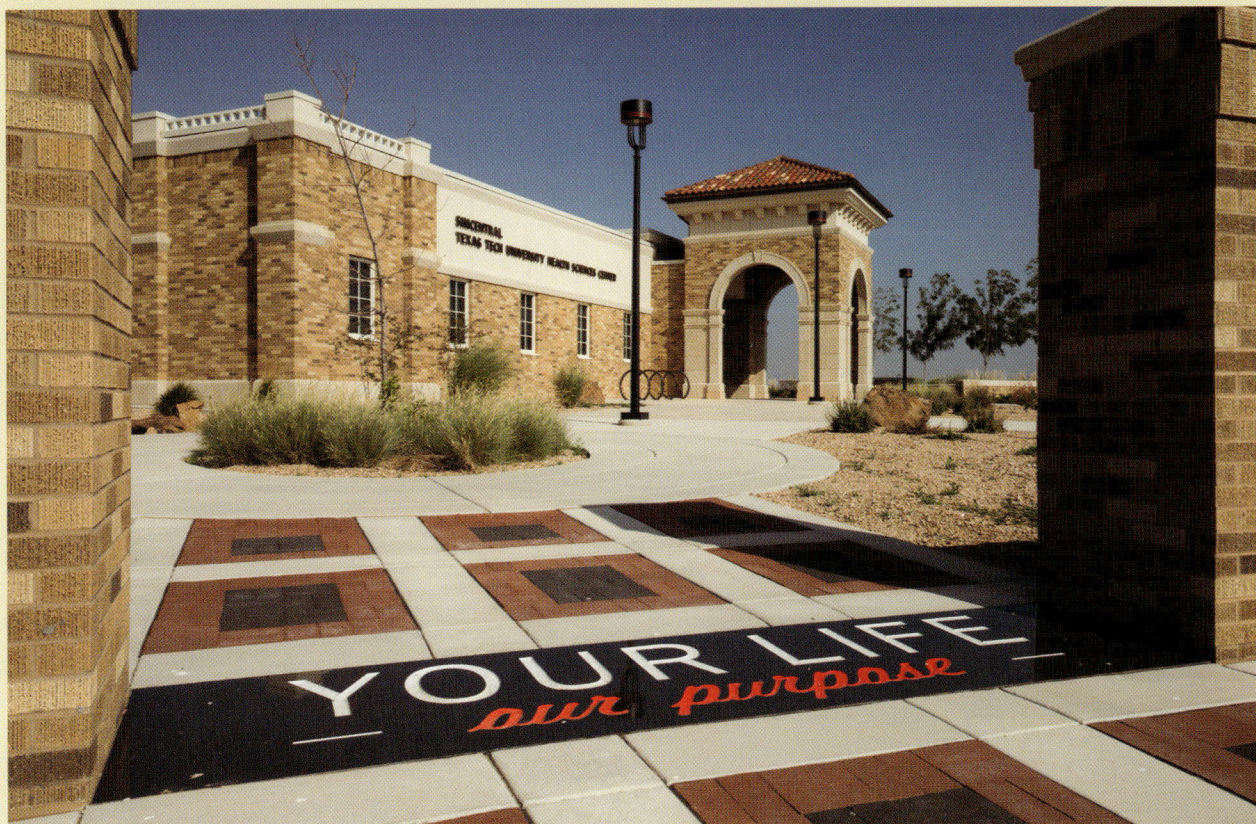

CHAPTER SIX

GRADUATE SCHOOL OF BIOMEDICAL SCIENCES

Brandt Schneider, PhD, Dean

From the moment its doors first opened in 1972, the Texas Tech University Health Sciences Center embraced training in scientific research, fostering creativity and discovery and showing students how to succeed as independent investigators. Mentoring student researchers began long before the official accreditation of the Graduate School of Biomedical Sciences in 2004. In 1972, the GSBS existed within the School of Medicine and its faculty held Texas Tech University appointments. "We started with a handful of faculty teaching medical students in Drane Hall, with our graduate students holding TTU affiliations for many years. It was a wonderful time, with a closeness between faculty and academic departments that came from the camaraderie of working together to essentially create a product and fend off the sharks vying for our closure and the money that might bring to other Texas schools," recalled Barry Lombardini, PhD, and a founding faculty member.

After several years of Texas Tech University support for the GSBS graduate program, a process began that would ultimately lead to an independent Graduate School of Biomedical Sciences. Associate Dean Barbara Pence, PhD, was instrumental in drafting the new official mission and creating much-needed documentation for the new GSBS,

which became independent of the School of Medicine in 1994.

The early accomplishments of faculty and students fueled the growth of the GSBS. For 30 years, GSBS students have organized Student Research Week, which introduces the next generation of biomedical researchers and their work. They also invite distinguished national and international speakers to present discoveries on a specific theme. Beginning in 1998 and every year thereafter, the Graduate Student Association hosts a conference to showcase a wide breadth of research. The week includes exceptional student presentations, a research competition, a fundraising banquet, and keynote speakers of international acclaim, including several past speakers who were Nobel Prize Laureates and National Academy of Science members. The event has grown from 62 to 250 students and now includes students from all TTUHSC schools, including all campuses. In addition to the students' initiative, Thomas Tenner Jr., PhD, and a professor in the Department of Medical Education and Department of Pharmacology and Neurosciences, feels that the most impressive part of Student Research Week is the speakers selected for the event. "The common thread amongst them was the 'normalcy' of these great scientists," Tenner said. "The ability to have informal conversations between our

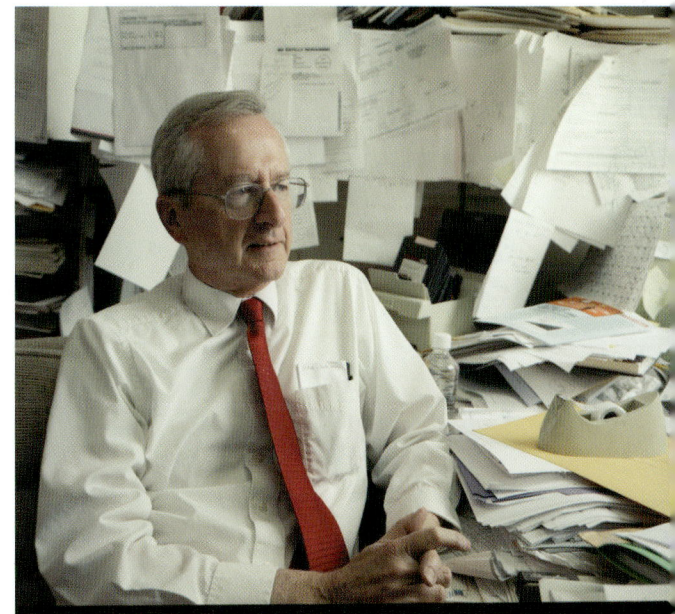

Barry Lombardini, PhD

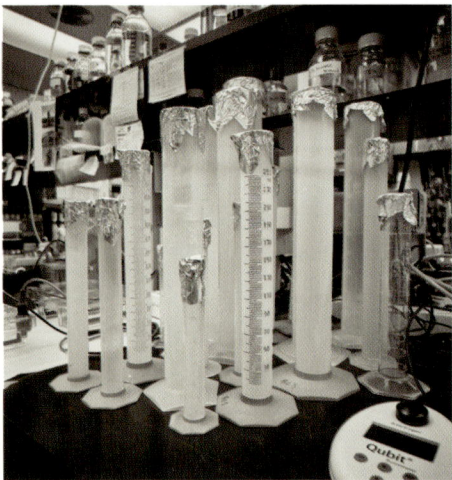

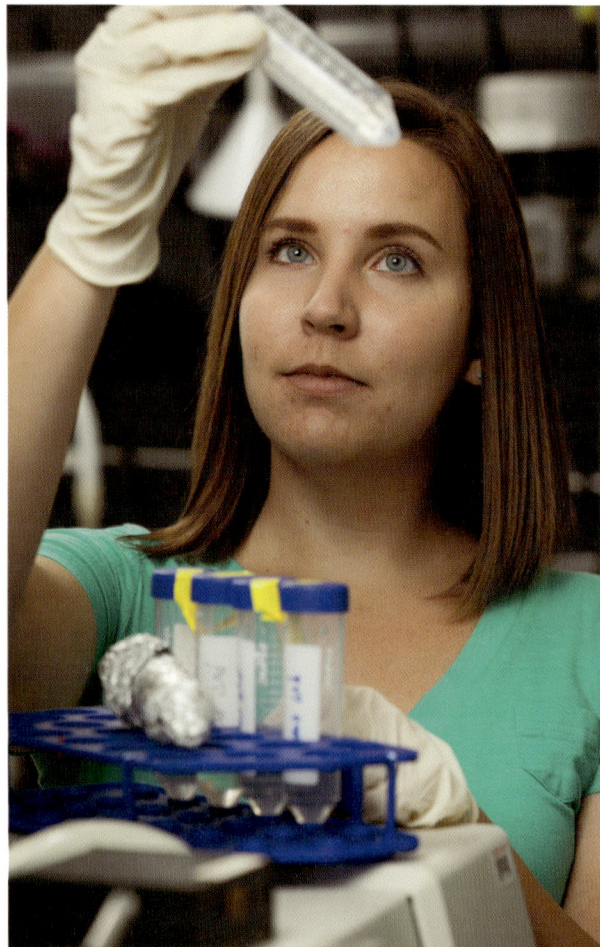

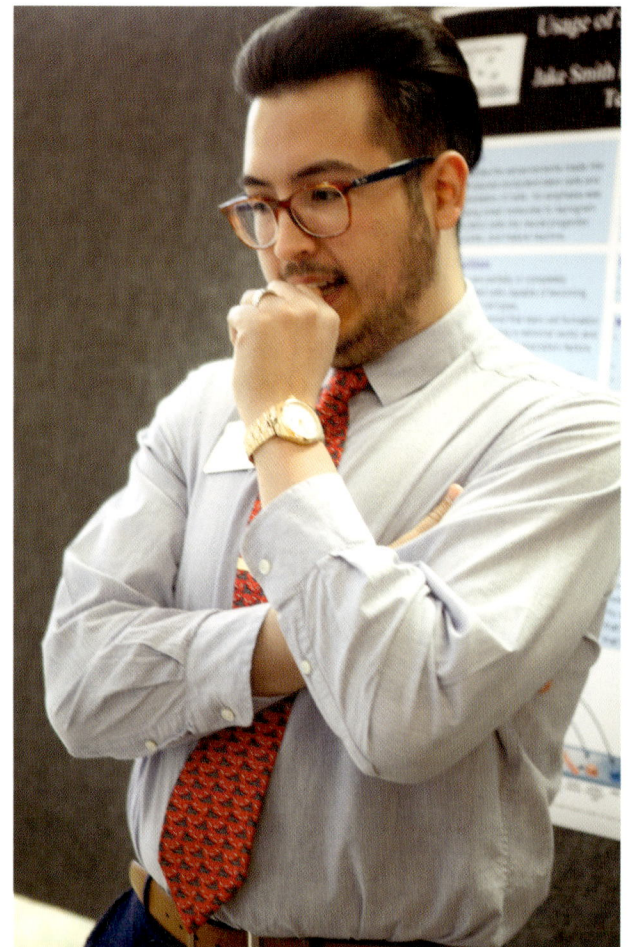

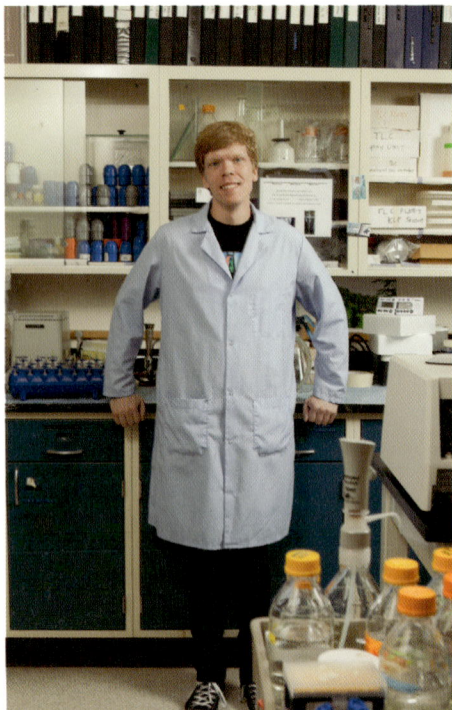

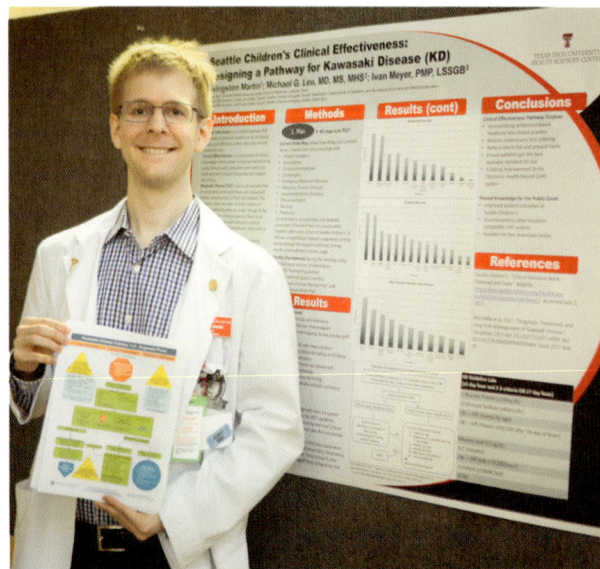

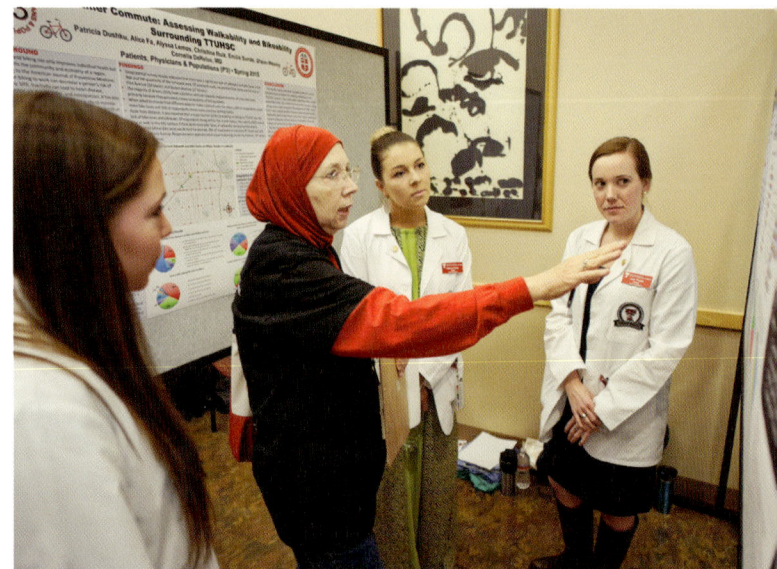

Schneider Lab

(TOP LEFT) Schneider Lab

(TOP RIGHT, BOTTOM LEFT, AND RIGHT) Research Poster Week

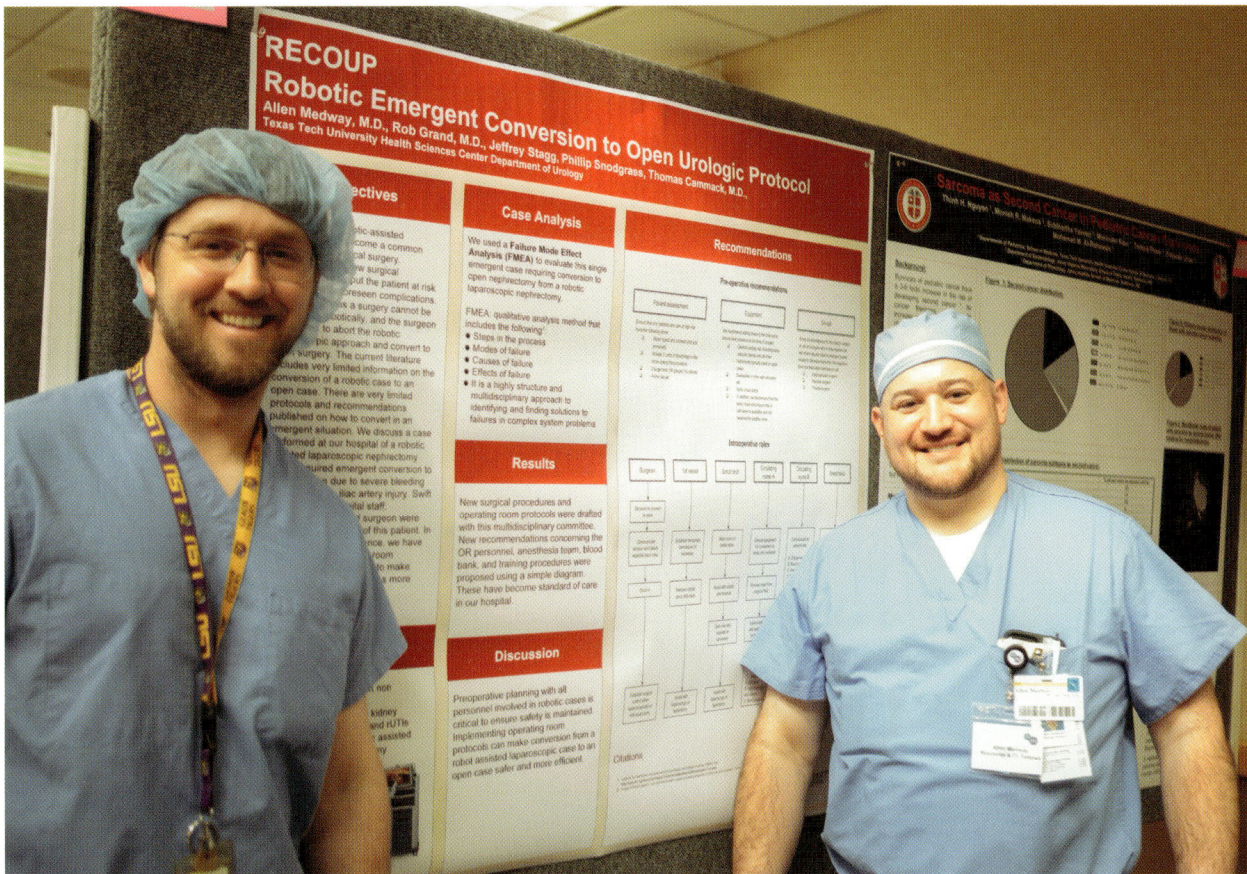

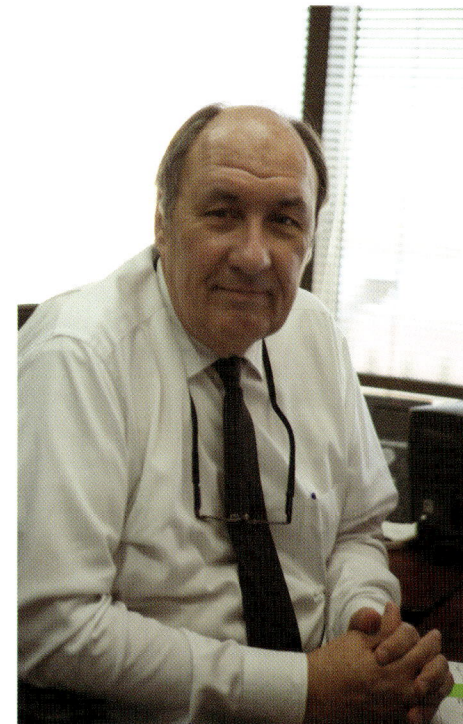

(ABOVE) Thomas Tenner, Jr., PhD

(LEFT TOP AND BOTTOM) Research Poster Week

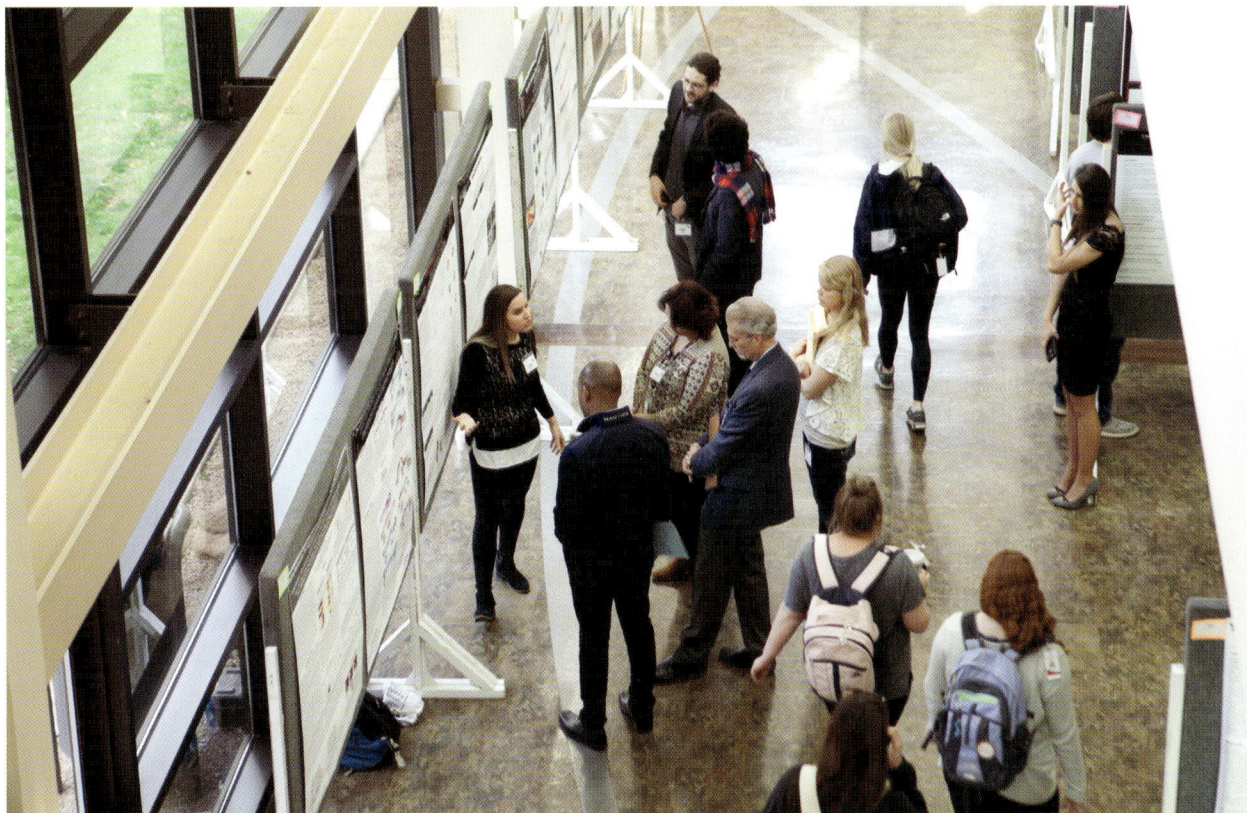

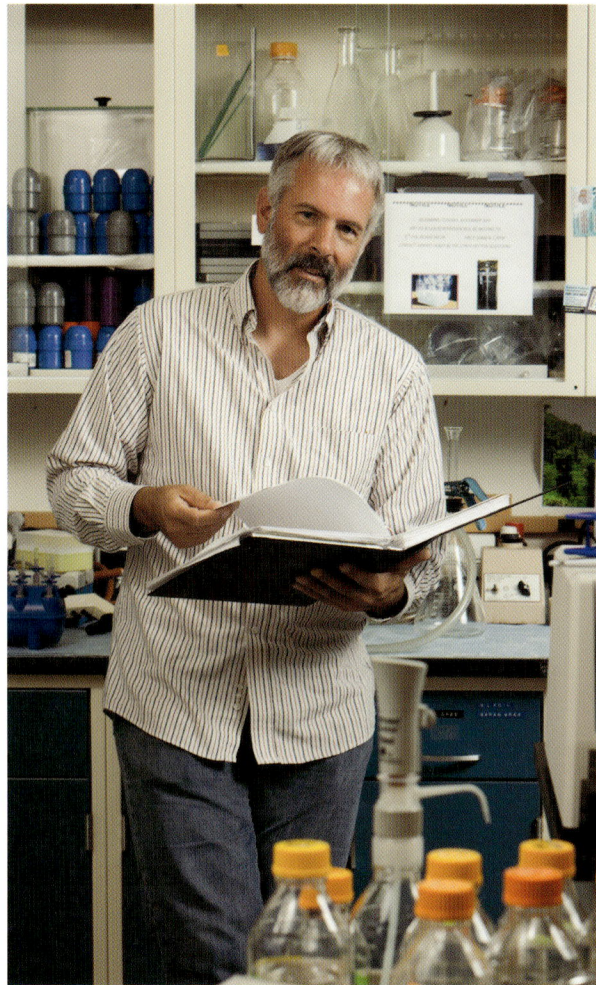
Dan Hardy, PhD

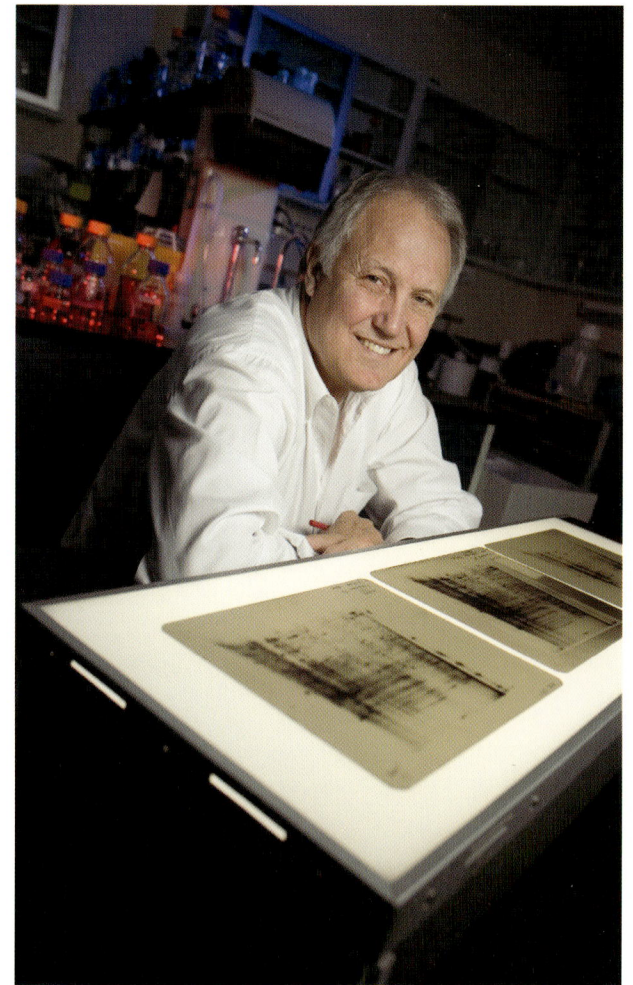
Doug Stocco, PhD

students and these guests has had an important impact on being able to realize that Nobel Laureates are human beings. They have provided encouragement as well as inspiration to our students, who, in very uncertain times, are just beginning their careers."

About the same time, GSBS created the Summer Accelerated Biomedical Research (SABR) program to expand the pool of excellent applicants. "During a meeting with faculty from the surrounding undergraduate institutions, it was mentioned that 'students need summer jobs and faculty need research associates' and so SABR was born," said Dan M. Hardy, PhD, a founding SABR member. It was that simple and now SABR attracts students from the area as well as from institutions of higher education all over the world.

Doug Stocco, PhD, and a professor of Cell Biology and Biochemistry known for groundbreaking steroidogenesis research, recalls how impressed he was with the collegial and collaborative atmosphere of GSBS when he first arrived in 1974. "It was not unusual to have excellent friendships with individuals from all of the basic science departments," he said. "The graduate students were a very important part of this family and they too interacted with the faculty and students from other departments." Later, as GSBS grew, the recruitment of graduates became a worldwide endeavor. "While the number and profile of the faculty and students changed significantly, the camaraderie between departments largely remained the same," recalled Stocco, who served as dean of the GSBS from 2011 to 2012. The Cell Biology and Biochemistry Department initiated a premedical sciences track within the Cell and Molecular Biology master's program based on a demand for anatomy instructors in schools of medicine and postbaccalaureate premedical training, which evolved into Graduate Medical Sciences.

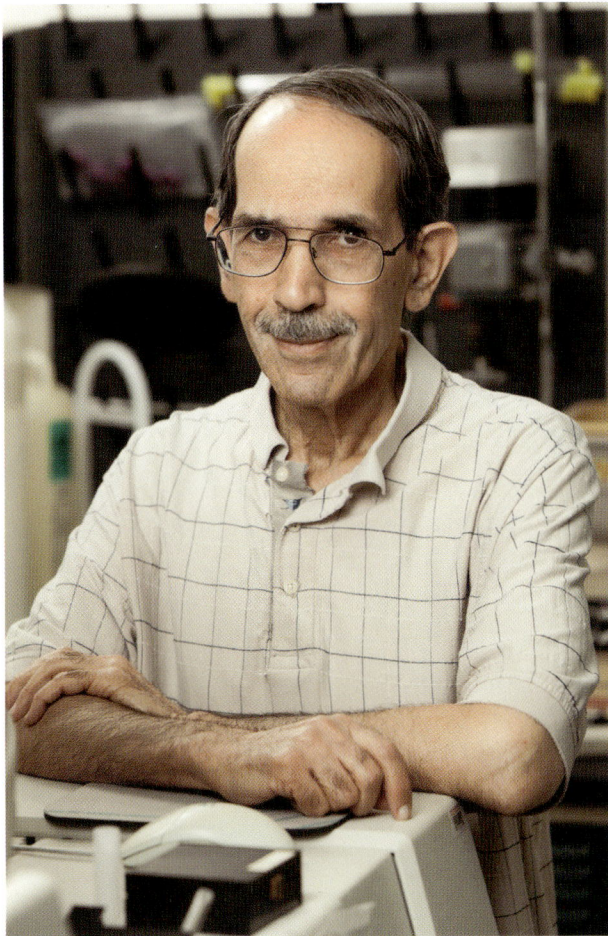

Abdul N. Hamood, PhD

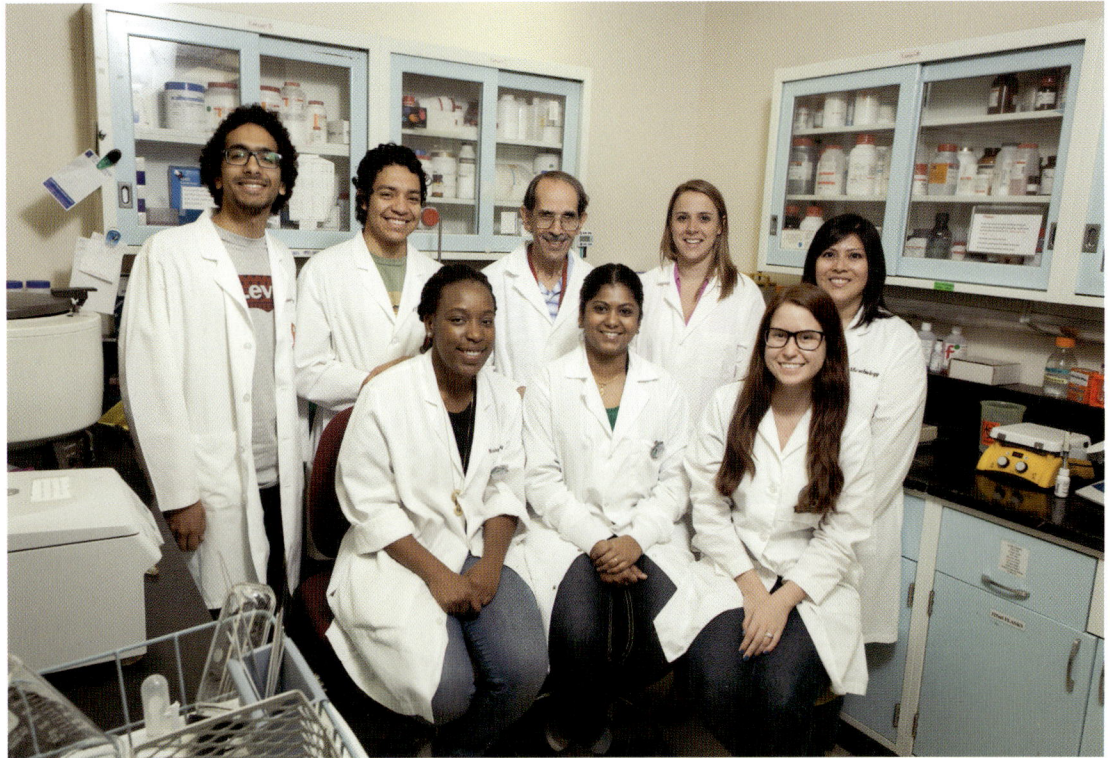

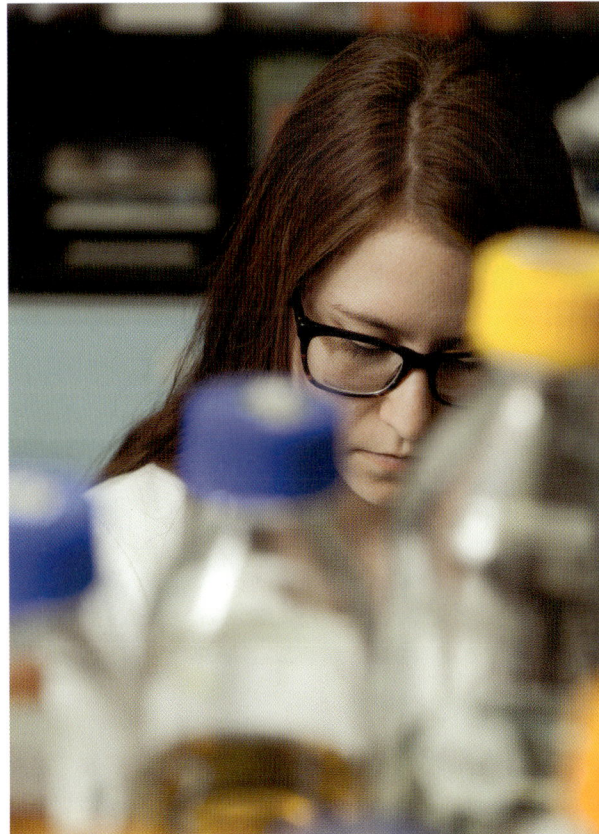

Hamood Graduate student researchers

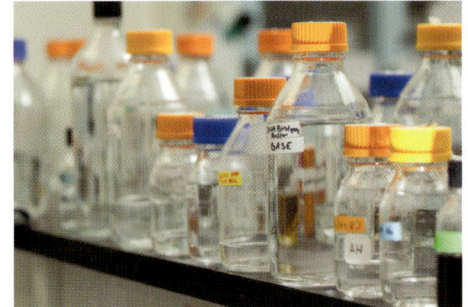

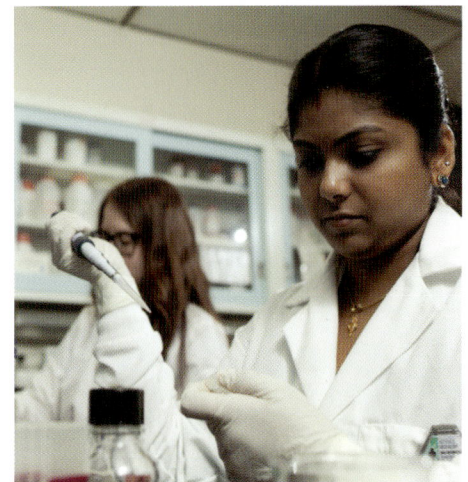

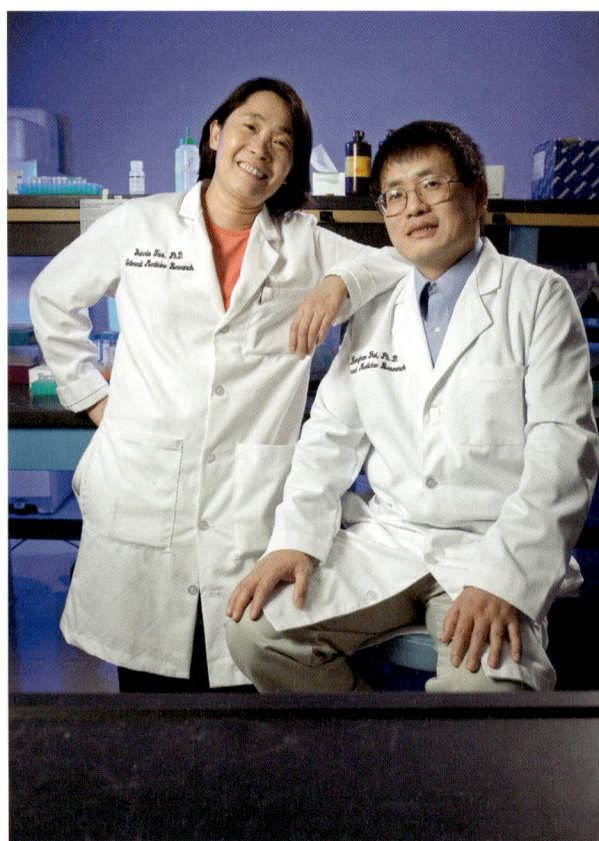

Amarillo researchers: Zonghan Dai, PhD, and Yunxia Tao, PhD

The leadership and faculty of the GSBS looked for opportunities to create academic and research programs putting students at the forefront of medicine and scientific advancement. When the TTUHSC School of Pharmacy opened its doors in Amarillo in August 1996, GSBS expanded and collaborated with the new school to create a new Pharmaceutical Sciences program. It was accredited in 1999 with the first degree conferred in 2001.

The new Amarillo members of the GSBS were immediately productive and have consistently graduated their students on a fast track, often with top dean's awards for their research. The first graduate, Dr. Sivakumar Vaithiyalingam, became a Chemistry, Manufacturing and Controls reviewer for the FDA and represents one of many career avenues available to GSBS graduates.

Dr. Tom Abbruscato, chair of pharmaceutical sciences and associate dean of the School of Pharmacy, explained: "The growth of the Amarillo Pharmaceutical Sciences graduate program was the perfect storm in 2000. A research goal of the Department of Pharmaceutical Sciences focused on faculty-mentored, graduate student research. It also helped that our program was attracting the attention of prospective graduate students due to the excellent job prospects in academia, industry, and regulatory agencies," said Abbruscato.

Another very successful master's degree program had its origin in a faculty retreat held by GSBS dean Joel Kupersmith, MD, in November 1999, when a conversation began on how to constructively grow GSBS. Daniel M. Hardy, associate professor in the Department of Cell Biology and Biochemistry, suggested they concentrate on biotechnology and collaborate with his colleague, David Knaff, Horn Professor of Biochemistry. Knaff was also chair of the Department of Chemistry and Biochemistry at Texas Tech University and director for the Center of Biotechnology and Genomics. Knaff's proposed master's program in biotechnology was accredited and implemented in 2001. The program proved timely because academic entrepreneurialism, then in its infancy, was about to explode into the scientific world and free-market system. The master's in biotechnology was an immediate success. As it expanded, the program provided faculty with additional hands-on research assistance. The program also offers two dual degrees, a JD/MS and MS/MBA. The resulting biotech graduates have gone on to rewarding careers.

John Hickox, the first biotechnology graduate, completed his MD at TTUHSC, becoming an ophthalmologist who is now positioned for biomedical entrepreneurial opportunities. Six students graduated the next year in the biotechnology program, including some who began their career in biotechnology companies. The biotechnology program expanded to Abilene in 2014 and gave students additional opportunities in biotechnology as well as in clinical labs through local hospitals.

In the past 10 years, applications and enrollment in the Graduate Medical Sciences (GMS) concentration has increased more than tenfold. Most GMS graduates are accepted to medical school where they excel. For example, it is not unusual for the School of Medicine class president to be a GMS graduate. In addition, several graduates are now in established teaching positions. Most recently, public health was added as an MPH program within the GSBS. Starting in the fall of 2018, students will have the option of face-to-face classes, techlinked classes, or online courses. The expansion was much needed in West Texas and included both the Abilene and Lubbock campuses. The development of this program and eventually a School of Public Health, is under the direction of Theresa Byrd,

Dr.PH, and chair of the Department of Public Health. "Having worked in the public health field for most of my career it was a dream of mine to start a public health program with a focus on community involvement and partnerships. Our community partners in West Texas have been incredibly open to working with us," said Byrd, who also is associate dean of GSBS.

Generous donations from a group of Abilene stakeholders created a state-of-the-art, new public health building in Abilene. GSBS admitted its first class of public health students in 2014 on the Lubbock campus and its first class on the Abilene campus in the fall of 2015. Public Health graduated their first class of students in May 2016. The MPH program consists of full- and part-time students with approximately one-third of the student body dually enrolled in the TTUHSC School of Medicine. The MPH program is a hybrid program, offered online or face-to-face and is expected to increase its enrollment to more than 100 students. The MPH can be completed totally online.

The genesis of the El Paso graduate program of biomedical sciences was developed similarly to the GSBS program in Lubbock. In January 2016, TTUHSC El Paso graduate school of biomedical sciences was accredited and became fully independent under the leadership of their new dean, Raj Lakshmanaswamy, PhD.

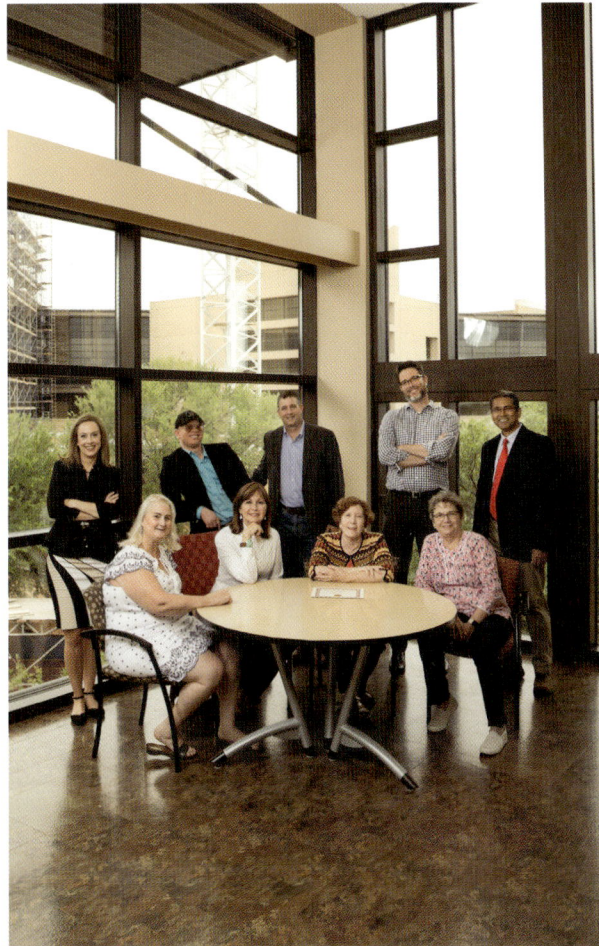

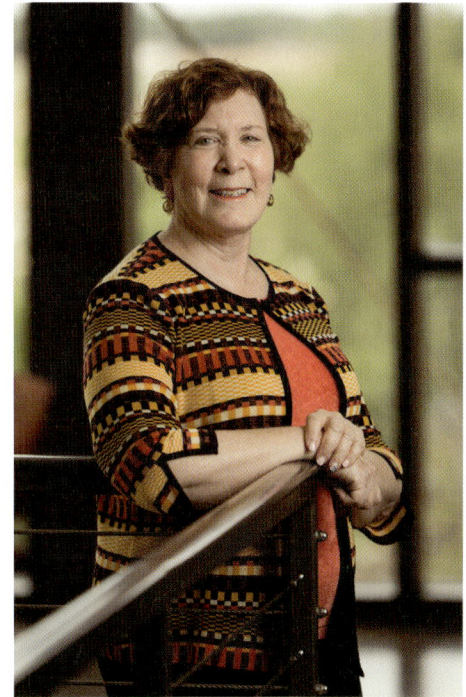

(ABOVE) Theresa Byrd, DrPH, MPH, RN, Chair—Department of Public Health.

(LEFT) Public Health Faculty, Lubbock

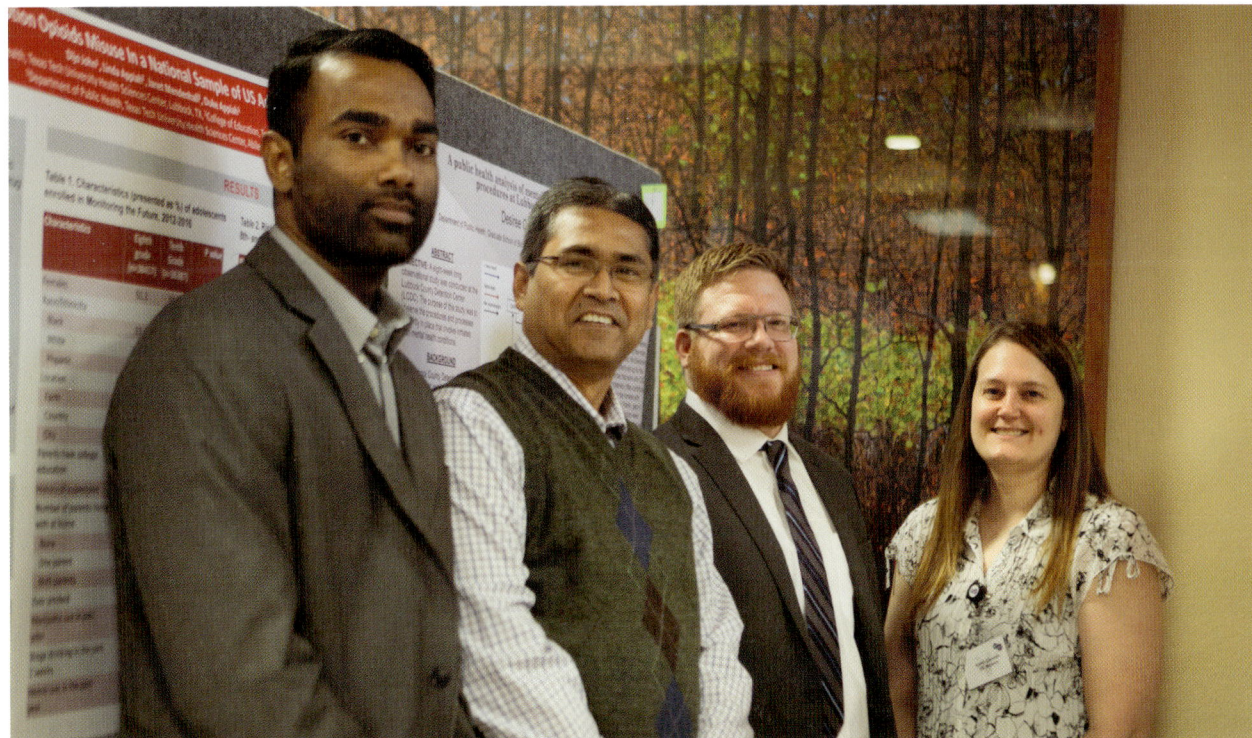

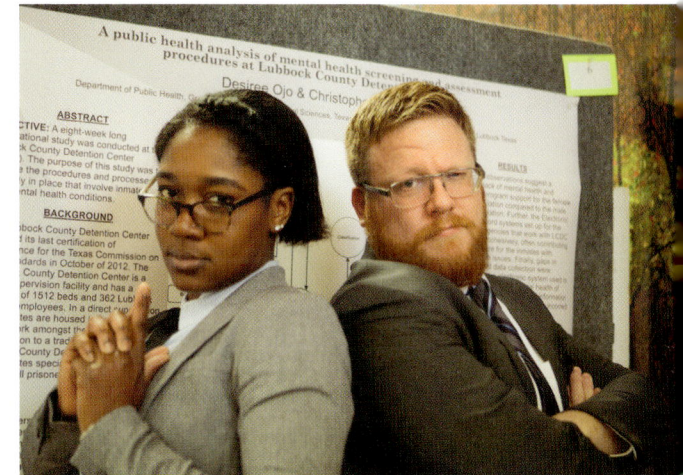

(LEFT) Hafiz M.R. Khan, PhD (second from left), and students at Research Week. Margaret Vugrin, Photographer

(ABOVE) Students at Research Week. Margaret Vugrin, Photographer

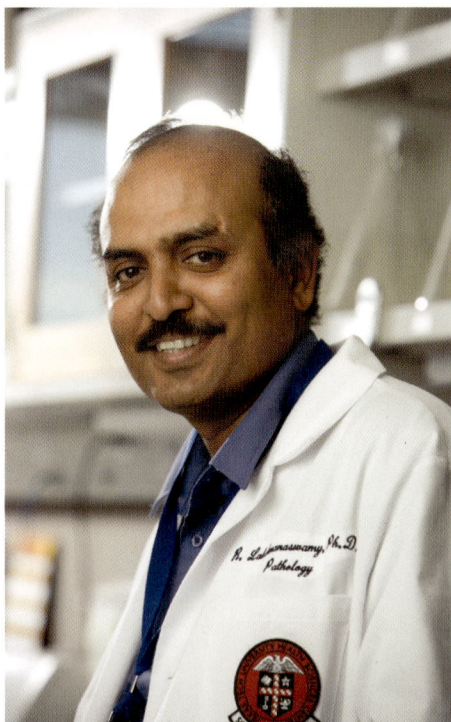

Dr. Raj Lakshmanaswamy, PhD

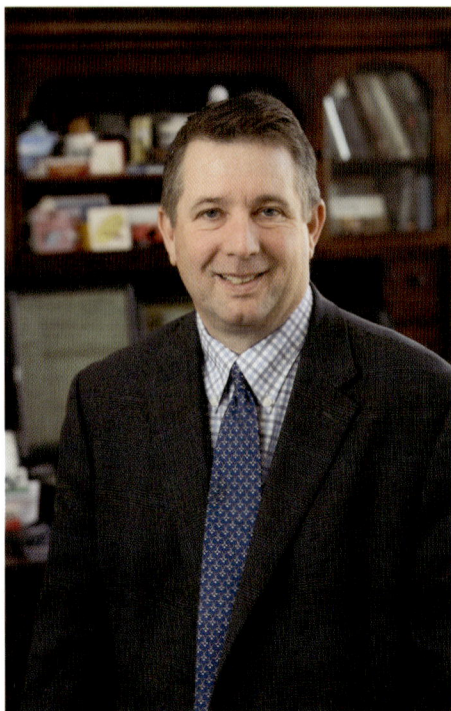

Brandt Schneider, PhD, Dean Graduate School
of Biomedical Sciences

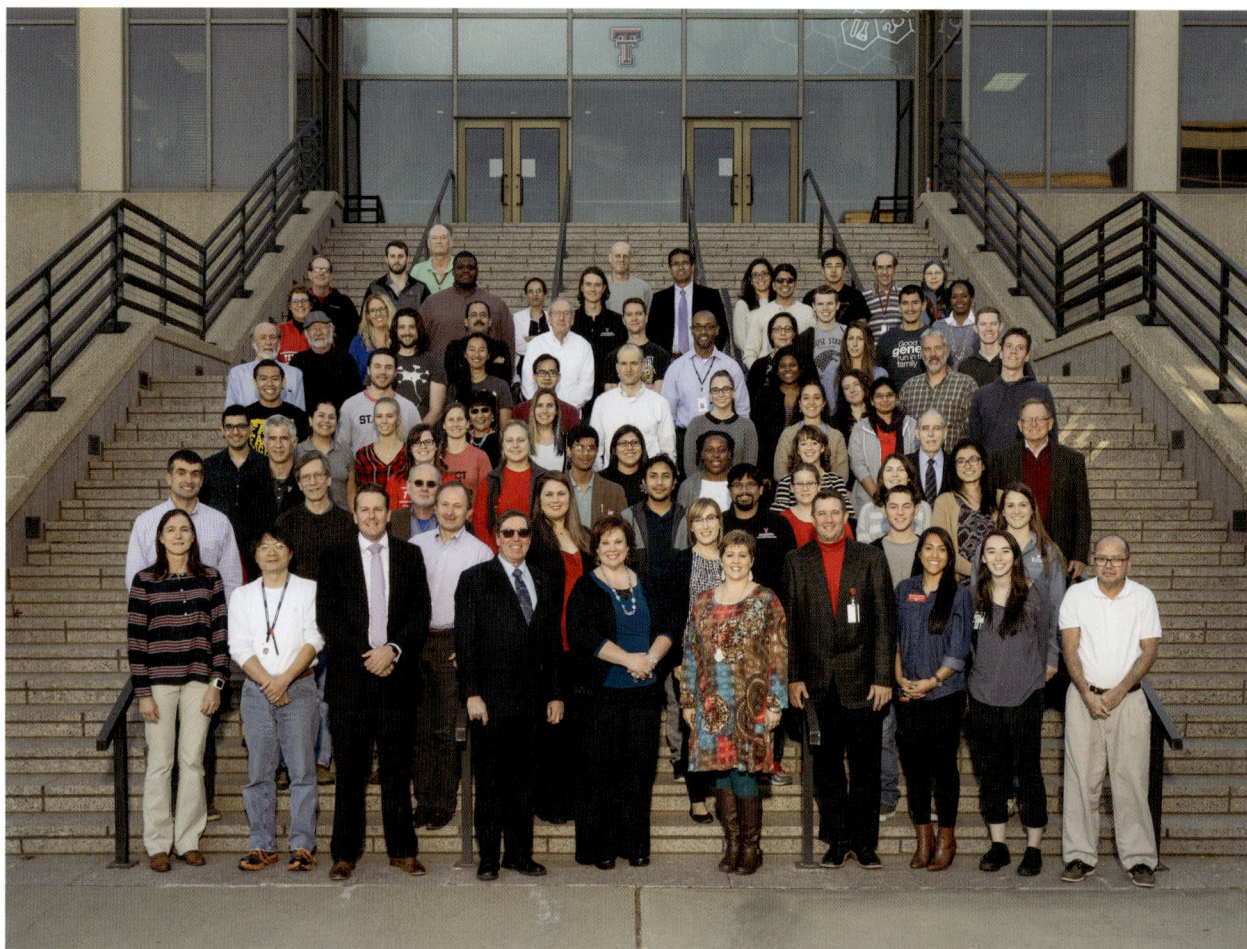

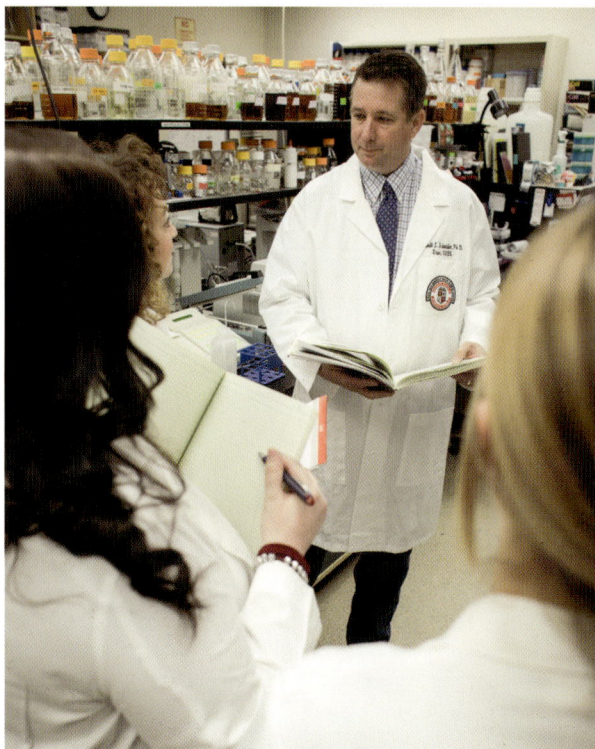

(ABOVE) GSBS faculty, staff, and students

(LEFT) Brandt Schneider, PhD, with students

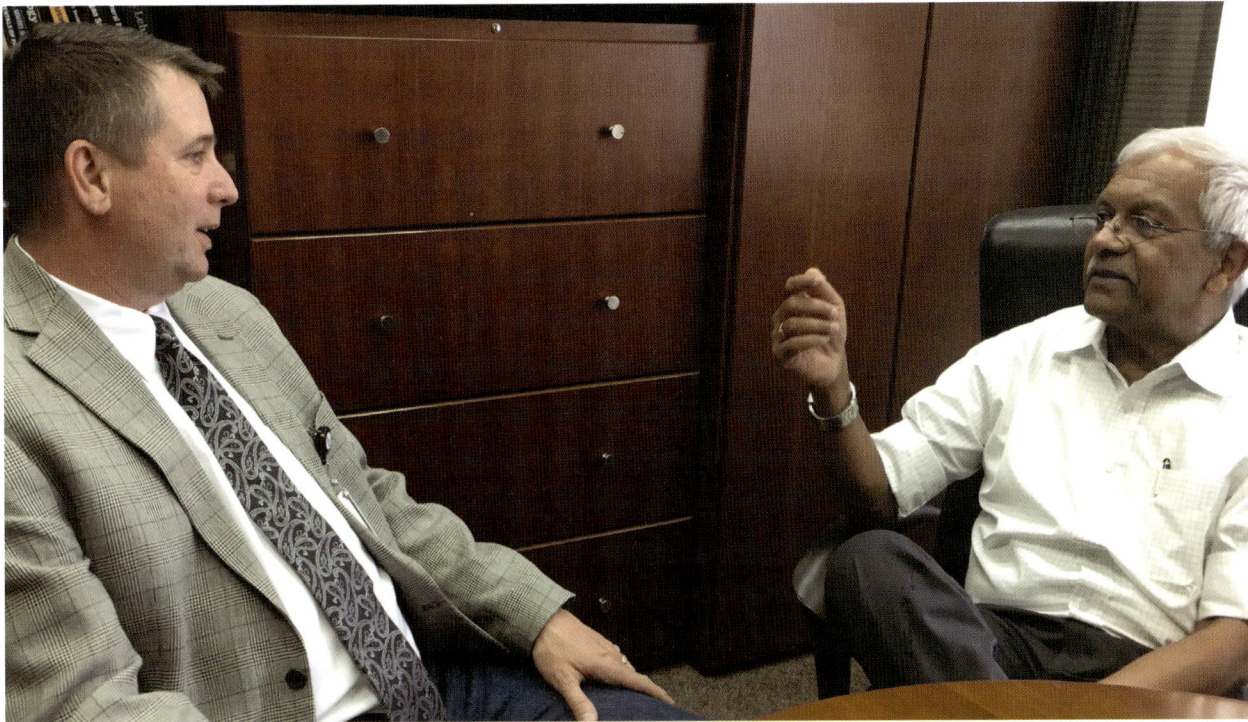

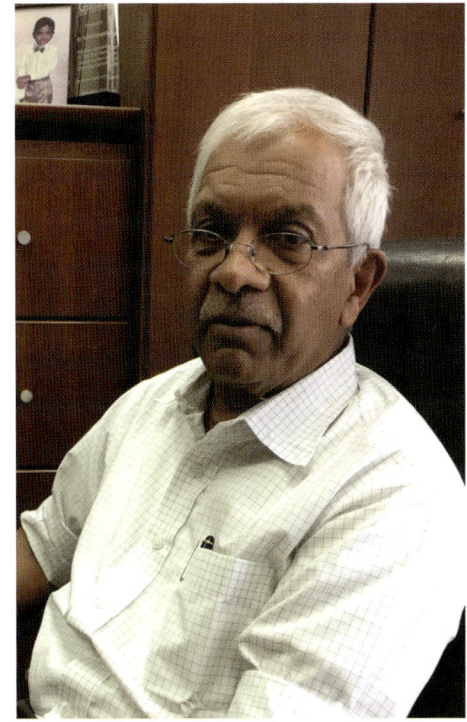

Today the GSBS has six graduate programs: Biotechnology (MS only), Biomedical Sciences (MS and PhD), Public Health (MPH only), and Pharmaceutical Sciences (MS and PhD). Program/concentrations at each location include:

Lubbock: Biochemistry, Cellular and Molecular Biology; Immunology and Infectious Diseases; Molecular Biophysics; Translational Neuroscience and Pharmacology; Graduate Medical Sciences (master's only); Biotechnology and Public Health.
Amarillo: Pharmaceutical Sciences
Abilene: Biotechnology; Public Health

In conjunction with the TTUHSC School of Medicine, the MD/PhD dual-degree program has graduated 14 students and has 16 students currently enrolled in the program. In 2015, GSBS implemented two additional dual-degree programs: MD/MS and the MD/MPH.

The school's enrollment has gone from 50 students in 1999 to 196 in 2015. The enrollment target for 2020 is 220 students. "Our students have been awarded more fellowships and travel scholarships than ever before, our student indebtedness is very low, our average time to a PhD degree is less than 5 years," said Schneider. "I am extremely proud of the values, integrity, and success of our students, and I greatly look forward to the continued growth and prosperity of our school."

(LEFT) Brandt Schneider, PhD, Dean, and Vadivel Ganapathy, PhD, Chair, discussing future research projects

(RIGHT) Vadivel Ganapathy, PhD, Chair of Cell Biology and Biochemistry, reflecting on latest experiment

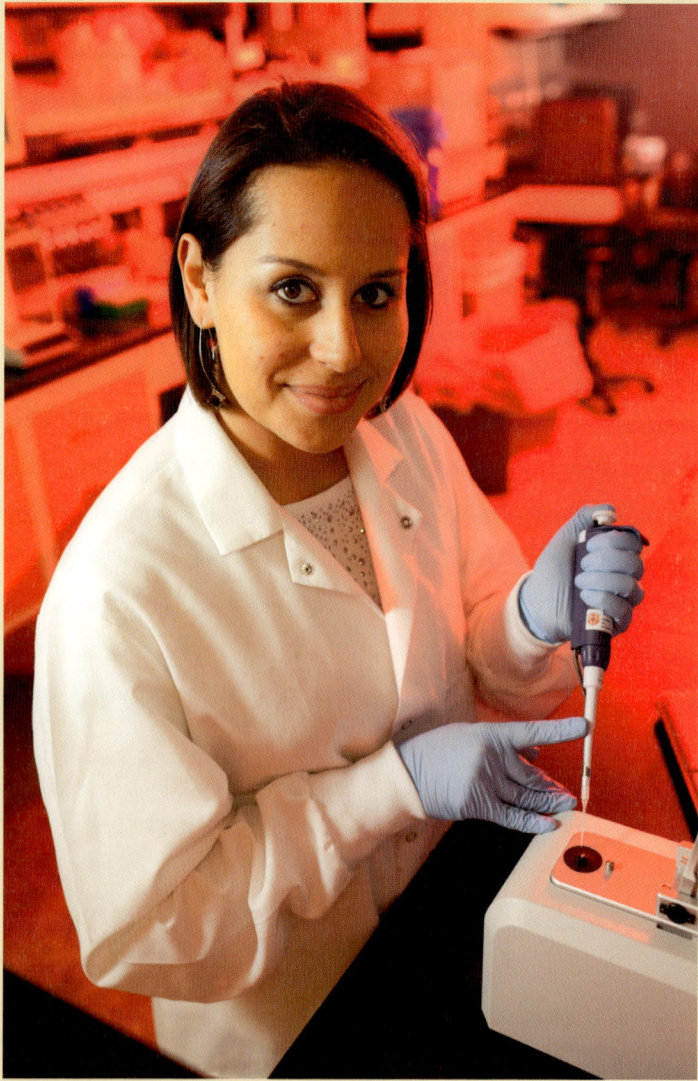
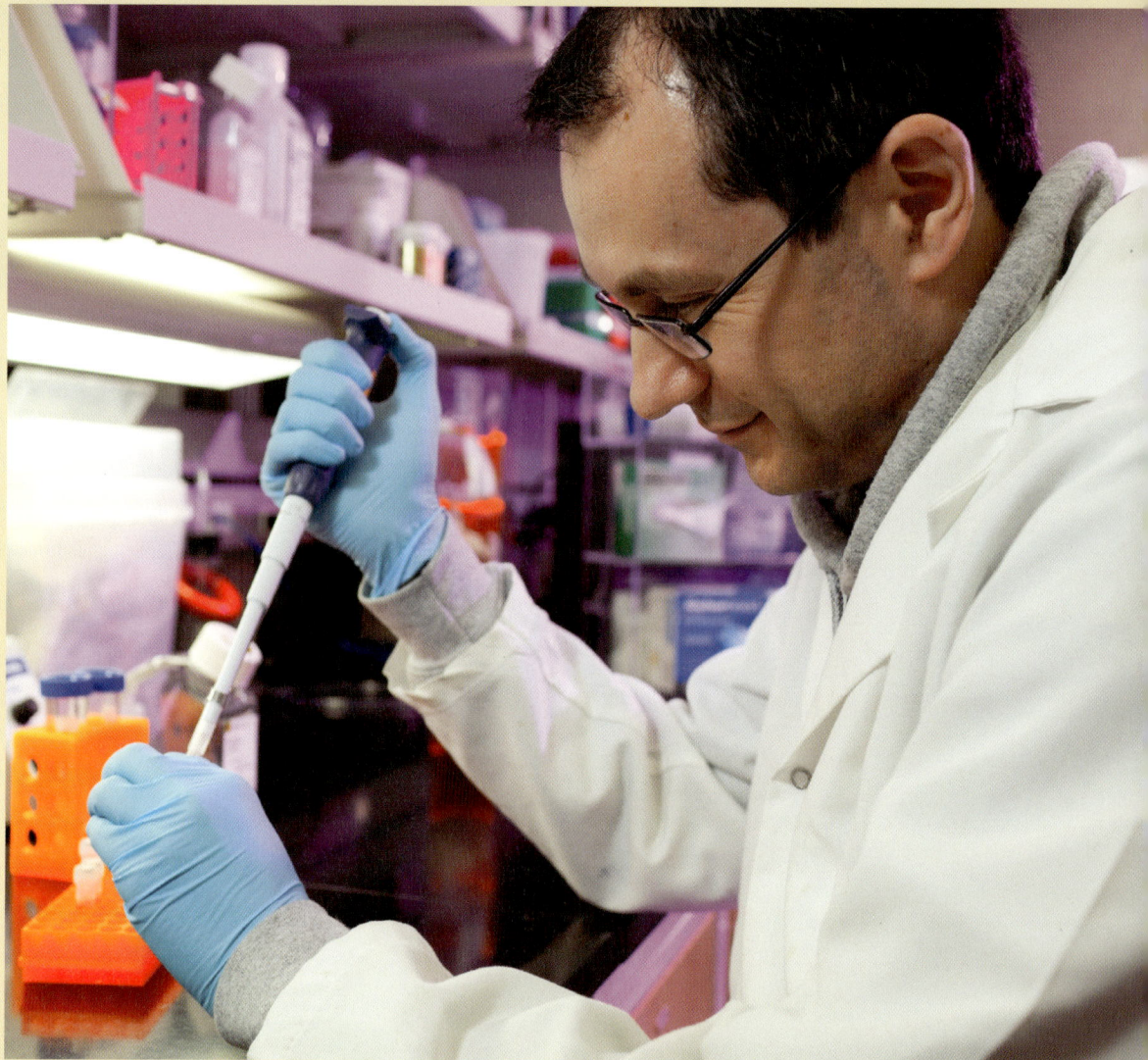

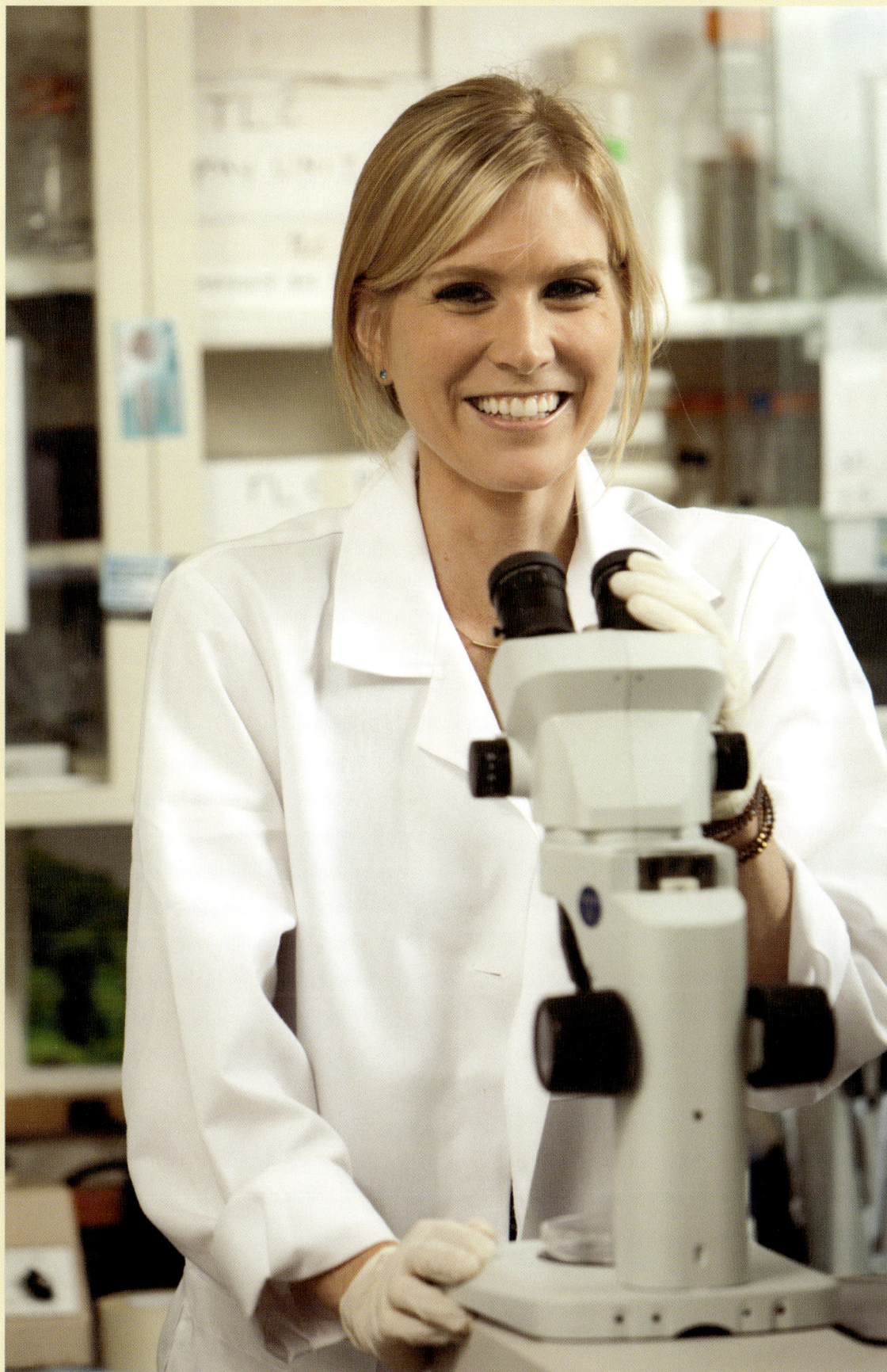

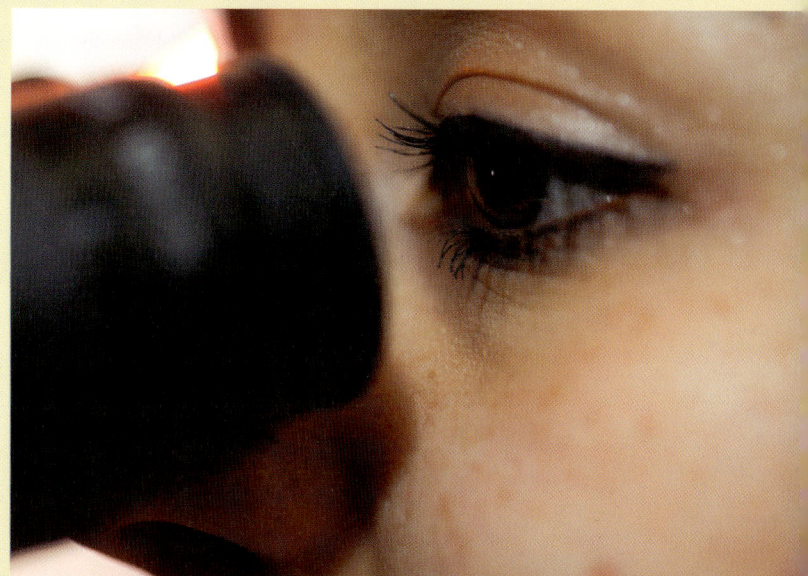

CHAPTER SEVEN

INSTITUTES AND CENTERS

Clinical Research Institute

Clinical research—translating basic research done in labs into new treatments and knowledge to benefit patients—assumed a new role at Texas Tech University Health Sciences Center in 2009. With Steven Berk, MD, dean of the School of Medicine, shepherding the process, the formation of the Clinical Research Center brought with it a new focus on investigator-initiated research. The shifting focus helped TTUHSC meet a then-new requirement for accrediting schools of medicine to place greater emphasis on scholarly research and raise the bar for recertifying residency programs. The institute's goal is to increase the number of investigator-initiated, clinical research projects done at TTUHSC and to increase faculty and trainee understanding of all aspects of clinical research. One way it does this is by providing clinical research courses and classes.

The new Clinical Research Center grew out of the TTUHSC Division of Clinical Research, which was formed in 2001 by Barbara Pence, PhD, and associate vice president of research, to engage primarily in industry-sponsored clinical research. This unit already employed highly trained and experienced nurse coordinators led by Cathy Lovett, MSN, RN. Lorenz Lutherer, MD, PhD, became the medical director.

The role of the Clinical Research Center expanded further the next year when TTUHSC president Tedd L. Mitchell, MD, asked Lutherer to assume responsibility for converting the center to an institute, which would encompass investigator-initiated clinical research in all schools on the HSC campuses. The Clinical Research Institute received formal approval in April 2011. The clinical research team in the Permian Basin campus joined the CRI in October 2012, with four coordinators on site supported by Gary Ventolini, MD, the dean of medicine. In 2013, the School of Pharmacy, led by Quentin Smith, PhD, began providing financial support to the CRI. Smith was named senior vice president of research in 2017 for the Texas Tech University Health Sciences Center. Smith serves as dean of the School of Pharmacy concurrent with his role as senior vice president of research.

The CRI resources are valuable to faculty with busy schedules and help partially offset the lack of protected time for research. There is no cost to investigators for CRI services due to the funding mechanisms in place. This system allows them to obtain pilot data necessary to support future research funding requests.

As the institute has grown and activities have expanded, the institute's staff has grown from six in the original Clinical Research Center to 18 in the current Clinical Research Institute. CRI personnel work with the investigators and trainees during each phase of a proposed

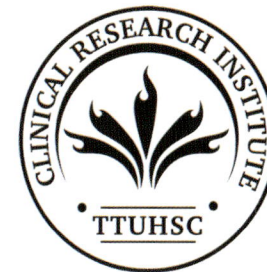

Clinical Research Institute Logo

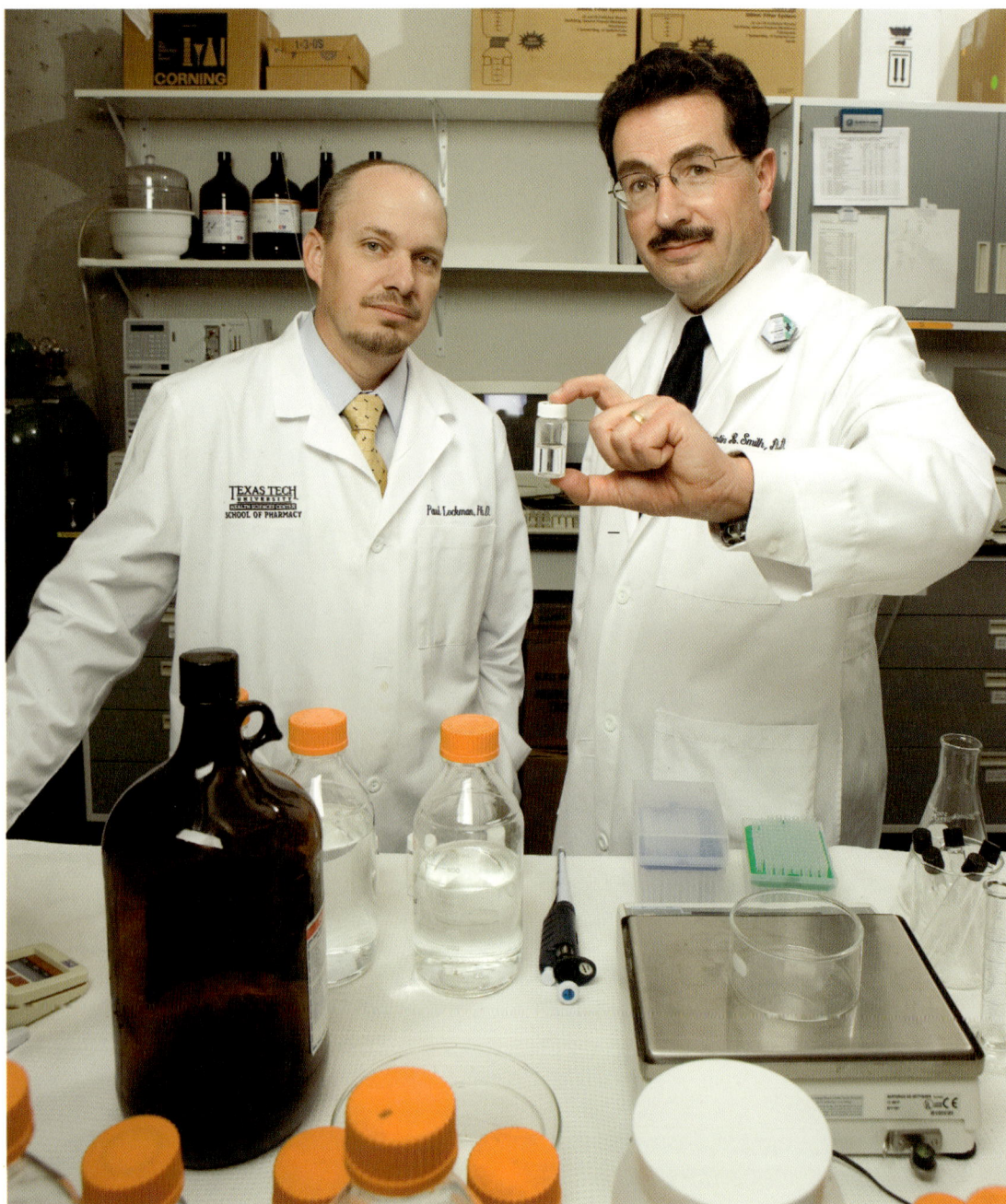

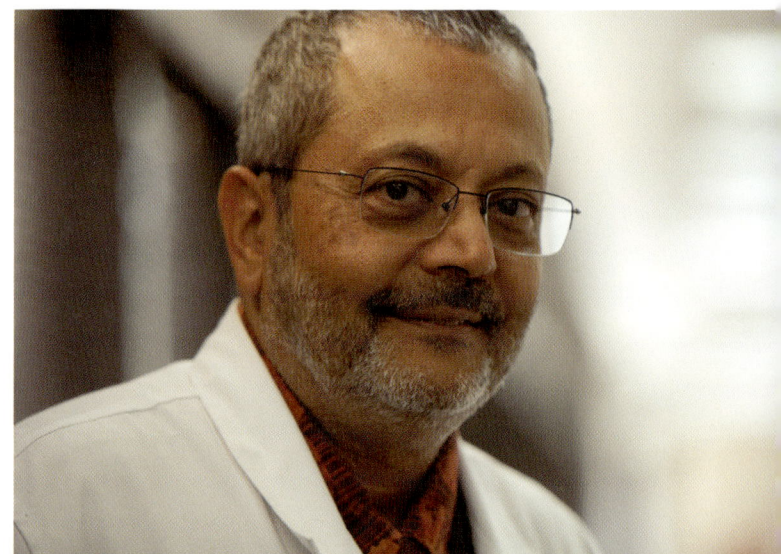

Alan Peiris, MD, PhD, Executive Director of Clinical Research Institute. Margaret Vugrin, Photographer

Quentin Smith, PhD, and Paul Lockman, PhD

study, including the development of a sound proposal that meets scientific and legal requirements as well as assistance in completing data analysis.

The CRI leadership consists of Executive Director Alan Peiris, MD, Assistant Director Thomas Tenner, Jr. PhD, and Managing Director Cathy Lovett, MSM. The executive director reports directly to the president and the provost. The directors have extensive experience with basic and clinical research.

The Garrison Institute on Aging

Sometime between now and 2020 there will be a first in human history. According to the U.S. Census Bureau the global population of human beings who are 65 and older will surpass those under five, and between now and 2050 the population 65 and over will more than double. So, when the leadership of Texas Tech University Health Sciences Center decided in 1999 to make healthy aging a strategic priority, the Board of Regents endorsed that decision and created the Institute for Healthy Aging, which was renamed in 2005, in honor of Mildred and Shirley L. Garrison and the $15 million endowment they provided.

The Garrison Institute on Aging (GIA) is the cornerstone of the TTUHSC's healthy aging initiative. It investigates the causes of neurodegenerative diseases such as Alzheimer's, prepares healthcare professionals for the growing demands of geriatric care, and educates seniors and their families through outreach programs on how to support healthy living.

In the beginning, Dr. Paula Grammas, PhD, led the institute, which received a multi-million-dollar grant from the U.S. Health and Human Services Administration on Aging. Grammas is an experienced vascular scientist, known for pioneering research into the role played by blood vessels and inflammation in the development of Alzheimer's and other neurodegenerative diseases.

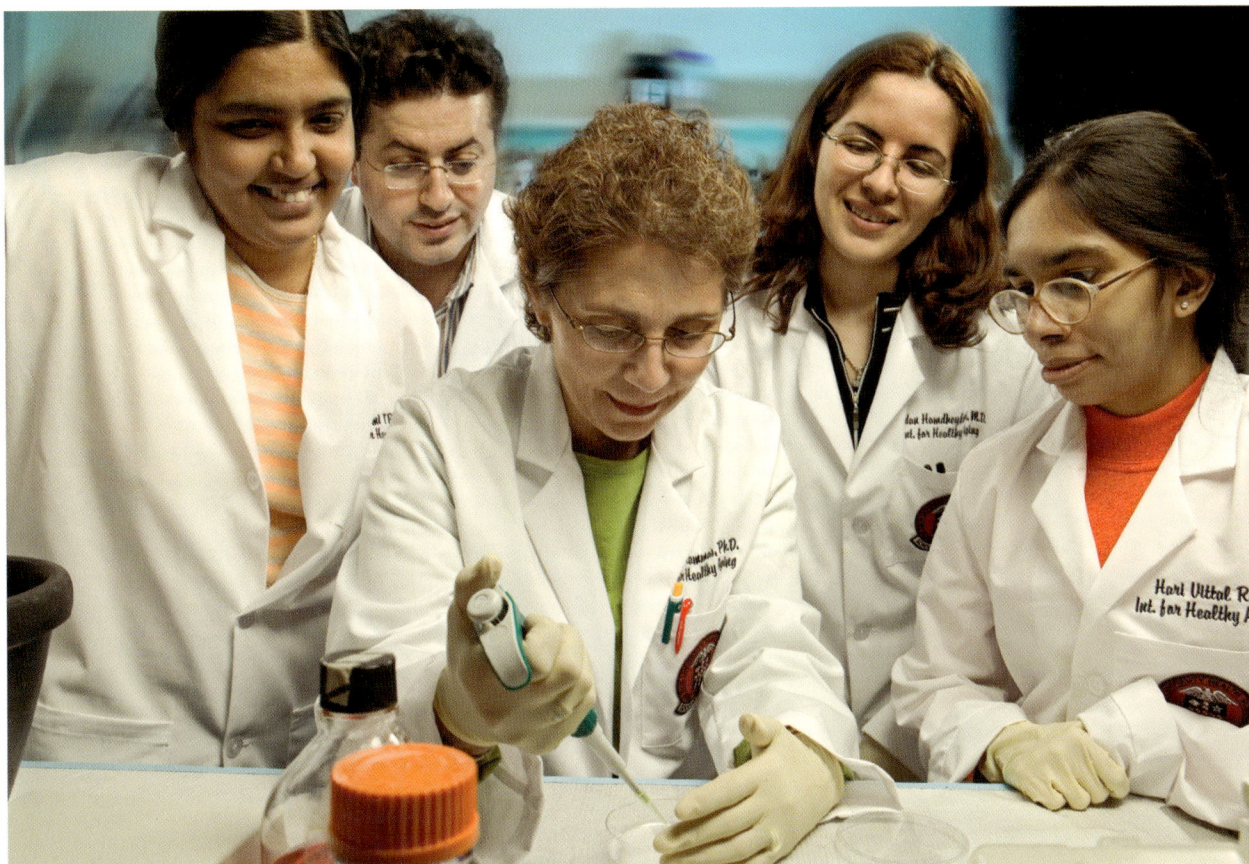

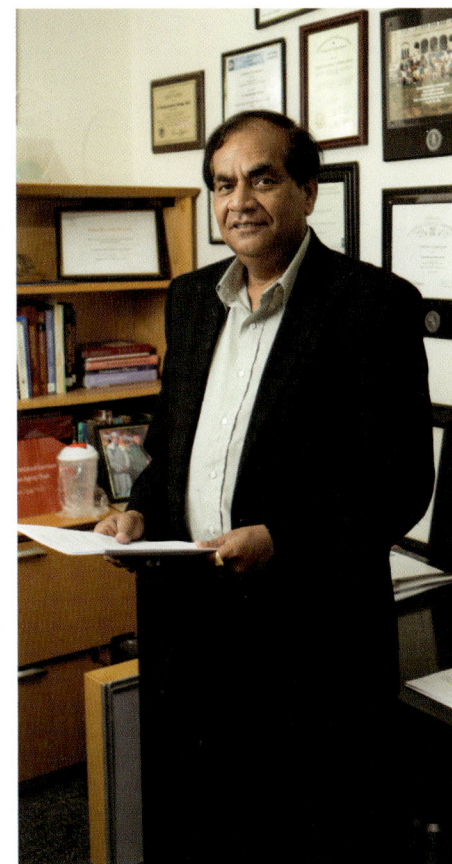

In 2006, the institute's researchers designed an investigation called the Cochran County Aging Study aimed at learning more about cognitive decline and various types of dementia among a multiethnic adult sample from rural communities in West Texas. In 2007, the institute created a Brain Bank that provided free brain autopsies to families. Tissue from these autopsies were made available to GIA researchers, and specimens without neurological disease were kept for comparison.

In 2015, the baton was passed to Hemachandra Reddy, PhD, who became executive director of the GIA. He came to TTUHSC from Oregon Health and Science University where his research on aging and neurodegenerative diseases was funded by the National Institutes of Health, the Alzheimer's Association, and pharmaceutical companies. Dr. Reddy expanded the institute's research and created three units, including one investigating a molecular and cellular basis for aging and neurodegenerative disease, a second for drug-based agents to prevent or delay onset of Alzheimer's and other dementias, and a third to identify biomarkers such as a protein that would indicate risk or prognosis of a specific neurological disease.

The Cochran County Aging Study expanded its scope and was renamed Project Frontier in 2009. Project Frontier is a longitudinal study that explores the natural course of chronic disease development and its impact on cognitive, physical, social, and interpersonal functioning. Its participants live in Cochran, Bailey, Parmer, and Hockley counties. Since its beginning, the data has been shared and analyzed by more than 80 researchers at 13 different institutions.

The institute sponsors a number of regular seminars promoting professional education, where investigators can share research findings on aging and age-related diseases. The institute's research team collaborates with investigators at Texas Tech University, at the TTUHSC School of Medicine, and other institutions, including Johns Hopkins University and Baylor College of Medicine. Garrison Institute researchers also train students in educational programs such as Student Scholars in Geriatrics,

(ABOVE LEFT) Paula Grammas, PhD

(ABOVE) P. Hemachandra Reddy, PhD, Executive Director and Chief Scientific Officer of Garrison Institute on Aging, Professor of Cell Biology and Biochemistry, Neuroscience/ Pharmacology, and Neurology

(BELOW) Project Frontier Logo

PROJECT
FR⌂NTIER
Texas Tech University Health Sciences Center

the School of Medicine Students' Summer Research Program, and the High School Student Scholars' Research Program.

In addition to research and education, the institute is involved in a number of community outreach programs. It supports caregivers for those with age-related diseases with practical resources for daily living, including health care, nutrition, exercise, and financial matters. It matches adults, 55 and older, with 600 active volunteers to provide them with companionship. It promotes physical and mental fitness through a number of programs, including the award-winning GETFiT Lubbock, a collaboration of local businesses and organizations.

Laura W. Bush Institute for Women's Health

The Laura W. Bush Institute for Women's Health was established in 2007. Its creation was a response to mounting evidence that women and men experience medical conditions and crises differently and yet many researchers and healthcare providers were treating women as "small men" and creating obstacles to accurate diagnosis and treatments for women. Associate Professor Marjorie Jenkins, MD, knew scientifically that sex and gender differences begin at a cellular level and continue through every system of the body.

In a quest to improve medical learning and health care, Dr. Jenkins and then-chancellor Kent Hance visited the White House in 2007 to discuss the need for a women's health institute in West Texas with the First Lady, Laura Bush. With Mrs. Bush's agreement, the Laura W. Bush Institute for Women's Health was established. Its three-part mission is to support scientific investigation, professional awareness to inform diagnosis and treatment, and outreach to provide education and personalized health care to girls and women throughout the state.

Scientific investigation that could lead to more personalized health care for was limited when the FDA barred women from participating in medical research as a "protected class." As a result, data were not typically available for women. From the beginning, the institute insisted researchers report individual data on male and female subjects at every level: cellular, animal, and human. It wasn't until 2015 that this important requirement was adopted by the National Institutes for Health. The Laura W. Bush Institute has provided scientists more than $2.5 million for groundbreaking research unique to women's health in

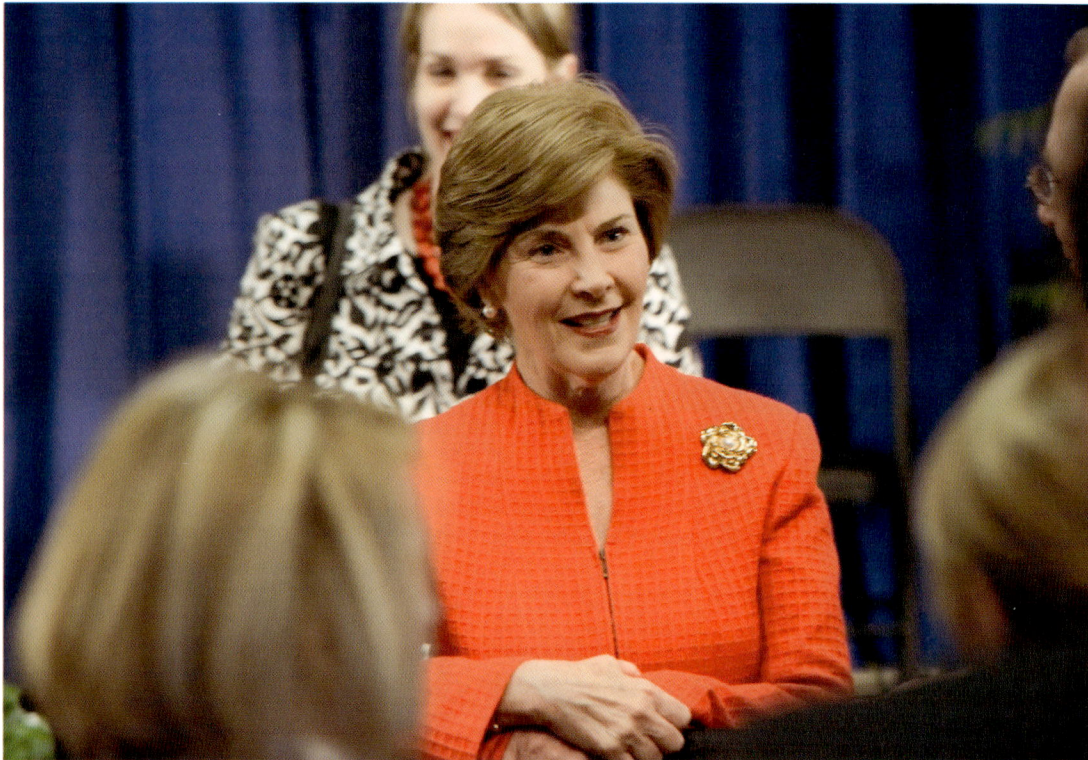

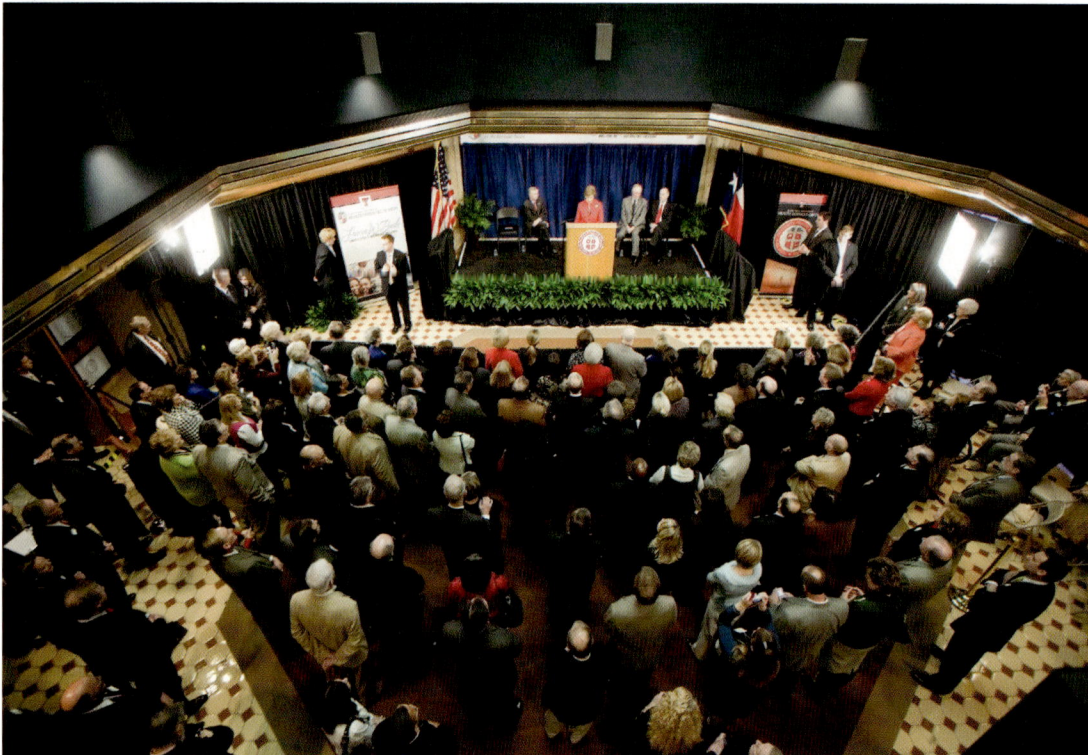

(TOP) Laura Bush meeting with audiences after her speech

(BOTTOM) Laura Bush speaks at the Laura W. Bush Institute for Women's Health

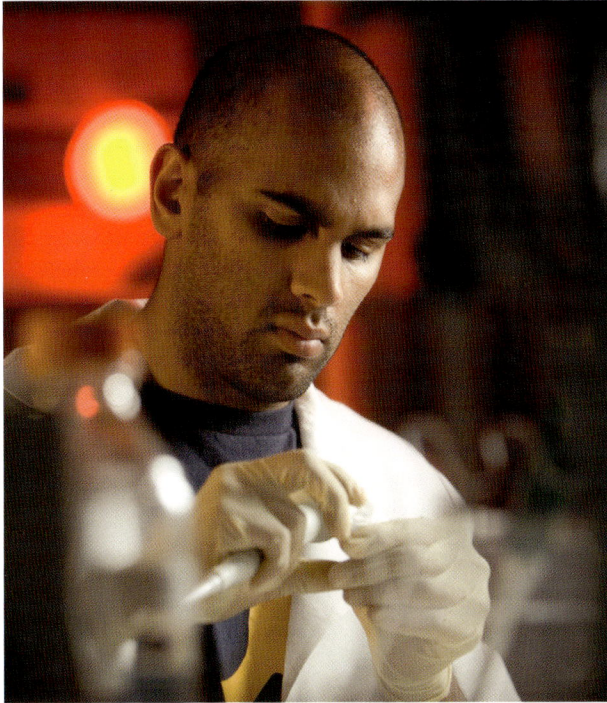

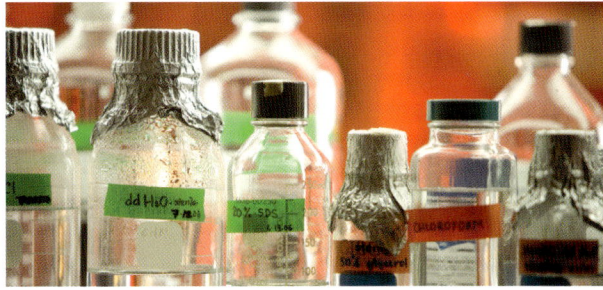

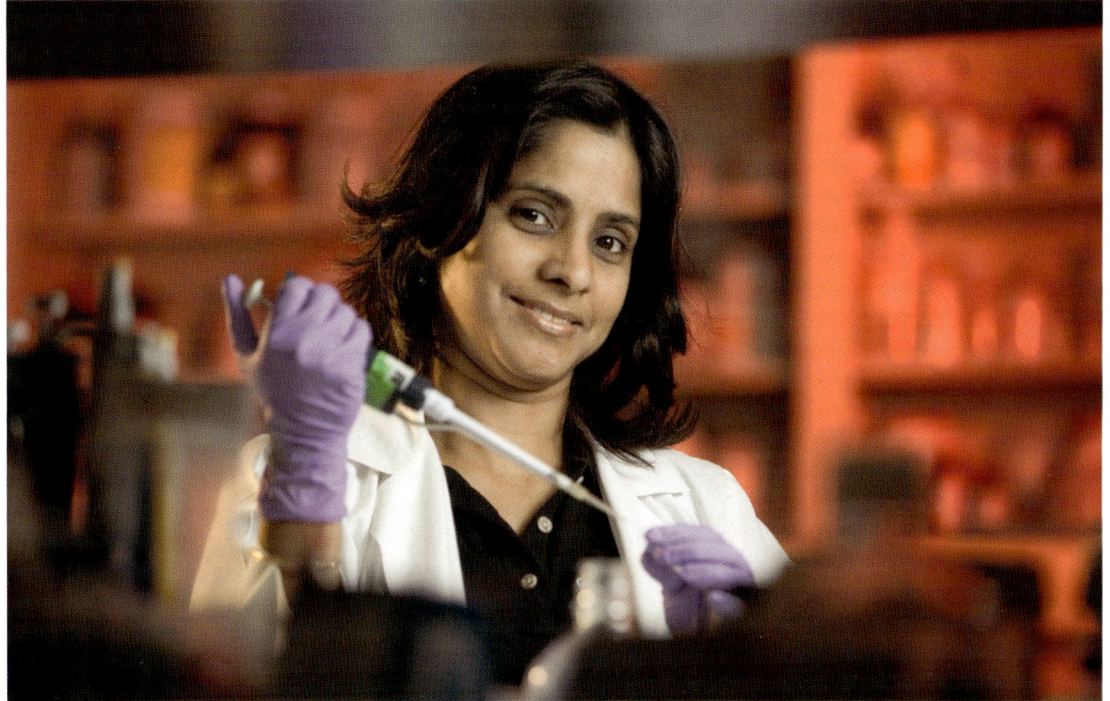

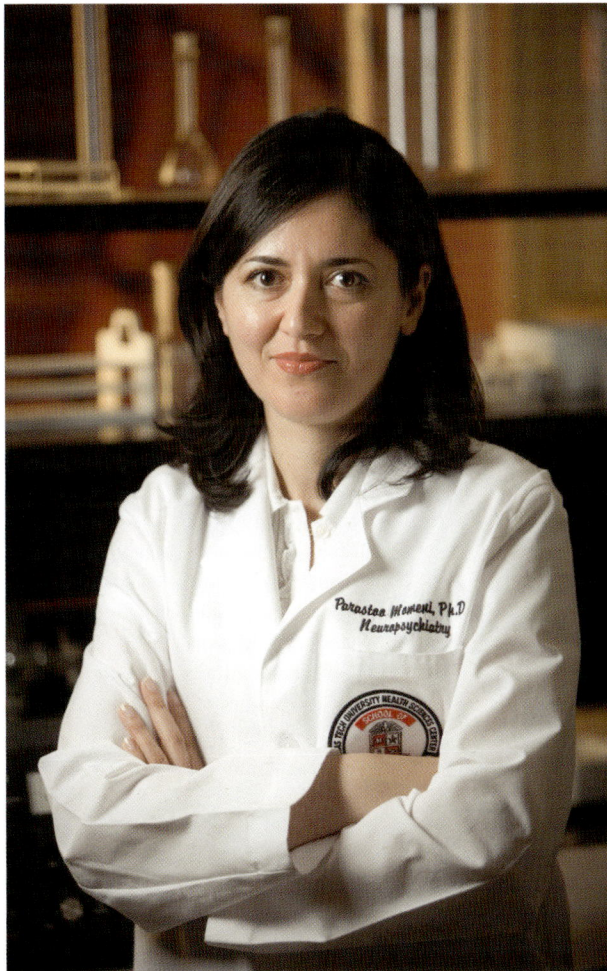

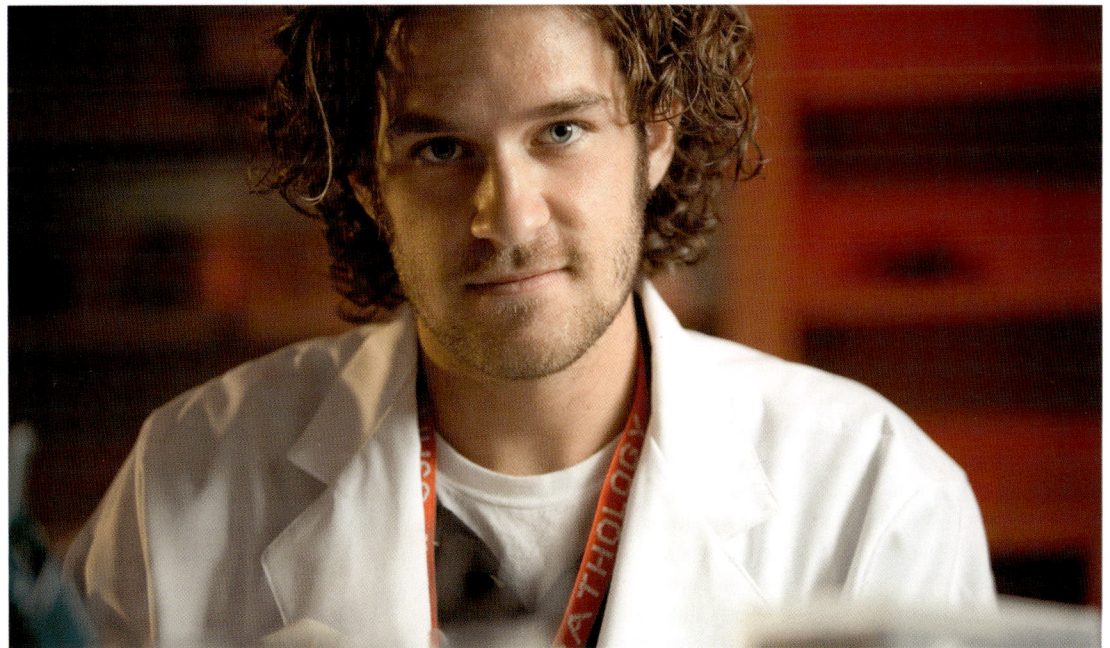

Researchers in Garrison Lab

the last 13 years. The Texas Tech University Health Sciences Center underwrites 80 percent of the operating expenses of the institute so the majority of donations goes directly to research.

To create personalized health care for women, "new information must become part of the curriculum taught in our schools," said Dr. Jenkins. So, in 2010, the institute developed a Sex and Gender Specific Health curriculum with open access to professors, students, and medical professionals across the country. It offers online access to a library of slides and interactive case-based modules. It has produced a library of videos for consumers and professionals and podcasts with research updates.

The institute's outreach within Texas has spread from Amarillo and Lubbock to include Abilene, San Angelo, Midland, and Dallas with health symposiums that educate and inspire women. With more than $7.5 million of support from the Cancer Prevention Research Institute of Texas in the last 10 years, more than 8,000 women have received breast and cervical cancer screening, HPV vaccines, and treatments. This resulted in 95 cancers being diagnosed and treated. The institute also operates the Infant Risk Center and the MommyMeds phone app where mothers can get information about the safety of pharmaceuticals, supplements, and herbs while they are nursing.

The institute promotes healthy living through its outreach to middle school– to college-aged girls across Texas.

Messages of personal safety, antibullying, good nutrition, healthy relationships, and self-care are conveyed through events like Girl Power and Girls Night Out. Through its research, professional training, and community outreach, the Laura W. Bush Institute for Women's Health is improving women's lives and answering the First Lady's challenge: "Whether women live in West Texas or across the world, we all share the need for answers to our unique health issues. Join us in the pursuit for women to live longer, healthier lives."

The F. Marie Hall Institute for Rural and Community Health

The F. Marie Hall Institute for Rural and Community Health, was founded under Patti Patterson, MD, MPH, former Commissioner of Health for the State of Texas. In 2003, the Institute received a three-year National Institutes of Health (NIH) grant called EXPORT (Excellence in Partnerships for Community Outreach Research and Training). James Spear, together with Patterson, supported a photographic project of the 108 counties in the TTUHSC coverage area, portraying visual examples of health disparities.

Currently, the Institute is led by Executive Vice-President Billy U. Philips, PhD, MPH, who has worked to meet the challenges of access to medical care in the 108

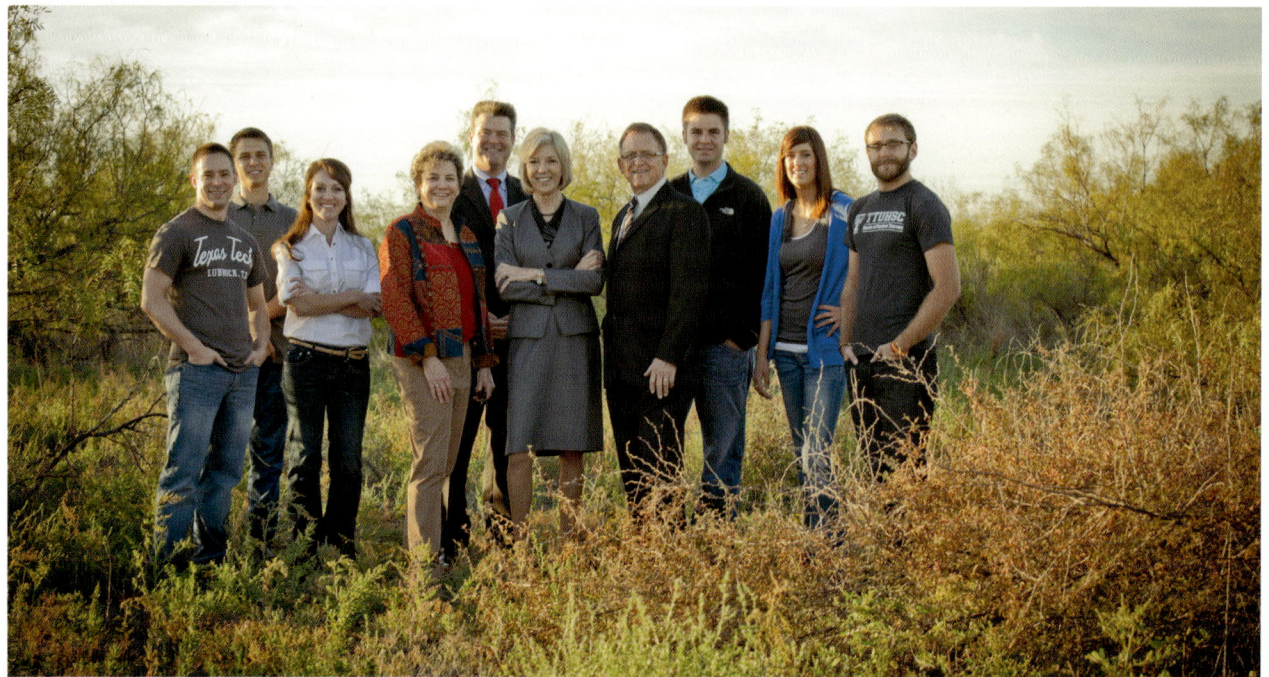

Billy U. Philips. Executive VP TTUHSC in Rural and Comm Health Lubbock, with Tedd Mitchell, MD, President TTUHSC, and Sharon Decker, PhD Director of The F. Marie Hall SimLife Center.

counties of West Texas. It connects young people to health education, which ensures future healthcare providers for West Texas and communities to health care and healthy results. It seeks ways to connect innovation to creativity and real-world applications of new knowledge and health technology to community needs and to shrink distances across the vastness of West Texas.

F. Marie Hall worked in banking and law, was a native of Big Spring, and lived in Midland. She created the FMH Foundation, which supports health organizations and the arts. She died in 2017 at the age of 80. She wanted all of West Texas to thrive—even people in small towns who didn't have the resources found in bigger cities. The people who work in "her" institute feel inspired by her vision—as one student put it, she was always "just one step beyond us. She has truly provided the means for us to go beyond ourselves."

Telemedicine is one program where residents of many rural communities can receive the specialty care they need while reducing the demands on individuals and families. Among other activities, the Telemedicine Clinic program works with 15 communities throughout the service region providing specialty consults for dermatology, cardiology, psychiatry, burn care, internal medicine, and more. These communities include School Based Health Care Clinics, FQHCs, and Rural Health Clinics. In addition, three of the TTUHSC campuses are equipped with telemedicine capability, allowing patients in El Paso, Amarillo, and Odessa to utilize the technology as well.

The Telemedicine Wellness Intervention Triage and Referral (TWITR) project started in Lubbock after the 2012 Sandy Hook Elementary School shooting and in 2018 was cited by Texas governor Greg Abbott as a model of how to deal with the rising violence in Texas high schools after the shooting at Santa Fe High School. TWITR leverages telemedicine services to intervene with junior high through high school students at risk for injury or harm to others or themselves in school settings. Students are identified and screened for risk-based behaviors in schools and are then provided psychiatric services by TTUHSC Psychiatry over a telemedicine link. Two telemedicine psychiatry sessions are provided through the project; students needing additional psychiatric services are then incorporated into the TTUHSC Psychiatry Clinic. Response to intervention is measured in terms of changes in grades, truancy referrals, and discipline referrals in the schools. TWITR's success has been noted

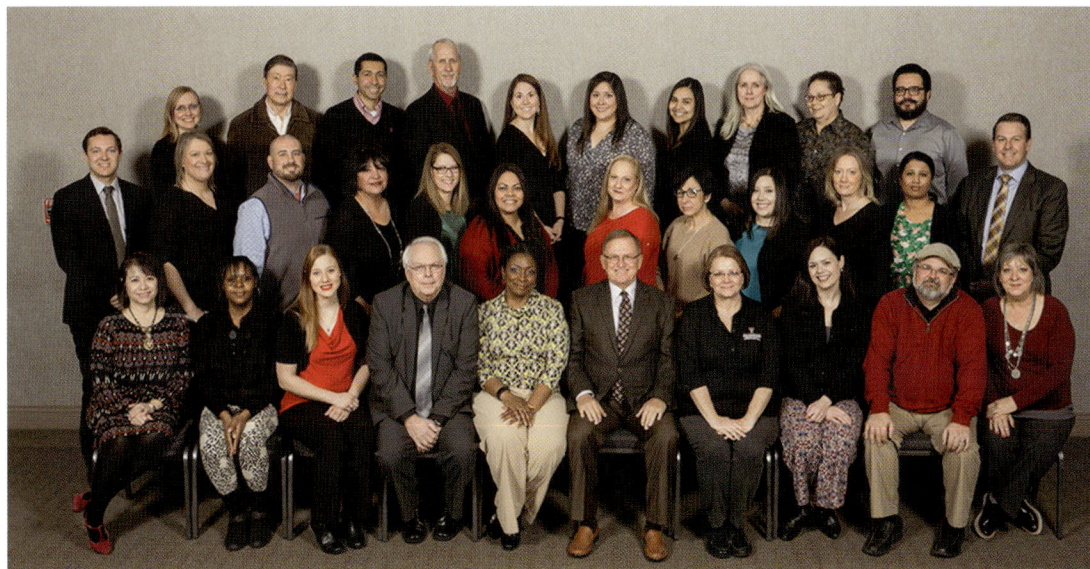

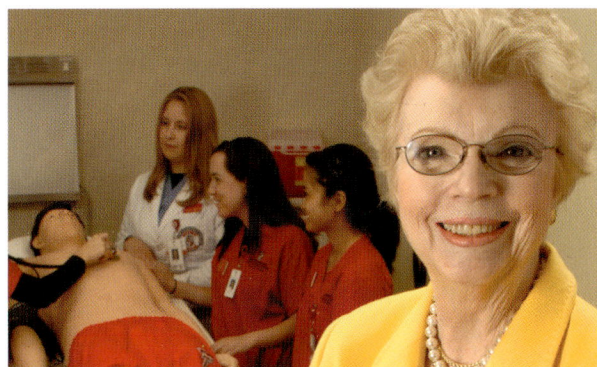

(LEFT) F. Marie Hall, Philanthropist

(ABOVE) Billy U. Philips, surrounded by members of the F. Marie Hall Institute for Rural and Community Health, which serves remote rural communities with the help of a multidisciplinary group of professionals.

through numerous publications and presentations and the program was awarded funding by House Bill NO. 13 for future expansion in other independent school districts around the state as an effort by Governor Greg Abbott to keep Texas schools safe.

Frontiers in Telemedicine is a one-of-a-kind program that trains medical staff and clinicians specific to telemedicine presenting procedures, technology, and business. The program focuses on competency-based learning and sets the standard for telemedicine training across the country. This was built on the original contributions of Jay Wheeler, MD, PhD, and J. Ted Hartman, MD, in the early 1980s. Students first complete the online portion of the course, then hands-on simulated learning, and finish with an objective structured clinical examination (OSCE) at the Frontiers in Telemedicine Lab in Lubbock.

The six West Texas Area Health Education Centers address the shortage of healthcare providers, improve

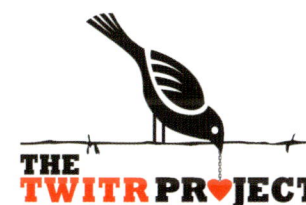

TWITR logo

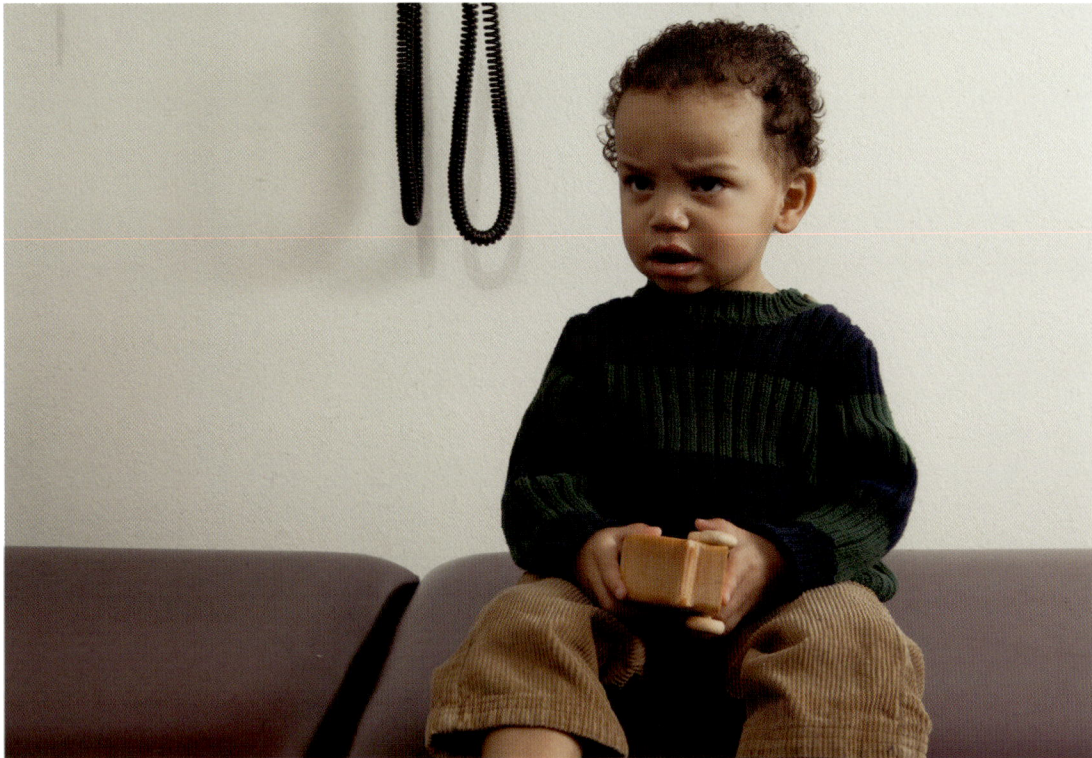

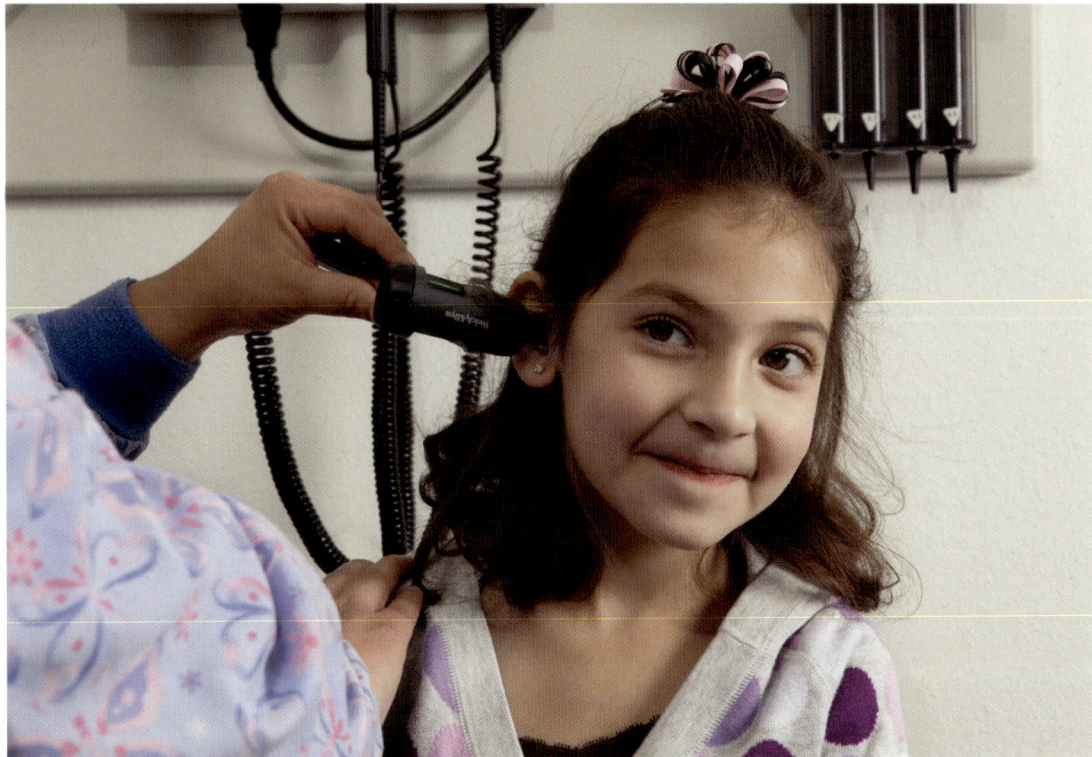

Telemedicine

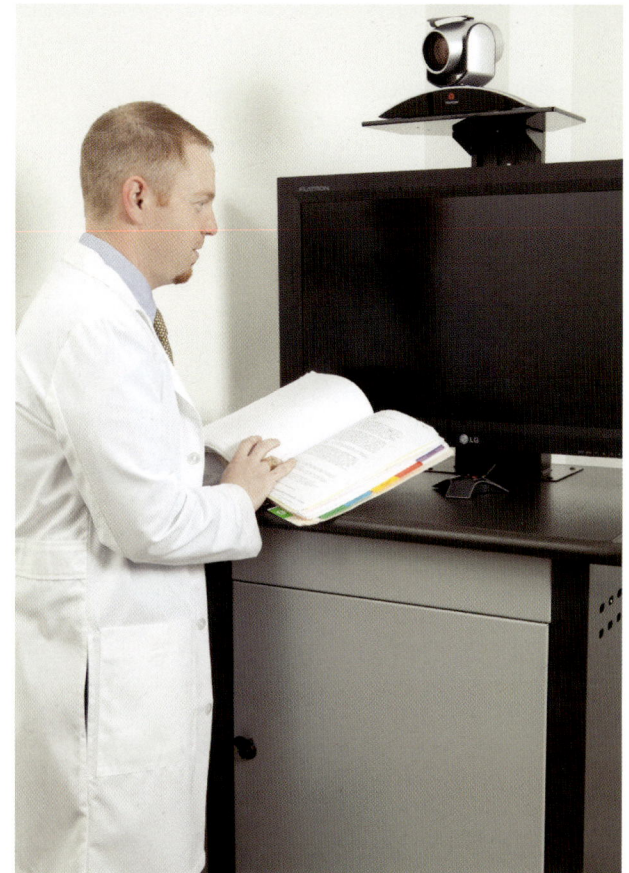

healthcare access in West Texas through education, and develop the healthcare workforce.

The Institute of Environmental and Human Health

TIEHH's history began in 1996 when Texas Tech University and Texas Tech Health Sciences Center proposed to form a joint venture to assess toxic chemical impacts on the physical—as well as the human—environment. The Texas Tech Board of Regents approved the program the following year.

TIEHH is the first of its kind among academic institutions at Texas Tech because it fused the resources of both universities. Ronald J. Kendall, PhD, was the founding director and instituted the Department of Environmental Toxicology.

This initiative employs a medical school and health sciences center interfaced with a comprehensive university, including the Texas Tech University School of Law, and represents an opportunity to address environmental and human health issues from many perspectives.

In 1999, TIEHH opened its research facilities at Reese Technology Center and currently occupies 12 acres of land 10 miles west of the main Texas Tech campus. The institute studies environmental impact on people, wildlife on land and in water, and more.

The Division of Human Health Sciences studies how environmental toxicants are connected to human diseases and develops ways to reduce those diseases. The institute is also home to the Admiral Elmo R. Zumwalt Jr. National Program for Countermeasures to Biological and Chemical Threats.

Starting as early as January 1999, discussions between Admiral Zumwalt (USN Ret.) and key administrators at Texas Tech University were focused upon the growing and realistic threat the nation faced from the potential use of biological and chemical weapon agents by domestic and foreign enemies of the United States.

This program is a permanent resource for the American public drawing expertise from academia, federal and state government, military, industry, and the private sector. The initial focus of the Zumwalt program was to further address research areas of need as identified by the National Research Council, including:

Pre-incident communications and intelligence
Personal protective equipment
Detecting and measuring chemical and biological
    agents
Recognizing covert exposure
Mass-casualty decontamination and triage procedures
Availability, safety, and efficacy of drugs, vaccines, and
    other therapeutics
Developing computer-related tools for training and
    operations

Southwest Institute for Addictive Diseases

The Southwest Institute for Addictive Diseases began in the 1970s to meet the teaching, training, and clinical service component of Texas Tech University Health Sciences Center's School of Medicine.

In 1986, the Texas Tech Board of Regents upgraded the program to institute status, adding research to its mission. The staff includes physicians, policy makers, research scientists, research assistants, professional counselors, and marriage and family therapists, as well as consultants and contractual employees. The institute's mission is to

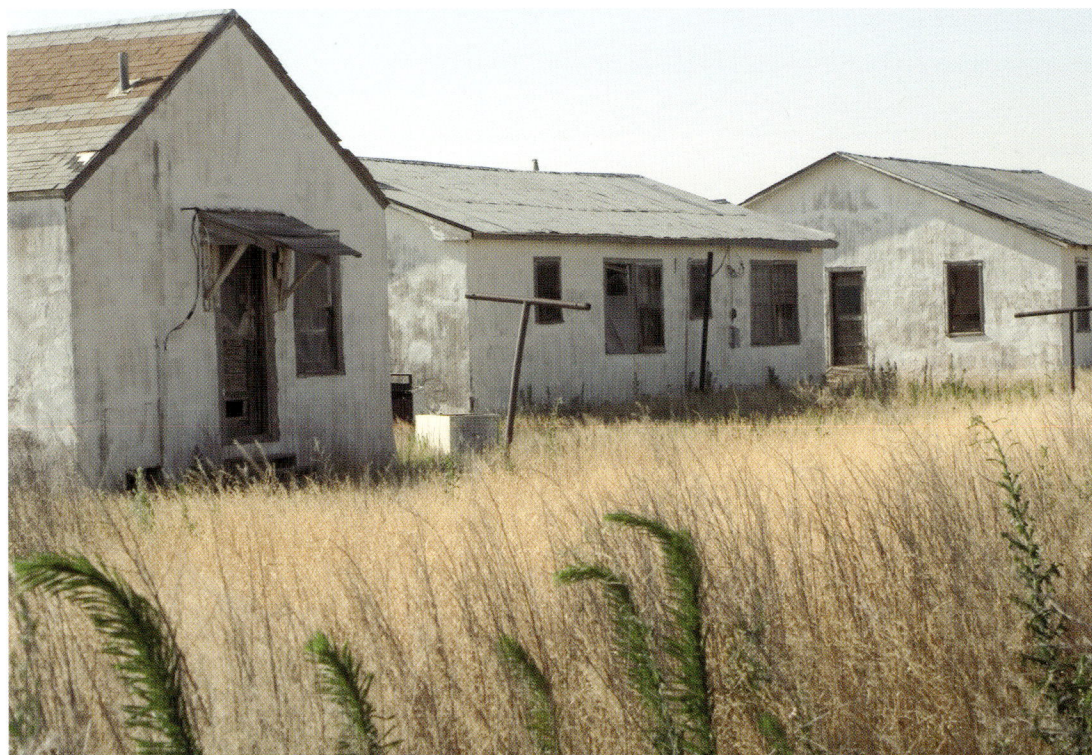

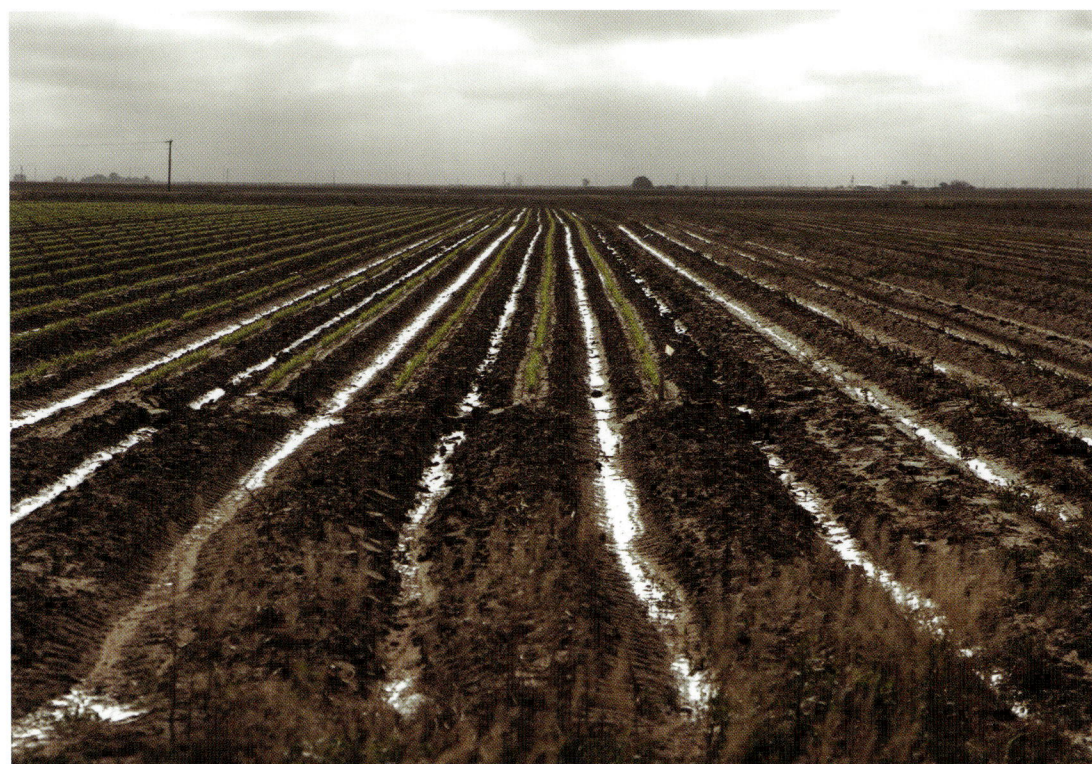

(TOP) Environmental Portrait—Farm workers' housing. Margaret Vugrin, Photographer

(BOTTOM) Environmental Portrait—Water on the furrows. Margaret Vugrin, Photographer

improve the quality of life of people with chemical dependency and mental health needs through comprehensive behavioral healthcare services and to provide opportunities for health professions training and research.

Texas Tech Mental Health Institute (TTMHI)

The newest institute began in 2018 to tackle an acute shortage of mental health care in West Texas and build on what was already being done on many Texas Tech campuses.

Keino McWhinney was appointed director of TTMHI, which is designed to offer a collaborative approach to mental health in which universities across the Texas Tech University System contribute their expertise to solve problems in the communities they serve and model solutions for the rest of the state and nation.

The institute will coordinate mental health efforts across the Texas Tech University System to avoid duplication and encourage collaboration; serve as a repository of systemwide knowledge on mental health; look for ways to apply research findings in clinical practice; and advocate integrating best practices into public policy.

The institute's first goal is to assess mental health needs and opportunities for the region in order to better understand current gaps in treatment and patient care.

TTUHSC Centers

BREAST CENTER OF EXCELLENCE

The Breast Center of Excellence (BCE) is organized around a multidisciplinary comprehensive care model, which is considered the gold standard by the National Accreditation Program for Breast Centers (NAPBC). Our multidisciplinary, sub-specialized approach to breast disease ensures that each patient with benign or malignant disease, or who is at risk of cancer, has access to clinical and paramedical specialists, using both knowledge specific to their specialized area of medicine and supportive care, to formulate an exact diagnosis and best treatment plan—in other words, an individualized care approach by a dedicated team.

CENTER FOR BLOOD-BRAIN BARRIER RESEARCH

The Center's mission is to discover and develop novel therapeutics that advance drug therapy in diseases affecting the central nervous system. The Center fosters research to characterize new drug targets based on understanding of

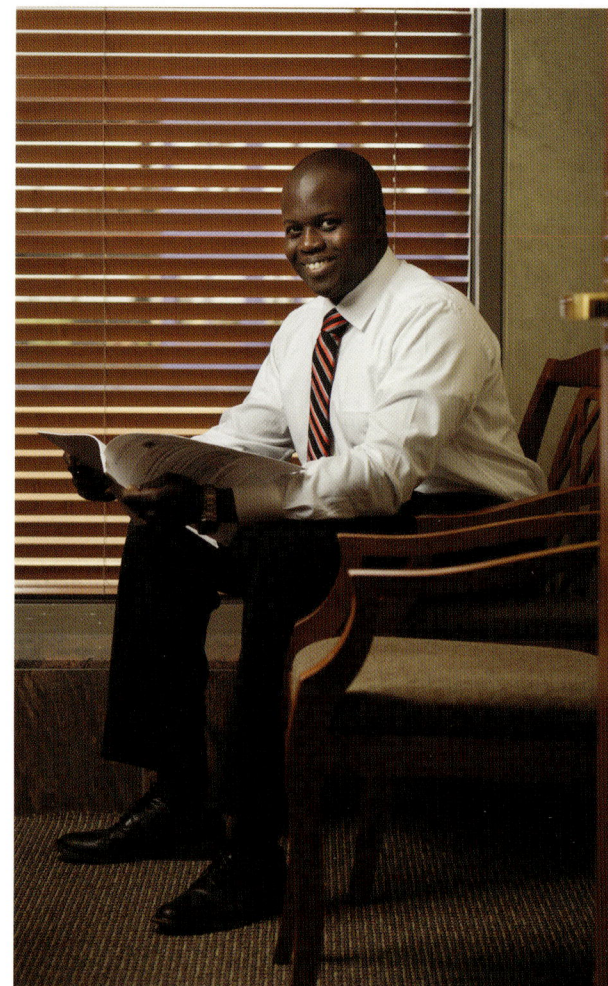

Keino McWhinney, MPP, Director, Texas Tech Mental Health Institute

both receptor and transport mechanisms and of metabolic pathways. By encouraging collaboration with colleagues across School of Pharmacy departments, the Center raises the pharmacy school's research profile, enhances the competitiveness of Center members for extramural funding and increases the attractiveness of the TTUHSC School of Pharmacy to prospective faculty members.

CENTER FOR ETHICS, HUMANITIES, AND SPIRITUALITY

When illness strikes, patients reach inside for sources of strength and explanation to sustain them through their crisis. These core sources may come from cultural, social, and spiritual values and beliefs and experiences which give meaning to life and create the patient's identity. Discerning these sources of meaning and identity, and the capability to connect with them in establishing a relationship are essential components of the clinician's task. Our focus is to humanize the practice of healthcare and address the challenges of the impersonal forces of biomedicine by studying and teaching ways in which compassionate care may be delivered in an ethically sound, spiritually sensitive, and culturally appropriate manner.

CENTER FOR IMMUNOTHERAPEUTICS RESEARCH AND BIOTECHNOLOGY

The mission of the Center for Immunotherapeutic Research is to improve the health care of people through the development and implementation of novel immune-based approaches and methods to detect and treat human diseases. Our goal is to grow translational and clinical research in immunotherapeutics at the School of Pharmacy through the establishment of a team of multidisciplinary and interdepartmental investigators working in a highly collaborative and technology-driven environment.

CENTER FOR MEMBRANE PROTEIN RESEARCH

The long-term goal of the Center is to advance our knowledge of the structure and function of membrane proteins in health and disease. The Center brings together a group of TTUHSC and TTU investigators interested in the broad field of membrane-protein research. After completing sequencing of the human genome, biomedical research has evolved into a combination of genomics, proteomics, and functional genomics. To a great extent, biomedical research in this century will be focused on prototypical proteins and protein families, including the determination of their structures, normal function, and roles in human disease. From this knowledge will emanate rational design of new pharmacological agents that open the way for novel therapeutic approaches.

CENTER FOR REHABILITATION RESEARCH

The Center for Rehabilitation Research (CRR) is an internationally renowned research, education, and clinical assessment center at TTUHSC that serves Lubbock and the West Texas region. The CRR is dedicated to improving the lives of people who have functional limitations caused by physical impairments. The CRR conducts research that emphasizes improving quality of life by both preventing disorders that lead to disability and restoring function. The CRR was established in 2002 as part of the School of Health Professions and is administered through the Department of Rehabilitation Sciences at TTUHSC.

CENTER FOR SPEECH, LANGUAGE, AND HEARING RESEARCH

The Center for Speech, Language, and Hearing Research (CSLHR) is embedded within the School of Health Professions, and is administered through the Department of Speech, Language, and Hearing Sciences at TTUHSC. The primary mission of the CSLHR is to promote education, research, and clinical practice in the areas of speech, language, and hearing. The Center's goal is to facilitate a collaborative effort among faculty in the programs of audiology, speech-language pathology, and rehabilitation sciences within the School of Health Professions and faculty from other programs within TTUHSC and Texas Tech University who have interest and expertise in normal processes, disorders, or the treatment of speech, language, swallowing, hearing, or balance systems.

CENTER FOR TROPICAL MEDICINE AND INFECTIOUS DISEASES

The Center for Tropical Medicine and Infectious Diseases (CTMID) is developing novel, rationally designed immunoprophylactics and immunotherapeutics for infectious disease pathogens, and training the next generation of basic scientists and clinical researchers. The CTMID promotes an environment that inspires passion with an emphasis on finding novel cures for diseases which recognize no human-made borders. Its focus is to the enrich lives of others by advancing knowledge through innovative research as well as educating and training students in this specialized area.

CENTER FOR EXCELLENCE IN EVIDENCE-BASED PRACTICE

The Center of Excellence in Evidence-Based Practice (CEEBP) is a Permian Basin initiative whose collaborative partners are the TTUHSC School of Nursing and the Medical Center Hospital. The mission of the CEEBP is to improve the care and safety of patients through the research, education, practice, and adoption of "best practice" as demonstrated through multiple avenues.

CENTER OF EXCELLENCE FOR TRANSLATIONAL NEUROSCIENCE & THERAPEUTICS

The overall goal of the Center of Excellence for Translational Neuroscience and Therapeutics (CTNT) is to serve as an incubator for the generation and dissemination of knowledge related to the neurobiology of clinically relevant disorders. CTNT strives to generate, facilitate, and coordinate multidisciplinary efforts to build bridges between basic science and clinical departments required for the development of novel and improved diagnostic and therapeutic tools and strategies. The CTNT advances our knowledge of mechanisms of nervous system functions and dysfunctions and neuropsychiatric disorders, which is essential for diagnostic and therapeutic advances.

CLINICAL PHARMACOLOGY & EXPERIMENTAL THERAPEUTICS CENTER

The Clinical Pharmacology & Experimental Therapeutics Center provides pharmaceutical expertise to conduct and support preclinical and clinical/translational trials, and post-marketing assessment of pharmaceutical drugs. The Clinical Pharmacology & Experimental Therapeutics Center consists of four core areas of focused research: the Pediatric Pharmacology Research & Development Core, the Experimental Therapeutics Core, the North Texas Clinical Pharmacology Cancer Core (funded in part by the Cancer Prevention and Research Institute of Texas), and the Pharmacoepidemiology and Clinical Outcomes Core.

COUNSELING CENTER AT TTUHSC

The Counseling Center at TTUHSC is an Employee Assistance Program. Our staff of trained professionals (all counselors are licensed by the state of Texas) is committed to providing quality counseling and assistance for individuals, couples, families, and work groups. Employers contract with us for confidential counseling sessions, all of which are provided at no extra cost. We strive to create and maintain an environment that enhances and encourages the positive self-image of the client and family, and preserves human dignity. Services are free (for 6–8 sessions) to those who qualify and completely confidential.

LARRY COMBEST COMMUNITY HEALTH & WELLNESS CENTER

Specializing in primary care and management of chronic diseases for all ages, the Larry Combest Community Health & Wellness Center is a Federally Qualified Health Center serving Lubbock and surrounding areas. Our Nurse Managed Center specializes in primary care and the management of chronic diseases such as diabetes, asthma, hypertension, and obesity. Care services are provided by Nurse Practitioners. The mission of the Larry Combest Community Health & Wellness Center is to provide access to comprehensive health services to those in need, to reduce or eliminate health disparities among high risk populations, and to integrate student clinical experiences and faculty practice in effective delivery of healthcare services.

THE SCHOOL OF MEDICINE CANCER CENTER

The Cancer Center at the TTUHSC School of Medicine was established in 2008 to provide a center of excellence for cancer research for the School of Medicine and the entire South Plains region. A major focus of the Cancer Center is conducting laboratory and clinical research that develops new anti-cancer drugs for both adults and children with difficult-to-treat cancers. The Cancer Center hosts the Operations Center for a clinical consortium, the South Plains Oncology Consortium, which conducts early phase clinical trials in adults and children with cancer. The Cancer Center also hosts the Operations Center and laboratories for the Texas Cancer Cell Repository, a Cancer Prevention & Research Institute of Texas (CPRIT)-funded collaboration to establish, bank, and distribute cancer cells from patients for use in studying the cancer biologies and novel therapies.

THE SCHOOL OF PHARMACY CANCER BIOLOGY CENTER

The mission of the Cancer Biology Center (CBC) is to advance understanding, prevention, diagnosis, and treatment of cancer by generating new knowledge in cancer biology and therapy and by participating in the application of this knowledge to translational and clinical cancer research.

SIM CENTRAL CENTER OF EXCELLENCE

SiMCentral is a collaborative initiative of TTUHSC, West Texas A&M University, and Amarillo College. The Center uses high fidelity human patient simulators to provide multi-disciplinary training opportunities to medical, nursing and allied health students and residents, as well as continuing education opportunities to the Texas Panhandle region. Simulation training provides opportunities to develop and enhance clinical and diagnostic skills through frequent participation in controlled clinical scenarios. The mission of SiMCentral is to provide multi-disciplinary education opportunities to improve patient safety and clinical outcomes by integrating clinical simulation and evidence-based training methodologies.

SURGERY BURN CENTER OF RESEARCH EXCELLENCE

The Surgery Burn Center of Research Excellence covers the entire spectrum of burn injury, from microscopic alterations at the cellular level to the clinical care of the whole person to the impact of burn injuries on society. This includes injury prevention, disaster planning, initial response and resuscitation, critical care, pain control, infectious complications, nutrition, surgical management, wound care, psychosocial issues and long-term rehabilitation. The Surgery Burn Center's objective is to develop research collaborations between clinical and basic science departments within TTUHSC, develop research collaborations between TTUHSC and UMC, broaden the impact of our scientific work through publications, presentations at national meetings and collaborations with outside institutions involved in burn research.

UNIVERSITY MEDICAL CENTER
SOUTHWEST CANCER CENTER

The UMC Southwest Cancer Center in Lubbock, Texas is a nationally recognized leader in the fight against cancer.

Founded in 1987 by Davor Vugrin, MD, a passionate medical oncologist who believes that cancer can be beaten using both the many tools that we have at hand now and those new ones being developed, but that first and foremost we must listen to the patient. The Cancer Center's multidisciplinary approach combines the expertise of Texas Tech Physicians with UMC's compassionate care and technological advancements. Comprehensive cancer treatment and care are available in one facility, close to home. The Southwest Cancer Center provides patients with a wide range of treatment options, as well as support services such as acupuncture, counseling, nutritional support, and more. What sets the Center apart from other cancer centers is that the oncologists, nurses, and other healthcare workers truly take the time to listen to the patients and respond with compassion. In doing so, the patient is empowered. Exceptional care today means hope for a cure tomorrow.

CHAPTER EIGHT

INNOVATIVE IDEAS

Institutional Educational Vision, Goals, and Objectives

To accomplish our goal of educating the best medical professionals to serve West Texas and beyond, the Texas Tech University Health Sciences Center School of Medicine has identified key objectives that address the knowledge, skills, behaviors, and attitudes needed for students to acquire the degree of doctor of medicine. These objectives are designed to achieve the six core competencies as designed by the Accreditation Council for Graduate Medical Education. Upon completion of all required courses and clinical educational experiences, the student will be able to practice the following:

Patient care that is compassionate, appropriate, and effective for the treatment of health problems and the promotion of health.

Medical knowledge of established and evolving biomedical, clinical, and behavioral sciences and their application to patient care.

Practice-based learning and improvement. The investigation and evaluation of patient care practices, appraisal, and assimilation of scientific evidence, and improvement of patient care practices.

Interpersonal and communication skills—the ability to effectively exchange information and collaborate with patients, their families, and other health professionals.

Professionalism—the behaviors of a competent, compassionate, and ethical physician.

System-based practice—the larger context and system of health care including effective use of resources in the system to provide optimum health care.

One of the original charges for the Texas Tech University School of Medicine—before it was named Texas Tech University Health Sciences Center—was to create innovative answers to healthcare challenges. This can be done inside and outside of the classroom.

It's been happening for half a century and outlined below are some excellent examples.

Telemedicine Wellness, Intervention, Triage, and Referral

The Telemedicine Wellness, Intervention, Triage, and Referral project (TWITR) was created to identify students at risk for committing school violence and intervening with those students.

The model uses licensed professional counselors who go into schools with shortages of mental health personnel and in locations with scarce mental health resources. Because the goal is always to try and keep students in school, if appropriate, telemedicine services are leveraged to connect students in schools with psychiatric services at TTUHSC.

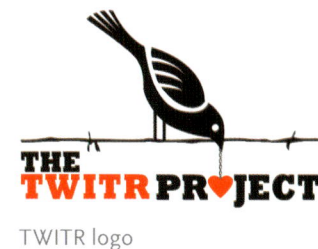

TWITR logo

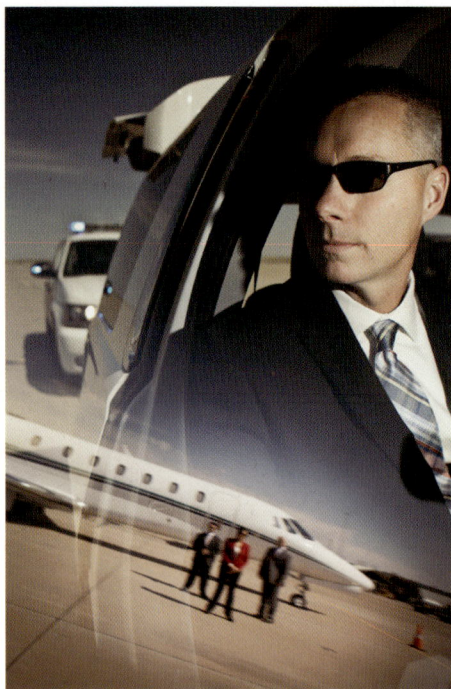

Jason Cooper, Lead, Dignitary Medicine

TWITR's success has been noted through numerous publications and presentations and the program was awarded funding by House Bill No. 13 for future expansion in other independent school districts around the state as an effort by Governor Greg Abbott to keep Texas schools safe.

Executive Medicine Program at TTUHSC/Permian Basin

Preventive medicine has been around for decades and was started by Dr. Kenneth H. Cooper of the world-renowned Cooper Clinic in Dallas almost 50 years ago. In recent years, preventive medicine in the form of executive medicine has grown in popularity throughout the country. The premise is taking proactive steps by exercising daily, eating a healthy diet, and taking the right steps to transform your lifestyle to one that's healthier. The program is designed to give appropriate health care to executives or to those looking to change to a healthier lifestyle.

The program started in September 2015 with the inspiration coming from President Tedd L. Mitchell, who had been the chief executive officer at the Cooper Clinic in Dallas. Timothy Benton, MD—chairman of the Department of Family and Community Medicine at the School of Medicine at the Permian Basin—became the program's managing physician. Dr. Mitchell recruited Kiko Zavala, MBA, from the Dallas Cooper Clinic in May 2016 to design, implement, and manage the operations of the Executive Medicine program.

The program is still in its infancy and testing phase. The Executive Medicine's Executive Exam program has the potential to influence West Texans to be healthier and become more proactive with their health. The Executive Exam is an easy, personalized way to take an in-depth look at one's health in less time than a normal work day.

Dignitary Medicine

West Texas sees its fair share of celebrities and dignitaries. It may be a new, fresh face of country music, a television or film star, or perhaps a visiting high-profile professional athlete. For the most part, emergency medical personnel travel with them. But this may not always be the case for political or governmental dignitaries who visit.

Jason Cooper, a 2006 graduate of TTUHSC's School of Health Professions, approached President Mitchell with his concerns about the lack of medical preparations and how he and other physician assistants with emergency medicine backgrounds could provide those services. Cooper said he also explained the importance of having trained personnel available for medical needs. Additional conversations between Cooper and Mitchell led to the beginning of a program to provide dignitary medical support services for local police and federal security teams.

"One of our guiding principles is serving our communities, to see our presence in the areas we serve," said Mitchell. "This type of program gives us an opportunity to provide a unique service for this area and to showcase the talent we have in our faculty and staff. It is a bold example of our mission to serve."

In 2014, Cooper was at an event with then–Texas gubernatorial candidate Greg Abbott and struck up a conversation with a member of Abbott's Midland security detail. The plainclothes agent was looking for an automated external defibrillator, and he and Cooper began talking about the need to have medical professionals available during such visits. The pair exchanged business cards. A couple of weeks later, Cooper received a call from the Midland Police Department, and they began to formalize a structured plan to include medical professionals in the security details of these types of visits, a practice becoming known as dignitary protection medicine.

Dignitary protection medicine is an evolving area largely built on the experience of White House, State Department, and other physicians who have traveled extensively with dignitaries, according to an article published in 2012 in the *American Journal of Emergency Medicine*. It stems from an increase in international travel of business executives and political dignitaries, particularly in regions that are socially unstable or have minimum medical services. According to Cooper, dignitary protection medicine programs are emerging nationwide and TTUHSC is a part of the national dialogue about this new emerging field.

The primary objective is to protect the dignitary from medically related threats. It includes several steps. A medical threat assessment determines emergency contact information, environmental risks such as exposure to weather, hospital locations, infectious disease risks, and preexisting medical conditions of the dignitary. Logistics and supplies are reviewed, including needed medications and emergency supplies. Additionally, evacuation procedures are reviewed, accounting for travel time to the nearest hospital, anticipated road construction, and weather alerts, according to the *American Journal of Emergency Medicine* article.

Thinking in 3D: Introduction to Medical Imaging and 3D Modeling Elective

This fourth-year School of Medicine elective started in the fall of 2018. The impact of 3D printing on health care is going to a big part of the future and the new Methodology Lab, housed in the Preston Smith Library, will increase its presence at TTUHSC.

Devices and implants tailored to the individual, pills designed to release a customized drug cocktail at defined intervals, 3D-printed tissues that will accelerate the pace of pharmaceutical research, and, within a few decades, 3D-printed organs for transplant will all be available.

Research and development of 3D-printing applications for health care is continuing at a rapid pace. Students entering the university are already familiar with and expect access to this technology. TTUHSC must proactively meet such expectations as well as provide them with a sound foundation in the fundamentals of 3D printing and beyond.

The Methodology Lab will increase experiential teaching and learning opportunities, interdisciplinary interaction, cross-pollination of ideas, and collaboration by gathering creative individuals already pursuing innovative projects in an active and collaborative hands-on learning environment, where students, faculty, and researchers can tap into their own creativity and imagination in their areas of specialization.

Correctional Managed Health Care

An increase in crime rates in Texas in the 1980s and 1990s prompted lawmakers to "get tough on crime." Accordingly, additional state prisons were constructed to house more prisoners, and the prisoner population expanded from 46,000 to 157,000. This created an immediate need in the prison system for more healthcare services.

In 1993, the Texas Legislature created a committee that established a partnership between the Texas Department of Criminal Justice (TDCJ), Texas Tech Health Sciences Center, and the University of Texas Medical Branch to provide quality, cost-efficient health care for offenders.

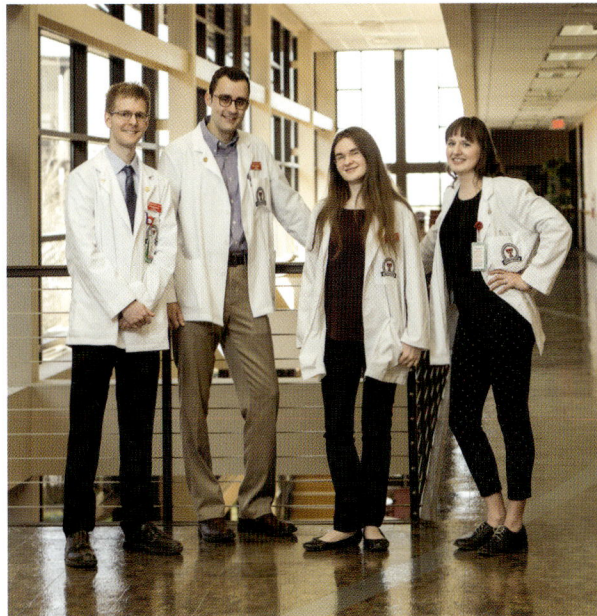

(TOP LEFT) TTUHSC SOM Technology Club Officers

(BOTTOM LEFT) Kate Serralde, from library, instructing student on 3D mechanics. Margaret Vugrin, Photographer

(BELOW) Resin creations. Margaret Vugrin, Photographer

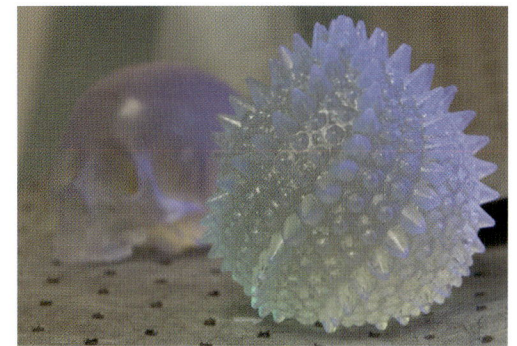

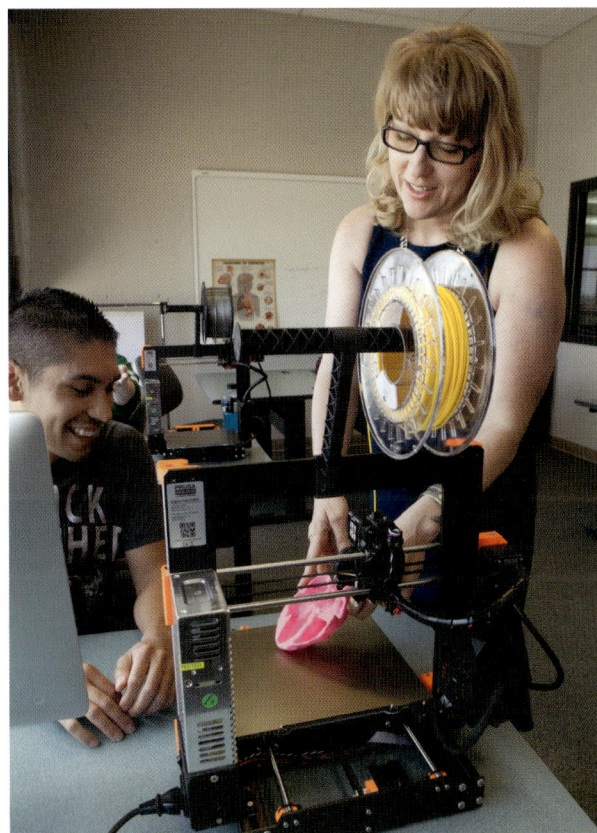

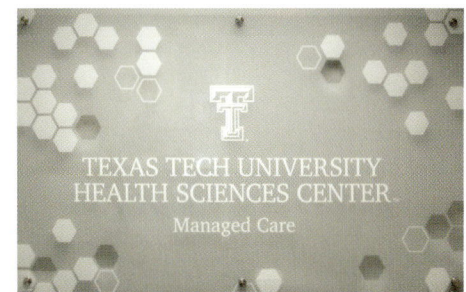

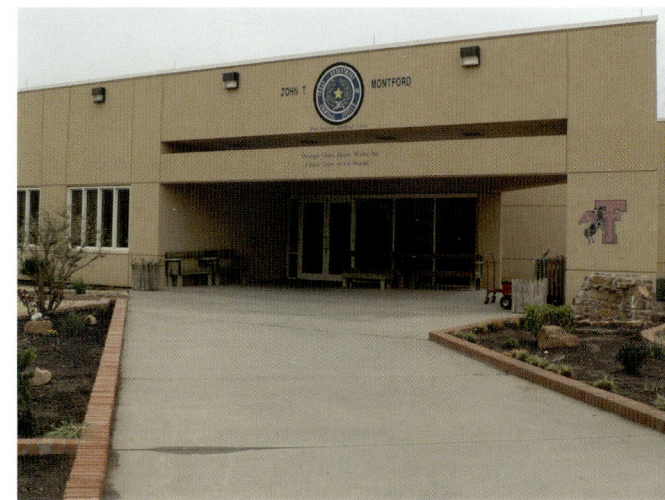

(MIDDLE) Montford Unit

(BOTTOM) Correctional Managed Healthcare

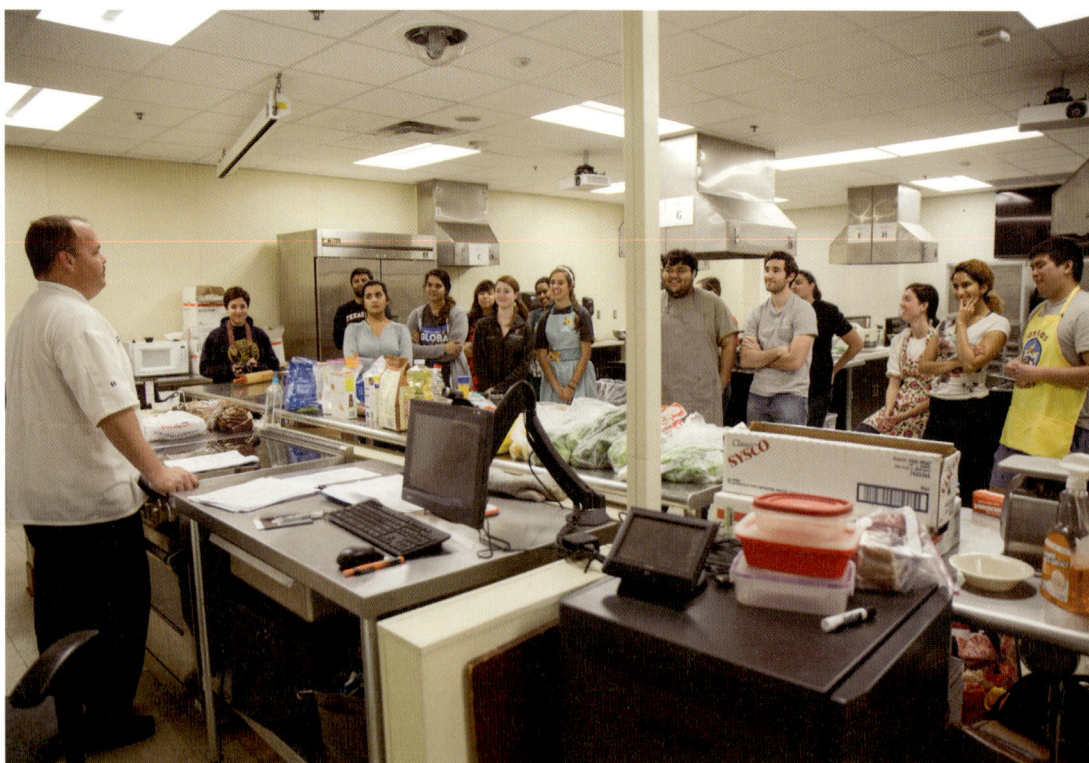

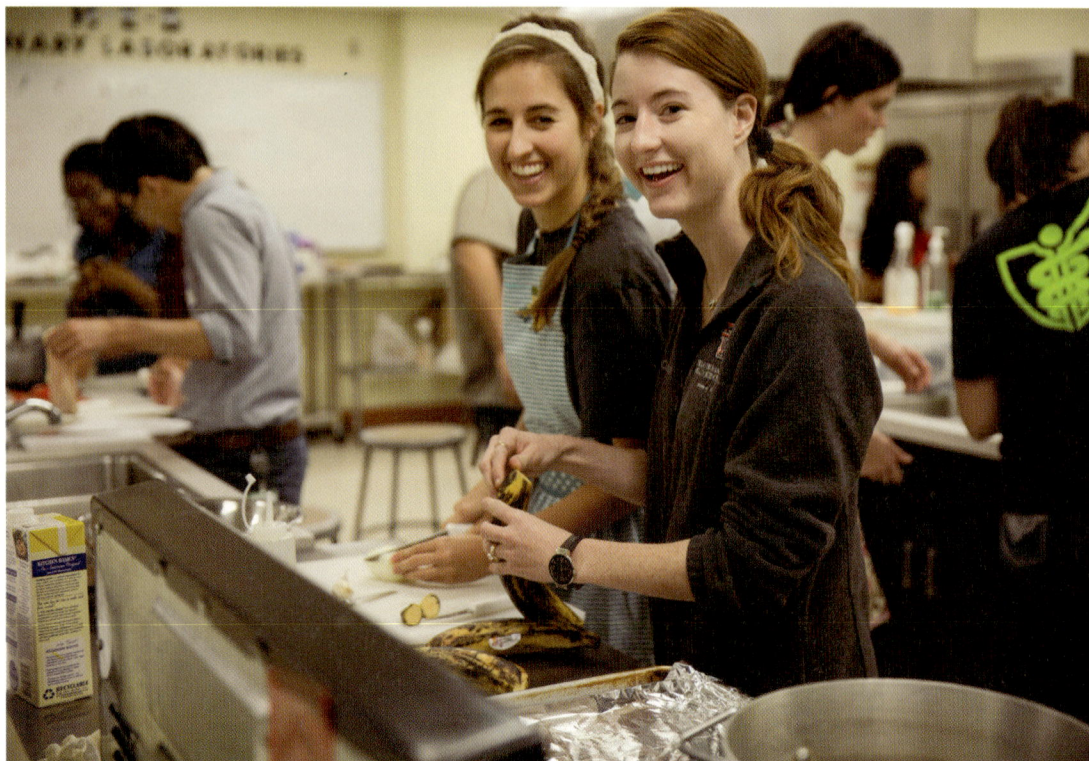

Culinary Medicine SOM Elective

Prior to this partnership, Texas was known for having one of the most inhumane criminal justice systems in the nation, with deplorable conditions and poor health care. As a result, the healthcare system was under federal oversight for numerous violations of offenders' eighth and fourteenth constitutional amendments. By 1999, due to this collaborative partnership, Texas was liberated from federal oversight.

Jim Laible became the first executive director of TTUHSC Correctional Managed Health Care in 1993. In addition to onsite medical services in 17 geographic locations, the program manages the Montford Regional Medical Facility, the most complex prison-based medical unit in the state of Texas. This Lubbock-based medical/surgical facility, which opened in 1996, is co-located with a 550-inpatient psychiatric facility that opened in 1995. Managed Care and TTUHSC clinical departments provide more than 20,000 annual behavioral health and primary and specialty care services to offender patients throughout the sector via an extensive internal 48-site Telemedicine network. The TTUHSC Amarillo School of Pharmacy has also played a pivotal role in the TDCJ offender healthcare contract by providing pharmaceutical management at all units.

In the 25 years since its inception, this creative and innovative Correctional Managed Health Care partnership has not only provided quality and cost-efficient offender health care but was a pioneer in and continues to be on the cutting edge of correctional telemedicine and the Electronic Health Record.

Equally noteworthy, as prisons are frequently located in rural and remote areas, this program has bolstered revenue for many struggling rural community hospitals. The program has also been honored with several awards and recognitions.

Culinary Medicine Elective

In Culinary Medicine classes, medical students trade stethoscopes and white coats for an apron and cooking utensils. The recently added elective class was established by Sarah Jaroudi and Bill Sessions when they were both second-year medical students.

Jaroudi and Sessions saw a need for education about nutrition that was not in the curriculum. Lectures explore various nutritional concepts and labs are taught by chefs. Students create different interpretations of recipes surrounding a central idea so they can compare and contrast the techniques and nutritional content. The mission is to educate and train medical students to develop and maintain healthy habits and perspectives that will benefit themselves, their communities, and, most important, their patients.

Health Policy Elective

Over the course of the year students are introduced to healthcare policy, follow bills through the legislative process to statutes, and then follow the statute to rulemaking at the agency level. They learn advocacy from different perspectives and are able to discuss the governance of public health agencies. Their knowledge and expertise will make it possible for them to make a difference in how the legislative process can be influenced from the healthcare professional perspective. This course has been offered since the fall of 2017.

Global Health

Faculty, staff, and students have been engaged in international initiatives since TTUHSC's beginning. These initiatives have included research projects with institutions abroad, faculty and student exchanges, school-sponsored service projects, and capacity-building initiatives. Over the years, TTUHSC faculty and staff have continued to share their expertise and knowledge with collaborative partners abroad, learning from each and working side by side with partners around the globe to promote education and healthcare delivery.

In 2007, under the leadership of then-president John Baldwin, MD, TTUHSC developed an increased focus on its role as a leader in the global health arena. The beginnings of the student-focused initiative were prompted in part by a grassroots movement lead by students and faculty with a passion for promoting the health and well-being of individuals far beyond the borders of West Texas. Patti Patterson, MD, has been a pioneer promoting programs addressing the needs of the poor, indigent and underserved. Many students from all areas of TTUHSC have participated in eye-opening trips to far off locations, where they were able to make a difference to the health of the various people they were meeting.

Under the leadership of President Mitchell, the Office of Global Health was created, spurring the initiation of

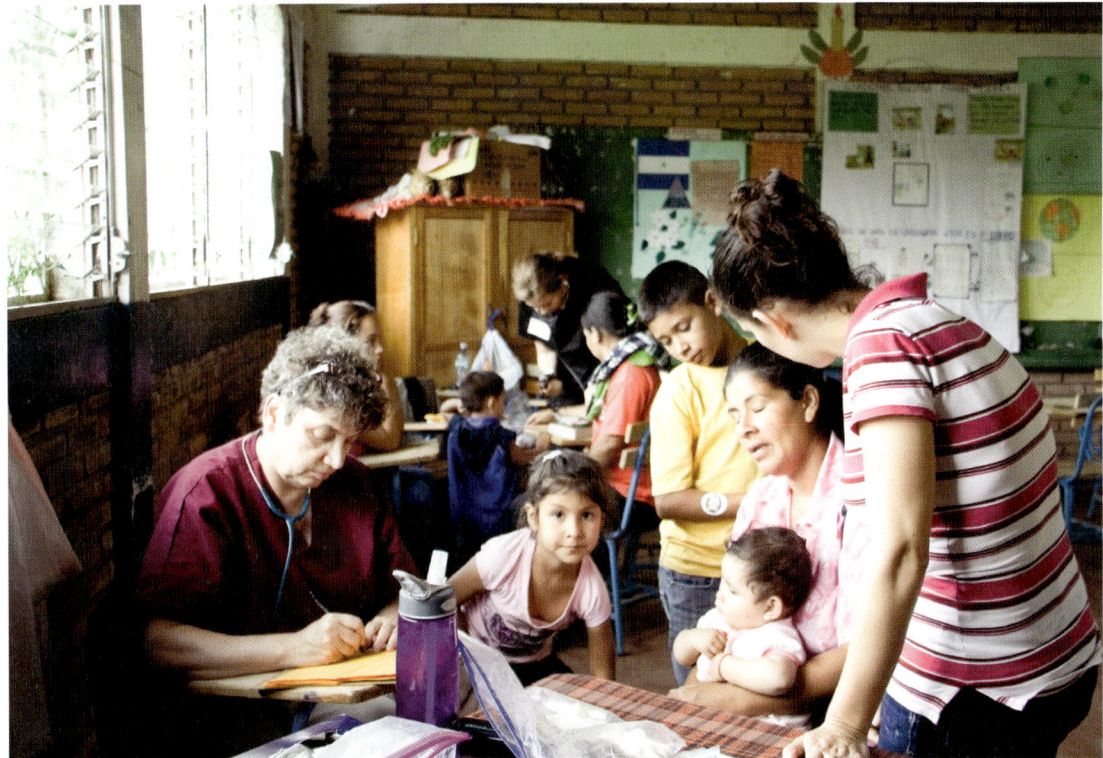

(ABOVE) Patti Patterson, MD, in Nicaragua clinic. Amy Moore, Photographer

(LEFT) Global Health Image. Whitney Boyce, Photographer

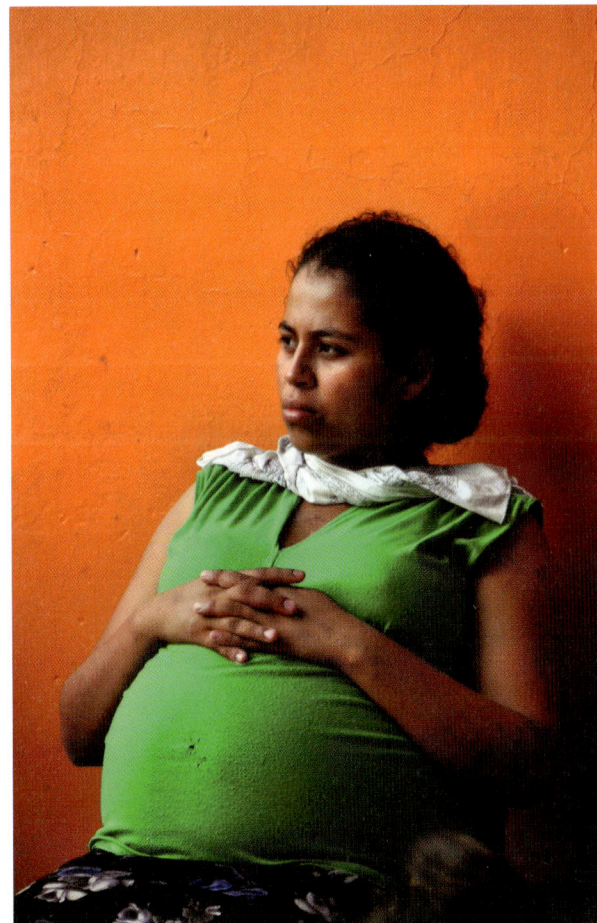

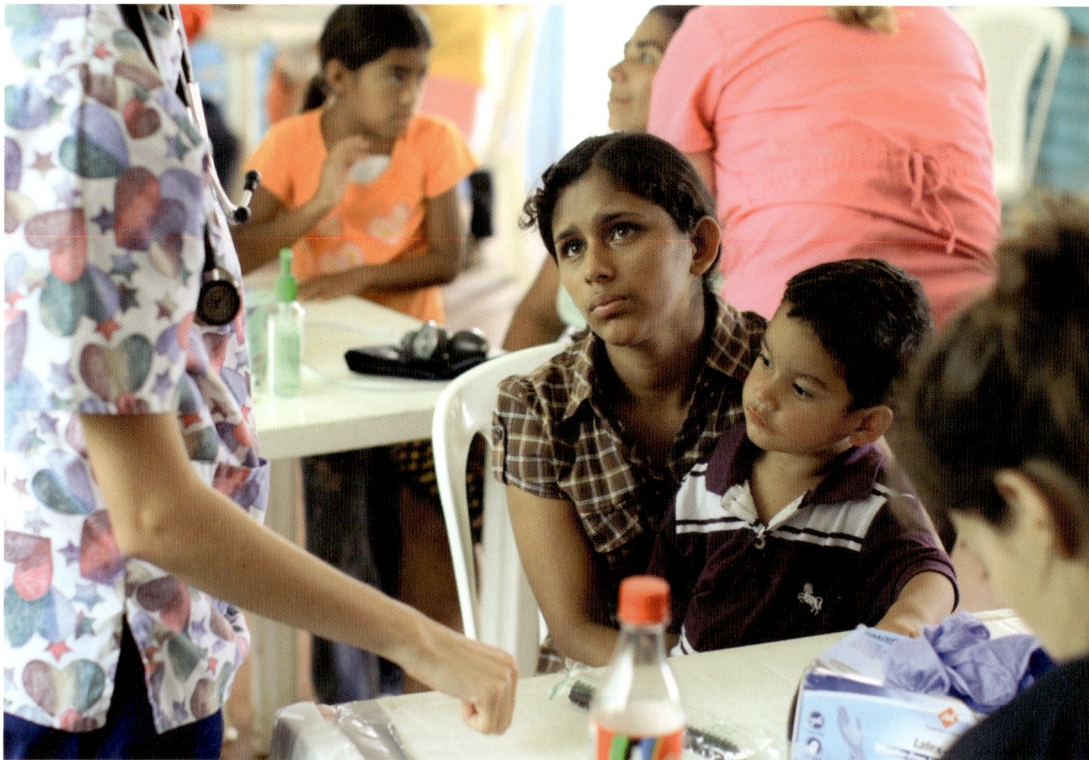

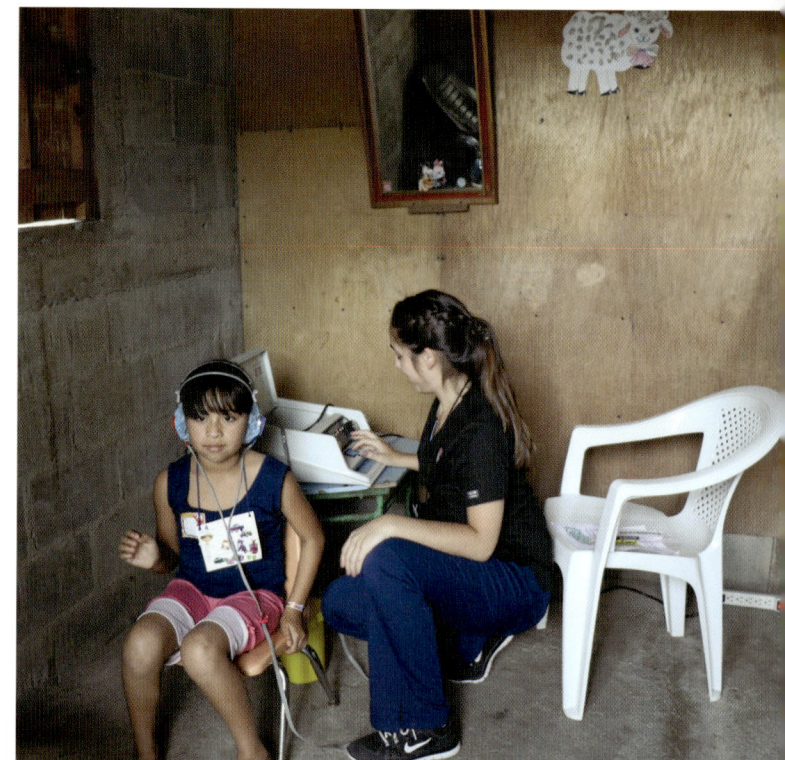

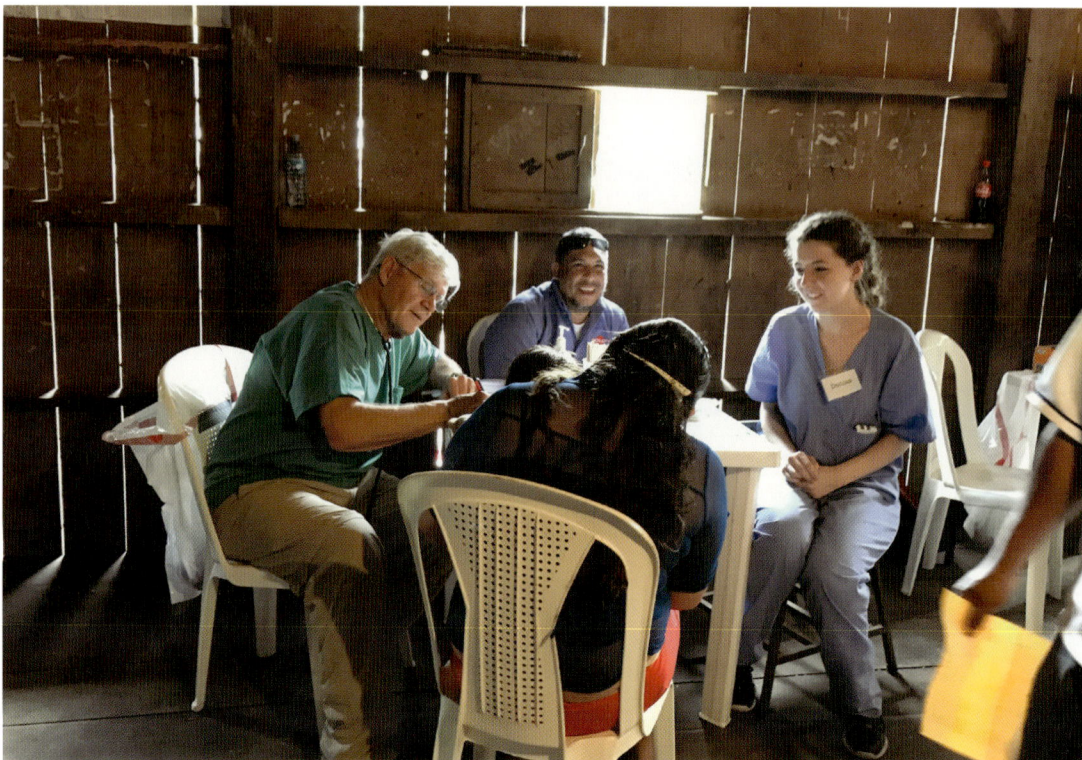

(TOP LEFT) Global Health Image. Amy Moore, Photographer

(TOP RIGHT) Hearing clinic in Nicaragua. Amy Moore, Photographer

(BOTTOM) Richard Lampe, MD, in Nicaragua Pediatric clinic.
Amy Moore, Photographer

more formalized collaborations abroad. The office serves as the primary resource for students interested in a global health experience. In addition to working with students, the office also supports faculty interested in global health initiatives, whether leading a group of students abroad, conducting education at universities abroad, or engaging in service projects that further develop community engagement and healthcare delivery.

Since 2010, TTUHSC's interprofessional teams, from all areas of the institution, have sent more than 700 students overseas. Affiliations with healthcare institutions have been developed around the world based on the outreach of the Global Health initiatives.

Workforce Overall Wellness Program

The award-winning employee Workforce Overall Wellness program (WOW!) at Texas Tech University Health Sciences Center has made great strides since its inception in 2012 at the request of President Mitchell. WOW! is an employee-focused program offering baseline screenings, education, and support on all TTUHSC campuses.

It consists of seven different areas:

Environmental wellness
Financial wellness

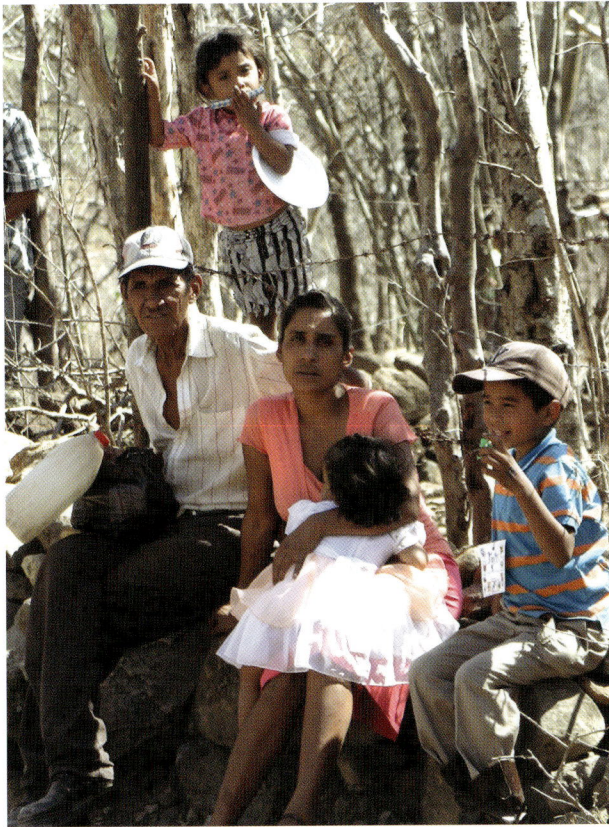

Global Health Images. Amy Moore, Photographer

Physical wellness (physical activity and nutrition)
Emotional wellness
Occupational wellness
Social wellness
Spiritual wellness

Challenges take place every month under these different areas to encourage positive lifestyle and behavioral changes for TTUHSC employees. One of the most popular challenges is the Get Fit Texas State Agency Competition. This challenge takes place January through March every year. Participation in this challenge far exceeds expectations as indicated by TTUHSC's top-five ranking out of all large (5,000 employees or more) state agencies.

Free onsite health screening and flu shots are provided each year for TTUHSC employees. They receive a full lipid panel, blood glucose, height, weight, body mass index, and weight circumference. All screening stations are run by TTUHSC medical, nursing, and pharmacy students. Results of the screenings help determine the program's focus for the next year.

The Center for Superheroes

The Center for Superheroes is the only mental health center in West Texas or Eastern New Mexico (our catchment area is 300 miles in any radius, with Lubbock as the central point of reference) designed to provide comprehensive medical, mental health, behavioral health, and developmental services for victims of childhood trauma and their families. The Center for Superheroes is one of only a handful of places in the nation that provide services such as this. Professionals from a variety of systems are trained (health care, therapists, the courts, law enforcement, child protective services, educators, and foster parents) in trauma-informed care. The center takes a multidisciplinary approach to treating and reducing the recurrence and long-term impact of child trauma.

The Center for Super Heroes provides evidence-based, scientifically supported treatments for the effects of child trauma such as Trauma-Focused Cognitive-Behavioral Therapy (TF-CBT); Treatment of Problematic Sexual Behaviors (PSB) for ages 3 to 18; treatment for physically abusive or neglectful caregivers such as Parent-Child Interaction Therapy (PCIT); and treatment of other related conditions (e.g., Behavioral Activation for Depression). All treatments have extensive empirical, scientific support for their efficacy and effectiveness. For example, TF-CBT has 20 randomized controlled trials (RCTs) and over 50 peer-reviewed studies demonstrating effectiveness. As multiple studies have demonstrated, those who work with trauma populations can be adversely impacted by this work; our approach entails addressing vicarious trauma effects and impairment for providers from multiple disciplines through the Trauma Stewardship protocol.

TTUHSC Libraries of the Health Sciences

Beginning in 1970, Charles W. Sargent, PhD, joined the faculty planning sessions already underway to create the Texas Tech University School of Medicine. Before coming here, he worked at the Lovelace Foundation for Medical Education and Research and did a stint at the National Aeronautics and Space Administration where he designed computer-based systems and participated in multiple NASA-related research projects. With this experience, Sargent came to Texas Tech as a forward-thinking librarian who understood medical libraries and the value of computer automation and organization. Accreditation

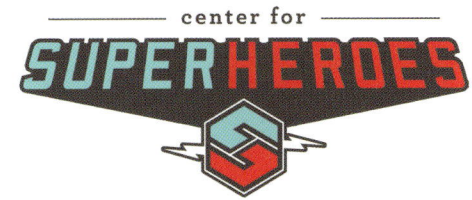

Center for Superheroes logo

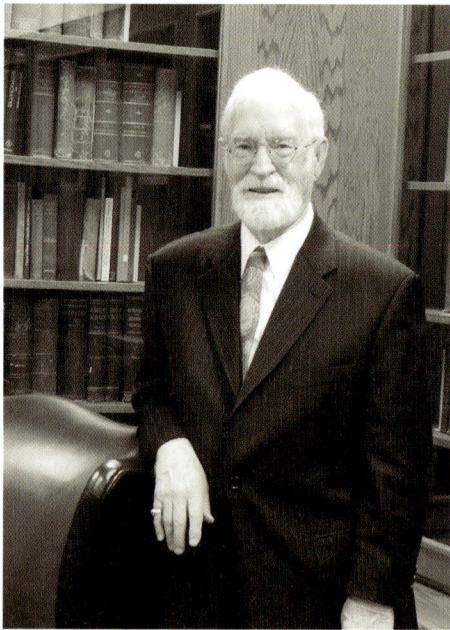

(ABOVE) Charles Sargent, PhD.
Margaret Vugrin, Photographer

(RIGHT) Rial Rolfe, PhD, and Richard Nollan,
PhD, MLS, Executive Director of Libraries.
Margaret Vugrin, Photographer

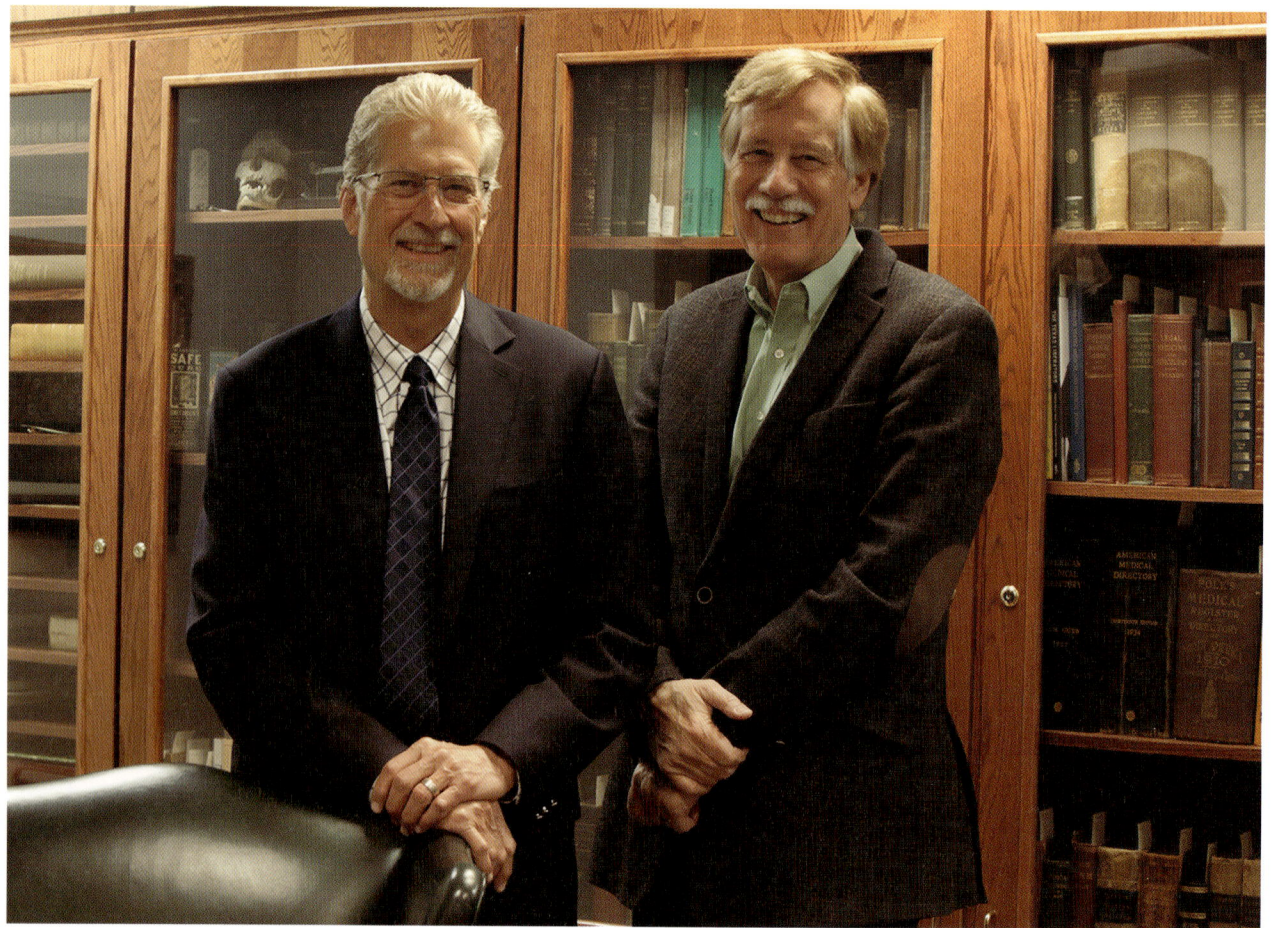

reviews from 1973 and onward noted the high level of excellence achieved in such a short amount of time.

An initial bequest of medical texts was made by May Owen, MD, of Fort Worth and her portrait hangs in the library. Sargent organized the print materials that were needed by the new school, including an impressive audiovisual collection and computer services. By 1982, the library had an automated circulation and acquisitions department and he could boast that the library had an electronic card catalog.

In addition to founding and organizing a medical library, Dr. Sargent created networks. He founded the Lubbock Area Library Association in 1982, which facilitated resource sharing among member libraries and discussions on common issues these libraries faced. He was also instrumental in organizing the South Central Academic Medical Libraries. This organization of library directors brought medical libraries together in Texas, Oklahoma, New Mexico, Arkansas, and Louisiana to share resources, to discuss and solve common concerns, and to leverage

agreements for shared information resources. Sargent retired in 1990 after a successful 18-year career, during which time he had established TTUHSC libraries in Lubbock, Amarillo, Odessa, and El Paso.

Richard C. Wood became the second executive director of the libraries. By this time, the libraries no longer served only the information needs of the School of Medicine but also those of the Schools of Nursing, Pharmacy, Allied Health (later Health Professions), and the Graduate School of Biomedical Sciences.

Wood built on Dr. Sargent's excellent work. The biggest change in Wood's 25-year tenure was the revolutionary inception of information technology and the personal computer. Print journals and books were steadily replaced with electronic versions of the same information, which led to a rethinking of the library and its role in the Health Sciences Center. Wood oversaw an increase in the library's resource budget of more than 440 percent and an increase in the number of professional and support staff from 46 to 64. New and emerging programs in medicine, nursing,

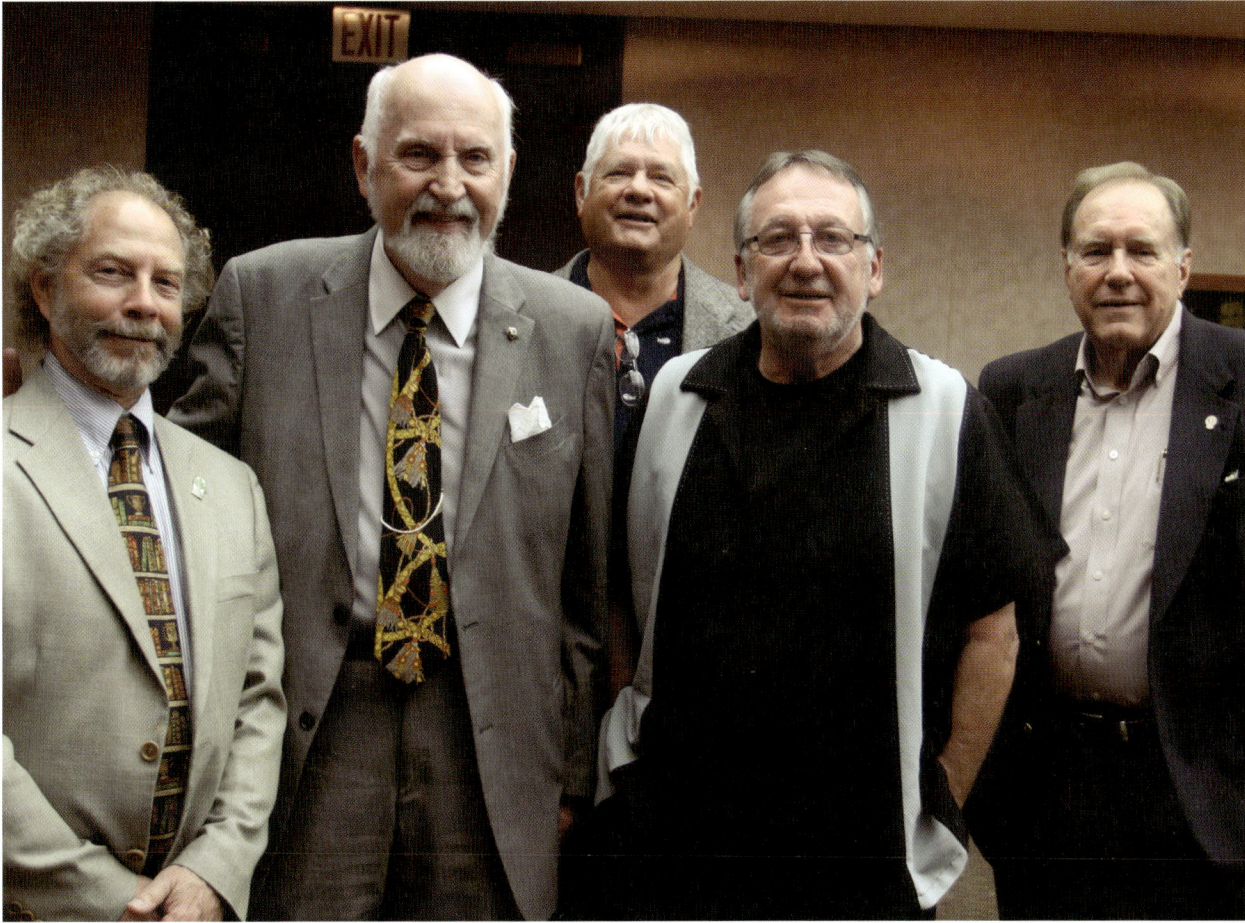

Richard C. Wood, Executive Library Director, at retirement reception with regional library directors. Margaret Vugrin, Photographer.

allied health, and pharmacy were reflected in the library's expanding services. The number of contracts to rural facilities increased as did the number of hours that the library remained opened. Teaching services all grew under his guidance as well.

In 1998 the library moved from its restricted location in the main Health Sciences Center building into a newly constructed library named after Preston Smith, the former governor of Texas who signed the legislation authorizing the creation of TTUHSC. After the move to the new location, Wood enticed J. Ted Hartman, MD, to volunteer his time, energy, and knowledge to organize archival papers of the many early members of TTUHSC faculty and administration. Hartman did this willingly and with enthusiasm.

One of the features of this new location is the inclusion of the rare book room. Over the years, as the library received donations, items were held and stored for a future rare books collection. Later, with the help of benefactors, Wood began adding significant works in the history of

medicine dating back to the mid-sixteenth century. These are works that otherwise cannot be found elsewhere in the West Texas region and are now available to be viewed by all.

In addition to the rare book collection, he collaborated with another library benefactor, James T. Wheeler, MD, to create a medical and pharmacy antique collection with hundreds of medical artifacts, including scarificators, bleeding bowls, transfusion equipment, pharmaceutical containers, mortars and pestles, and more. The items in this collection range from the seventeenth to the nineteenth centuries and are on display in the library.

Wood retired in 2015 and a year later Richard Nollan, PhD, MLS, was brought on board to lead the library into a new and bright future. With the construction of the new Pod D, which will directly connect the Health Sciences Center to the Preston Smith Library, Nollan is preparing for the library's renovation in space, collection, and services.

CHAPTER NINE

BUILDING OUR FUTURE

Under the leadership of President Tedd L. Mitchell, MD, the Texas Tech Health Sciences Center has grown in innumerable ways. This growth is evidenced in academics and research, service and outreach, and in its people and operations.

An academic example is found in the Scopus database, a bibliographic database that allows for the search of articles by affiliation. It lists 8,720 citations with authorship from TTUHSC campuses (Lubbock, Amarillo, and Odessa) from the 1970s to 2018. This is certainly not a comprehensive list but it gives one an idea of the amount of work that has been created by faculty and students and is being presented to a global audience. There are over 57 articles that have been cited more than 250 times. Twenty-two of these articles have been cited more than 400 times. Others are listening, reading, and responding to the research and academic work that is being accomplished at Texas Tech University Health Sciences Center. While there are many other academic examples that can be presented, here are two: The PhD program in Physical Therapy is number one in the nation based on student reviews for the last three years in a row. Of the first class of TTUHSC veterans studying for their BSN degree, 100 percent passed the nursing licensure exam on their first try.

Dr. Mitchell spoke recently about the "growing demand on universities to produce graduates skilled in integrative thinking and the ability to apply team-oriented approaches to addressing problems as well as to provide educational experiences that include personal and ethical development" ("2019 Values-Based Culture Field Guide," 4). To this end, Human Resources, working with many members of the TTUHSC family in all departments and on all campuses, helped to consolidate our joint vision into a team guide to lead the institution toward a new values-based working culture.

Service and outreach opportunities are available to students to expand their knowledge. Some of these are hands-on opportunities for research and clinical experience, including collaborations with the communities in which they are now living, gaining practical knowledge that is vital to their success. Patients are helped by the healthcare team in clinics and in hospitals throughout our region through these faculty clinics. Interprofessional teams work throughout the community in programs like the Barbershop/Cardiac disease prevention program, the student-run free Impact Clinic, and at the nurse-managed Larry Combest Community Health and Wellness Center, a federally qualified health center. These clinics/hospitals provide access to comprehensive health services to those in need, to reduce or eliminate health disparities among high-risk populations, and to integrate student clinical experiences and faculty practice in effective delivery of healthcare services. This past year the Combest Center had approximately 28,000 visits from those in high-risk populations.

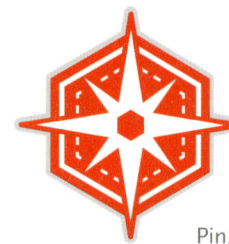

Pin/Logo

VALUES BASED CULTURE

ONE TEAM
Unite and include diverse perspectives to achieve our mission

- Empower and energize one another to create positive growth
- Collaborate through open communication
- Hold ourselves and each other accountable by giving and accepting constructive feedback
- Foster a fun and healthy environment that encourages team spirit
- Recognize and celebrate contributions and achievements

KINDHEARTED
Exceed expectations with a kind heart, helping hands and a positive attitude

- Assume good intentions
- Listen first to understand
- Treat all consistently with compassion, respect and an open mind
- Acknowledge each other with courtesy
- Respond rather than react

INTEGRITY
Be honorable and trustworthy even when no one is looking

- Be honest regardless of the outcome
- Make ethical choices in every situation
- Honor commitments
- Be transparent in your purpose, expectations and actions
- Protect and conserve institutional resources

VISIONARY
Nurture innovative ideas, bold explorations and a pioneering spirit

- Promote an innovative environment that embraces appropriate risk
- Be resilient and confident when faced with challenges
- Inspire continuous curiosity
- Demonstrate and inspire commitment to life long learning and personal development

BEYOND SERVICE
Create and deliver positive defining moments

- Anticipate the needs of each individual and respond with a generous heart
- Invest in the well-being, safety and success of *all* by going the extra mile
- Be solution-oriented, create the pathway to a win-win resolution
- Deliver excellence in everything we do

TTUHSC

9.1.18

Values-Based Culture

In order to support the growth in our population, the buildings of the TTUHSC Center also had to grow. Dr. Mitchell and his staff have been integral in the planning and organization of the numerous construction projects on the campuses. Recently completed construction includes: Amarillo: SimCentral—opened in September 2017; Midland: Psychiatry Clinic—opened on November 8, 2018; and Abilene: Public Health Building—opened in September 2016.

The Lubbock TTUHSC campus hosted the ground-breaking ceremonies for its many construction projects that are anticipated to open in the course of the coming year, 2019. These include: University Center—anticipated in March 2019; the Academic Event Center—anticipated in June 2019; West Side Expansion—anticipated in August 2019; and 4th Street Main Entrance—anticipated in February 2019. The Permian Basin campus anticipates the opening of its Academic Classroom Building in Spring 2019. Finally, Dallas's TTUHSC Building Phase 1 is complete, Phase 2's completion is anticipated in August 2019.

Texas Tech University Health Sciences Center has grown in all dimensions. Since 2009, over 16,313 degrees have been conferred on its students. With its 2018 enrollment of 5,083 students, many more degrees will be earned and conferred in the future. The goal of producing caring and compassionate healthcare professionals is now and will continue to be met in the future. As Dr. Mitchell stated in a recent convocation, TTUHSC is "Strong, Secure, and Robust" as it builds for the future.

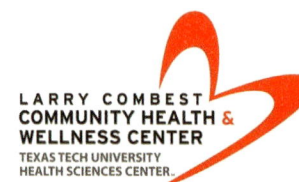

LARRY COMBEST COMMUNITY HEALTH & WELLNESS CENTER
TEXAS TECH UNIVERSITY HEALTH SCIENCES CENTER.

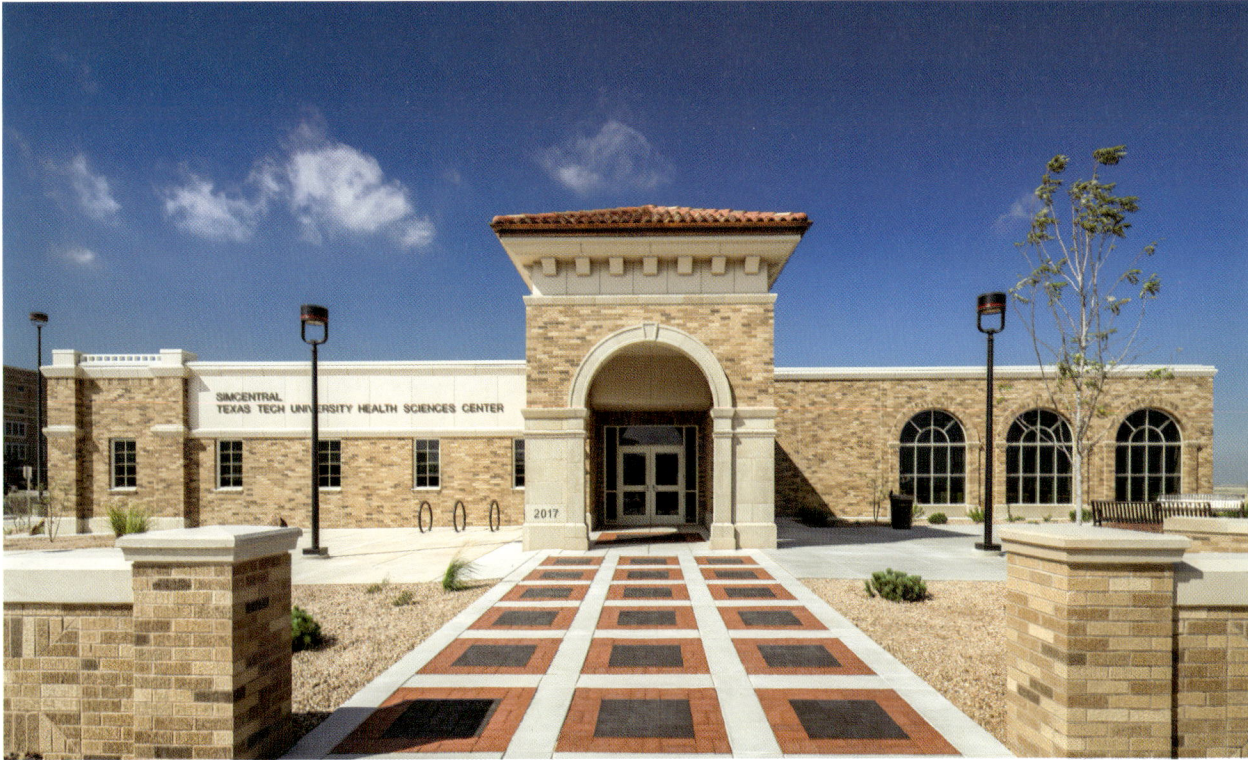

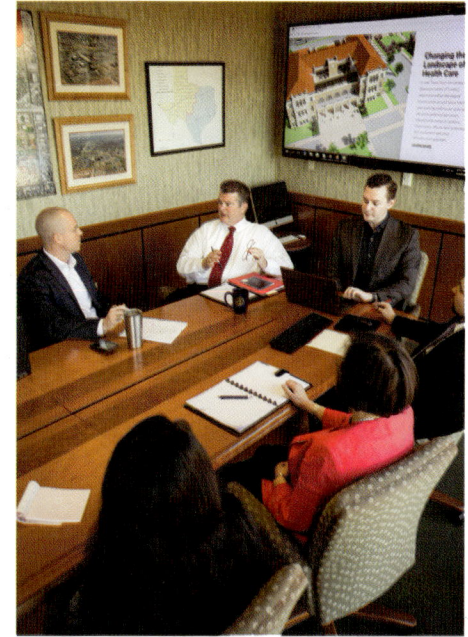

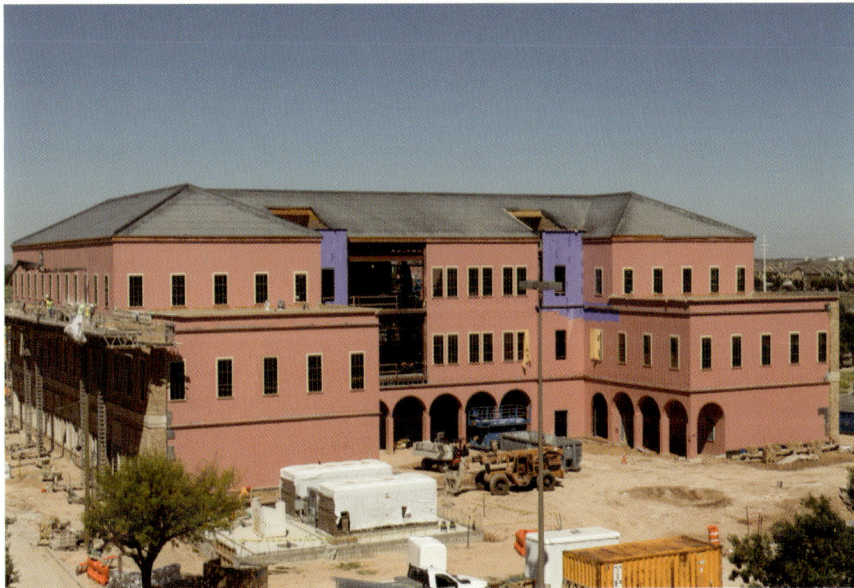

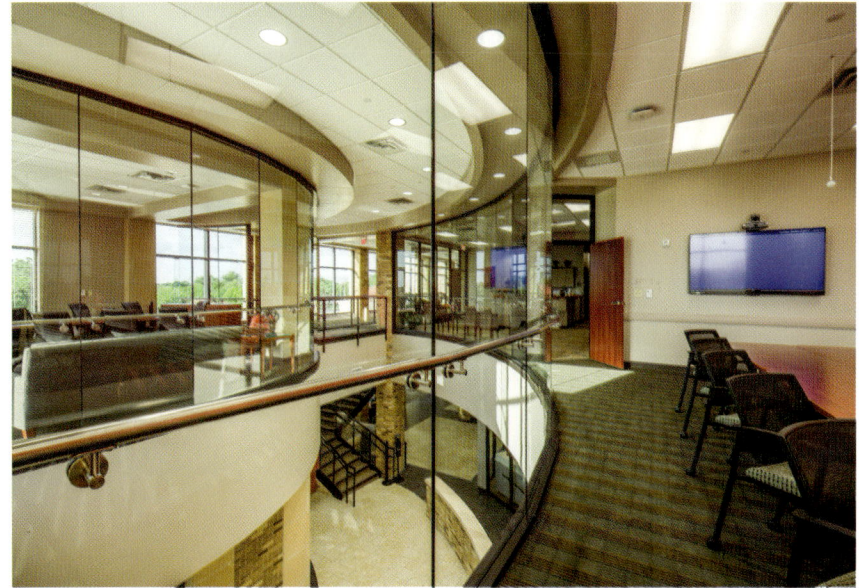

(TOP LEFT) TTUHSC SiMCentral AM. Courtesy TTU Facilities Planning and Construction. Contractor: Western Builders of Amarillo, Inc (Brandon Robertson—Project Manager) Architect: Dekker/Perich/Sabatini (Garrett Pendergraft—Lead Architect)

(TOP RIGHT) Tedd Mitchell, MD, and Staff—Justin L. White, Bryce Looney, Cole Johnson, Didit Martinez and Ololade Holmes—planning project for TTUHSC.

(BOTTOM LEFT) University Center under construction

(BOTTOM RIGHT) TTUHSC—Abilene. Photographer: Kevin Halliburton, AIA, www.Ice-Imaging.com, Architect: TLP/PSC, www.Team-PSC.com

(TOP LEFT) Dr. Mitchell at Lubbock Ground breaking ceremony 2017. Artie Limmer, Photographer, Associate Director, Institutional Advancement

(TOP RIGHT) J. Ted Harman MD, Dean Emeritus; 92 years old at Lubbock ground breaking 2017. Artie Limmer, Photographer, Associate Director, Institutional Advancement

(BOTTOM) TTUHSC—Lubbock groundbreaking 2017, Quentin Smith, PhD; Dan Pope, Lubbock Mayor; John Frullo, Texas House of Representatives for District 84; Robert Duncan, Chancellor TTUSystem; Brandt Schnieder, PhD, Dean GSBS; Tedd Mitchell, MD, President; and Mr. Elmo Cavin, Executive Vice President for Finance and Administration. Artie Limmer, Photographer, Associate Director, Institutional Advancement

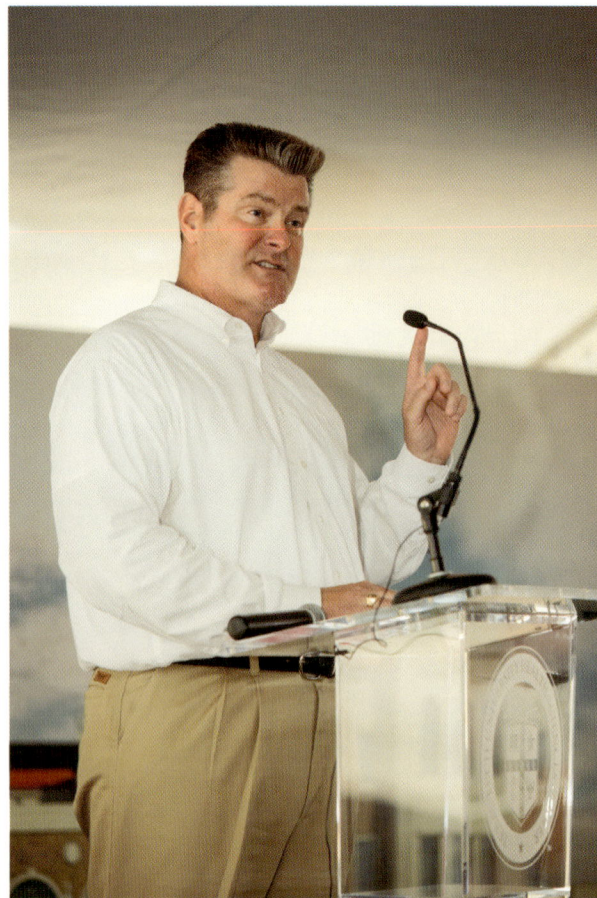

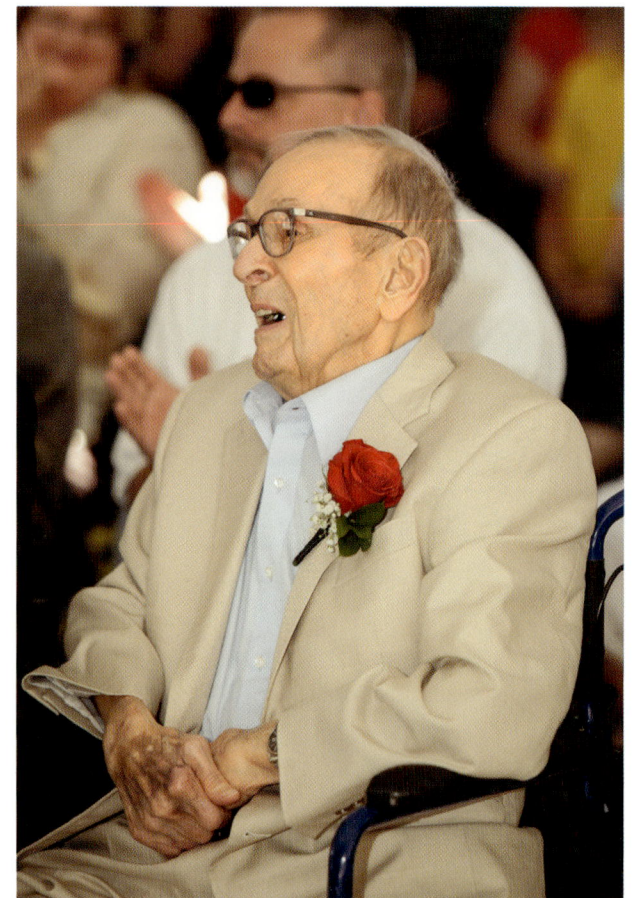

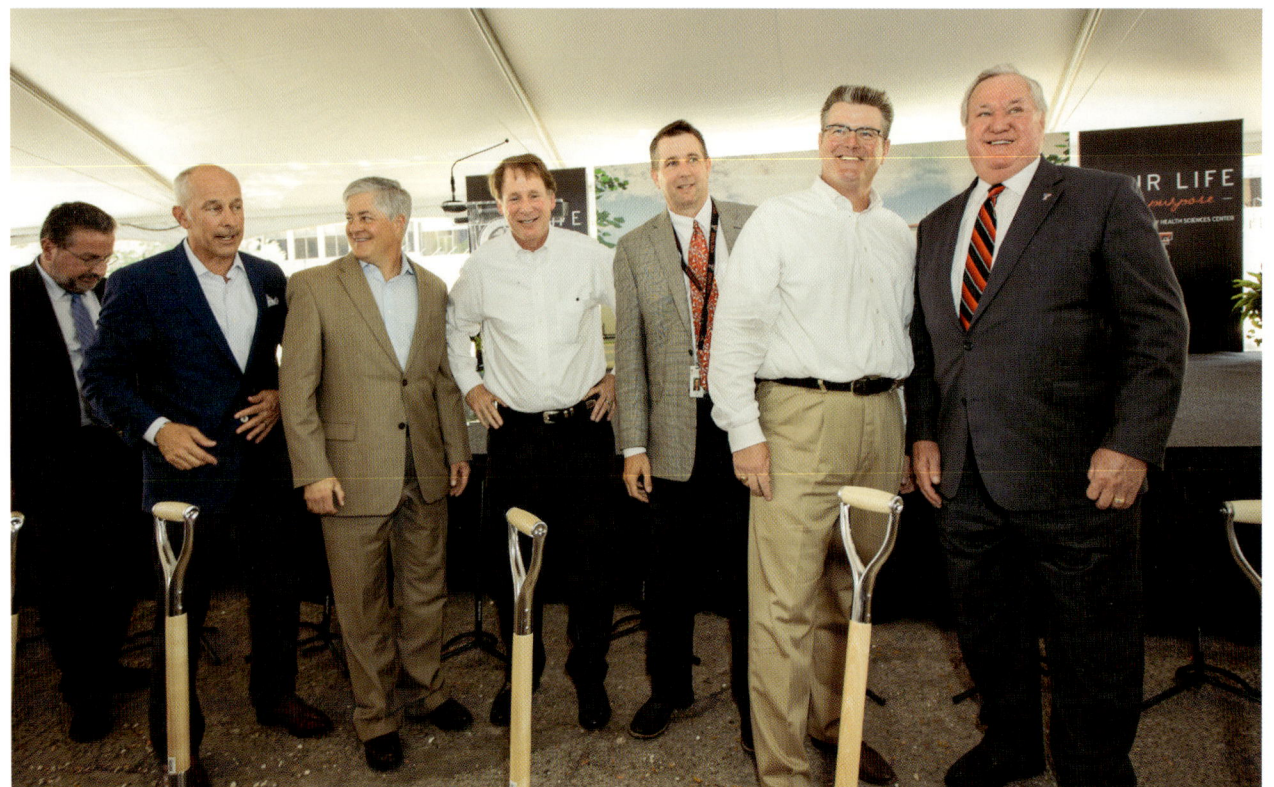

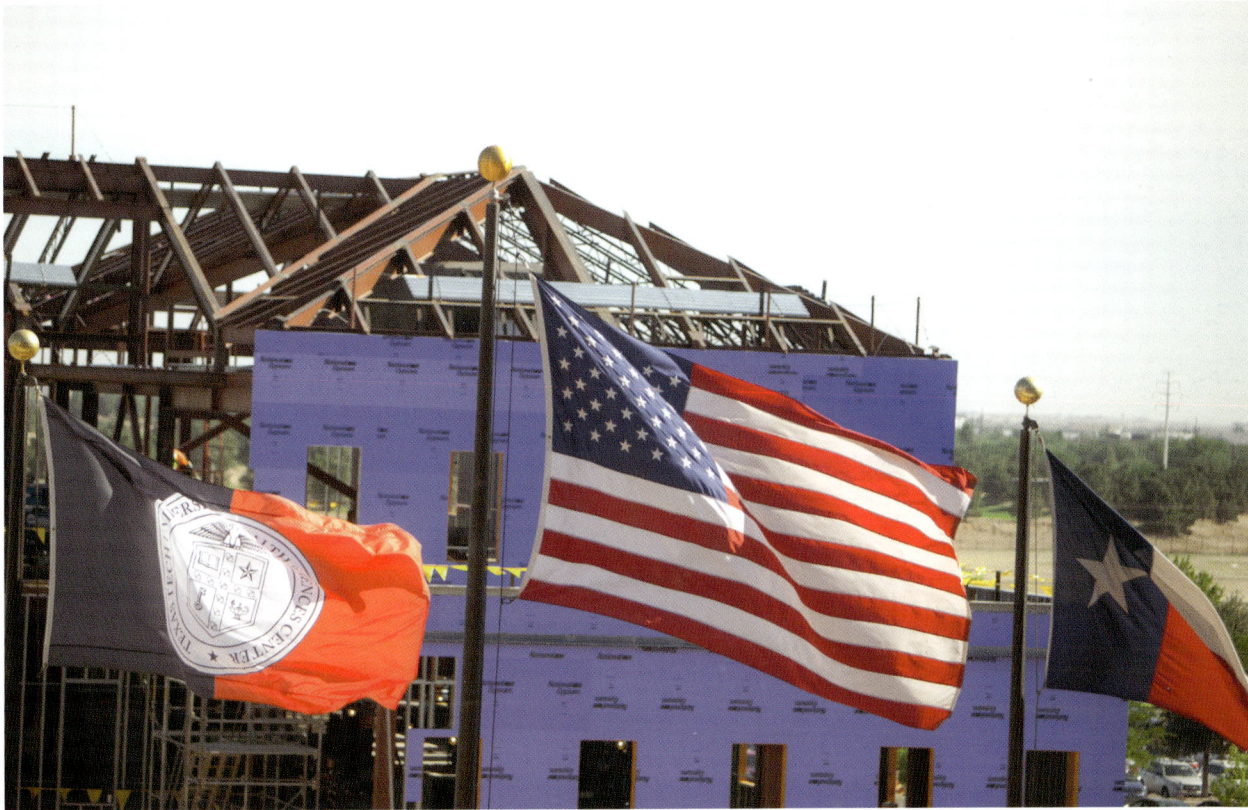

(TOP) Welcome Center and flags. Margaret Vugrin, Photographer

(BOTTOM) Martha Brown, Vice-Chancellor for Government Relations; Billy Breedlove, Vice-Chancellor for Facilities; John Michael Frullo, Sr., Member of the Texas House of Representatives for District 84; Tedd Mitchell, MD, President TTUHSC; and Charles Lee Perry, Member of the Texas State Senate from West Texas District 28 touring the construction site of the Welcome Center. Artie Limmer, Photographer, Associate Director, Institutional Advancement

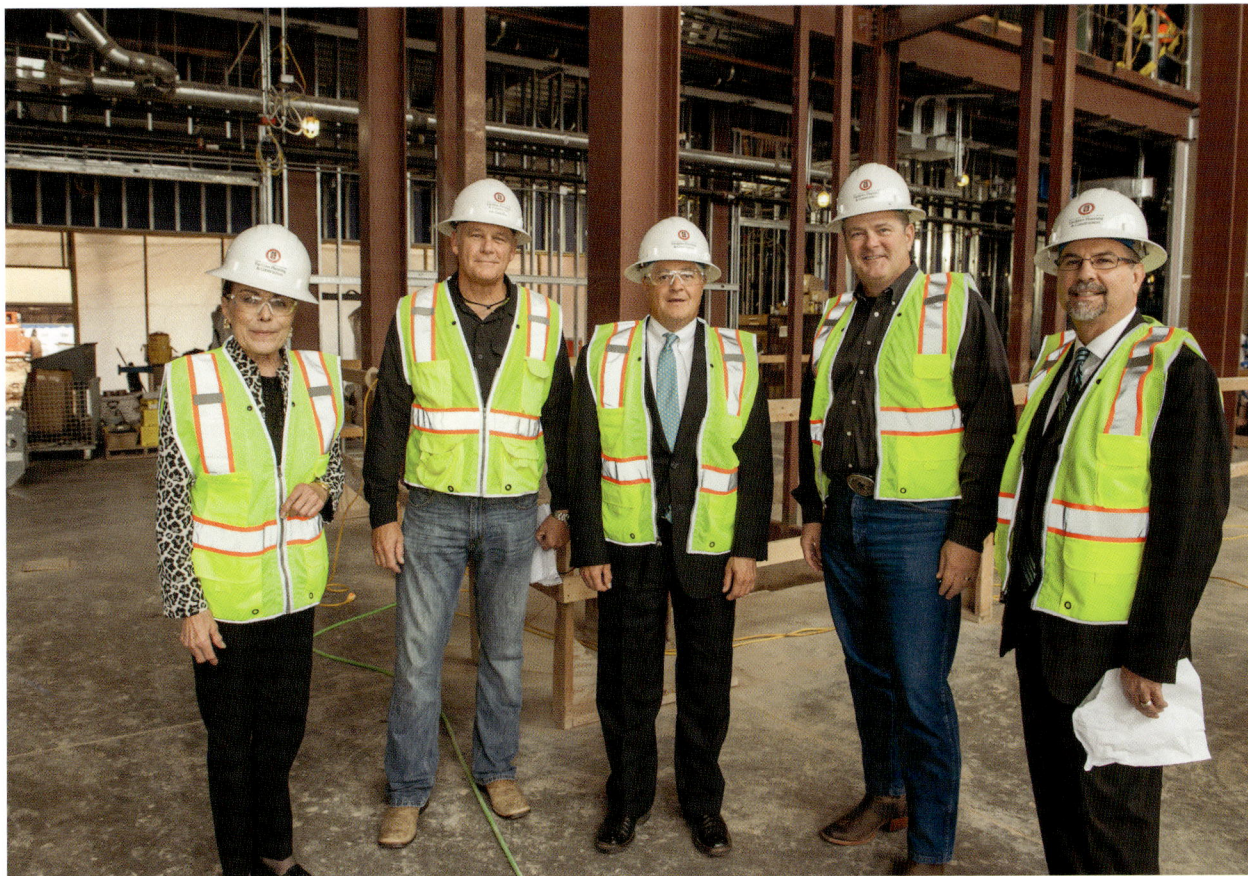

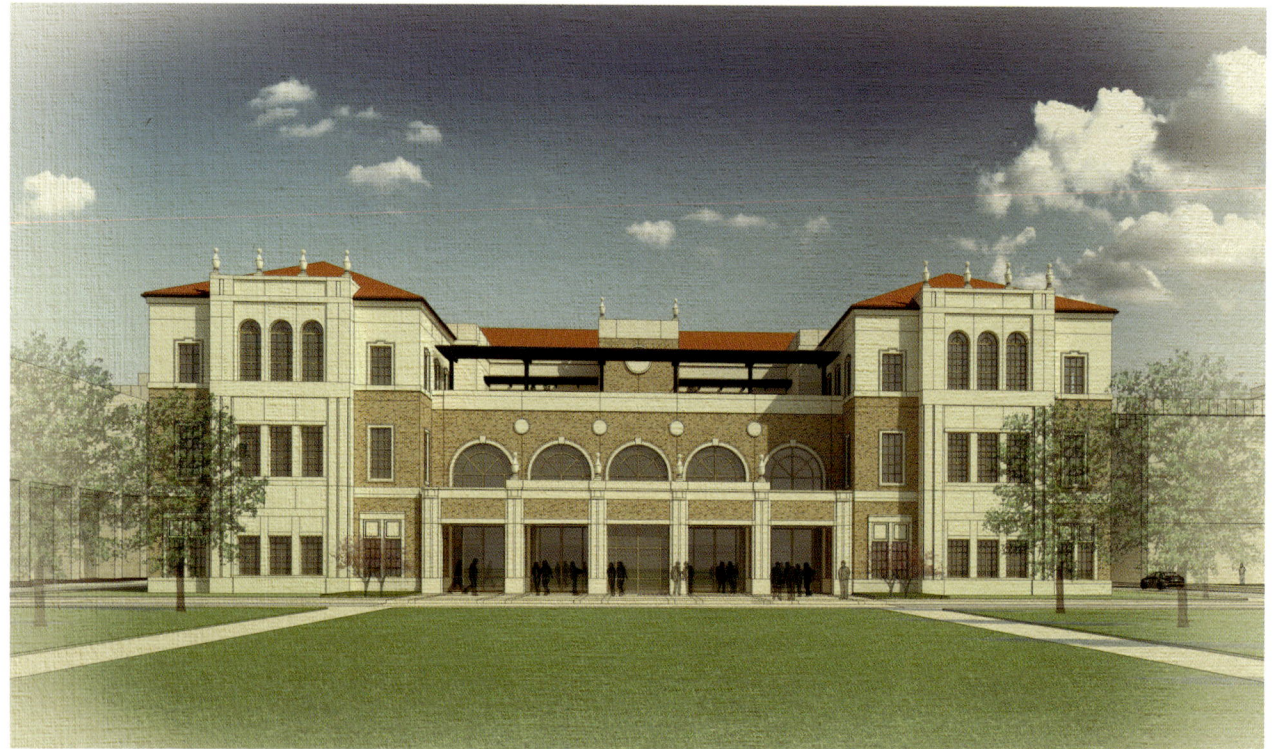

(RIGHT) TTUHSC Lubbock University Center. Courtesy TTU Facilities Planning and Construction. Contractor: Hill & Wilkinson General Contractors (Danny Elmore—Project Manager); Architect: Perkins+Will, Inc. (Dan Eikenberry—Project Architect)

(BELOW) TTUHSC Lubbock, Western Expansion. Courtesy TTU Facilities Planning and Construction. Contractor: Hill & Wilkinson General Contractors (Danny Elmore—Project Manager); Architect: Perkins+Will, Inc. (Dan Eikenberry—Project Architect)

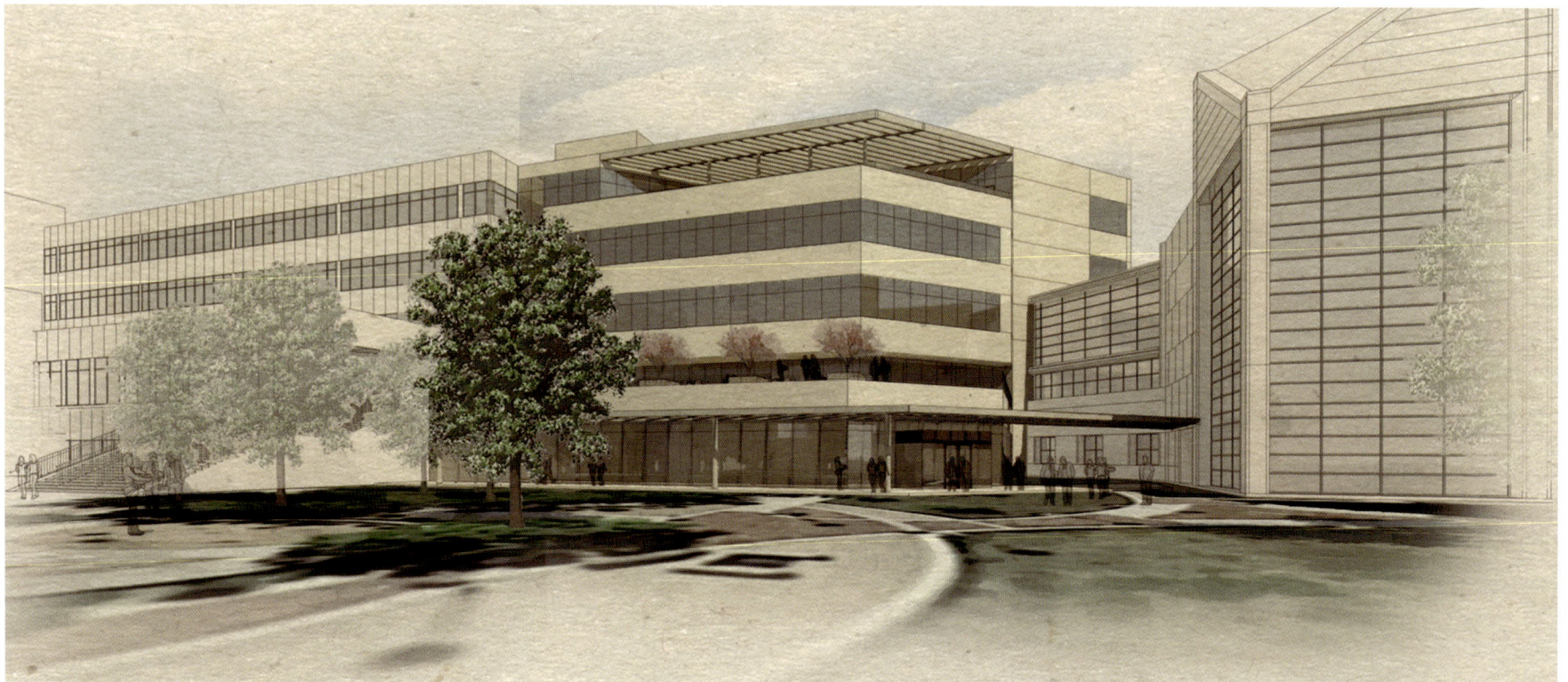

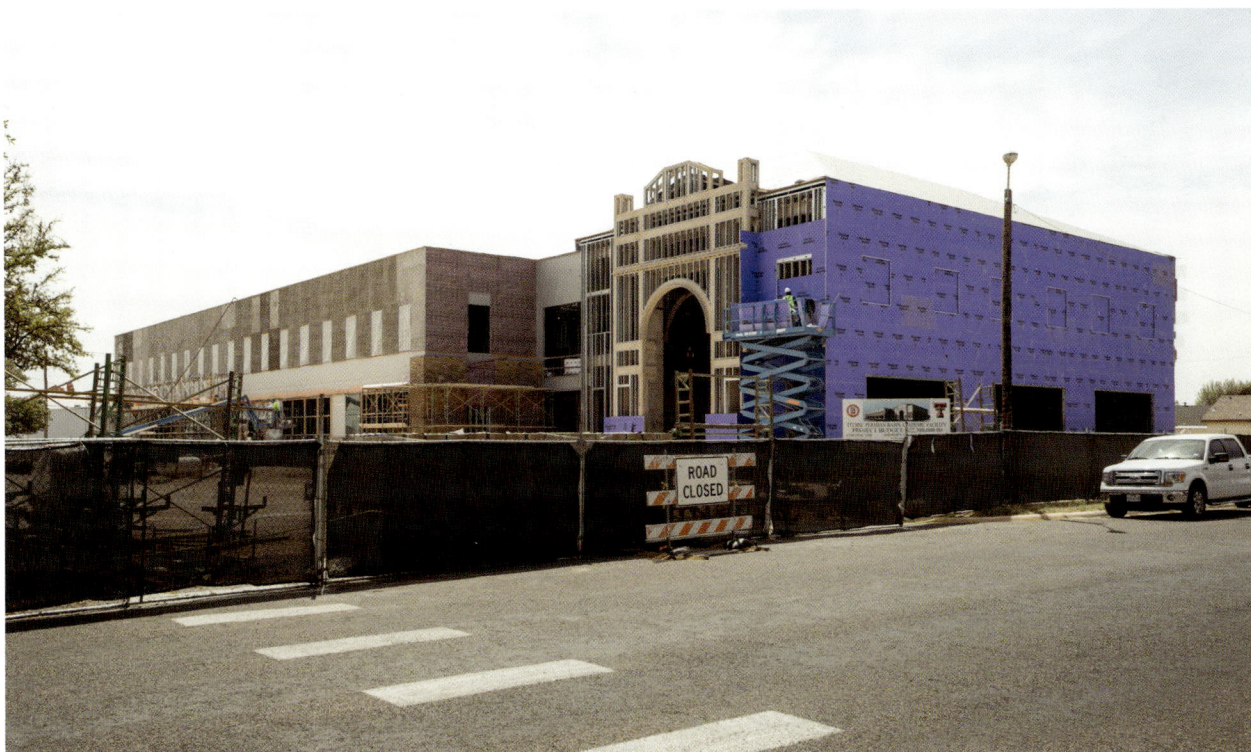

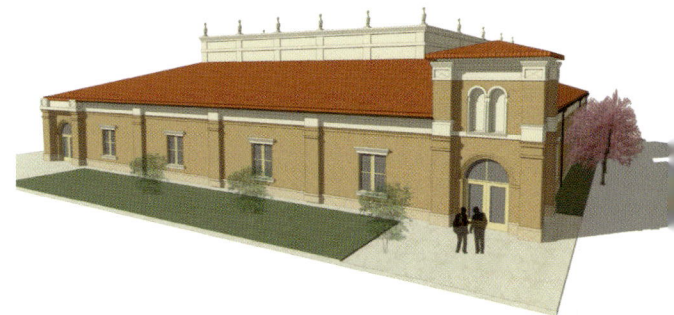

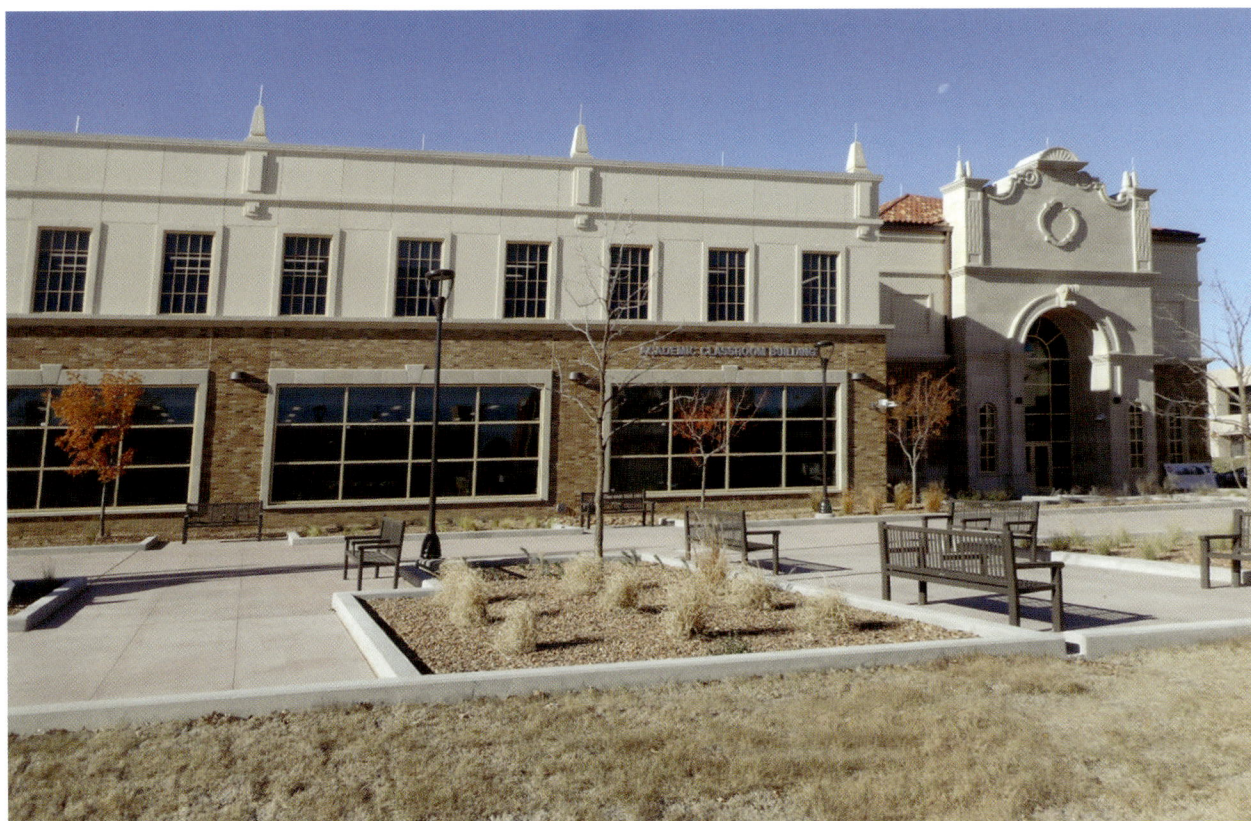

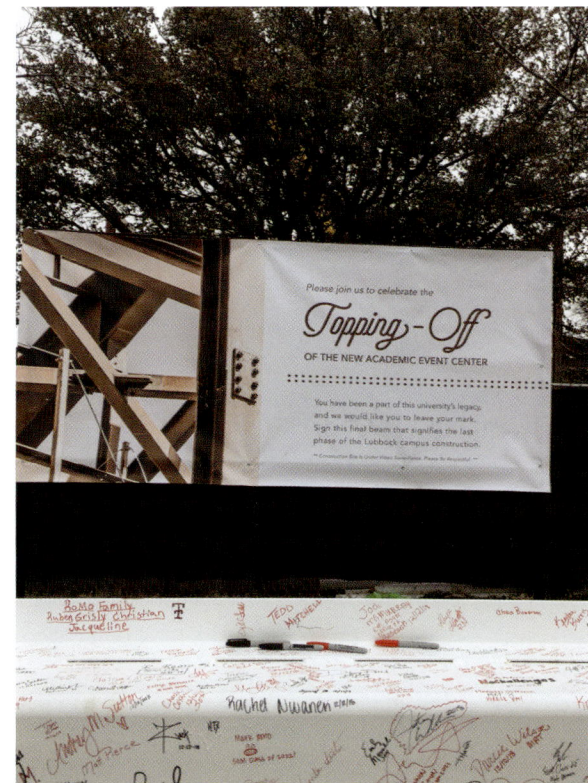

(TOP LEFT) TTUHSC, Odessa, Under Construction

(TOP RIGHT) TTUHSC, Lubbock, Academic Event Center. Courtesy TTU Facilities Planning and Construction. Contractor: Hill & Wilkinson General Contractors (Danny Elmore—Project Manager); Architect: Perkins+Will, Inc. (Dan Eikenberry—Project Architect)

(BOTTOM LEFT) TTUHSC, Odessa, Nearing Completion. Courtesy TTU Facilities Planning and Construction. Contractor: Flintco, LLC (Brandon Sweeter-Project Manager)

(BOTTOM RIGHT) Topping-off Ceremony, Academic Event Center. Courtesy TTU Facilities Planning and Construction. Architect: FKP/Cannon Design Architects (Ardis Clinton—Vice President)

CHAPTER TEN

CONTINUING OUR PROGRESS

When we think about the future, we focus on the technological innovations it brings. Given the rapidity with which discoveries are made today, this makes sense. In fact, with technology developing at such a break-neck pace, it's hard to imagine what our world will look like in another 50 years. When we opened our doors a half-century ago, the pace of life seemed calmer. The world had not yet been introduced to the microprocessor, which would revolutionize computers. There were no emails, word processors, or digital cameras. Telephones were attached to walls, movies were seen in theaters, and knowledge was acquired by studying books and face-to-face interactions with professors. Information was housed in libraries and had to be gathered in person rather than by accessing the World Wide Web over a smart phone. Medicine was also simpler. "Intensive care" units were in their infancy, surgical techniques and tools were relatively primitive compared to the scopes used today, medications to treat both simple and complicated diseases were fewer and less effective, and even discovery researchers' tools were meager relative to the powerful technology available today. The same innovations that revolutionized the world transformed our ability to diagnose and treat diseases and augmented the ability of scientific researchers to make new discoveries.

Our university took advantage of such advances, utilizing technology to link our campuses for classroom instruction, to build some of the nation's best hi-tech simulation training centers for education, and to make rural West Texas "smaller" for patients by introducing telemedicine. Given the enormous size of our coverage area, there is no doubt that future technology will remain a critical part of our growth as an institution. Whether training students with media they are adept at using to make their experience more familiar and their learning more effective; seeking ways to make patients' interactions with providers easier and more "user friendly" utilizing technology (such as telemedicine); or outfitting our laboratories with the cutting-edge equipment necessary to aid our researchers in advancing scientific knowledge, we remain committed to investing in our university's future by investing in its technological assets.

However, it would serve us well to remember that there is a downside to placing too much emphasis on technology alone. Our mission is to "enrich the lives of others by educating students to become collaborative healthcare professionals, providing excellent patient care, and advancing knowledge through innovative research." This cannot be accomplished solely by drilling into our students the technical competencies necessary for their careers. It also requires that we cultivate in them a passion for serving others. This is actually the more difficult part of our task. In a world driven by technology, training healthcare professionals to balance their scientific knowledge with their humanity is critical. Yet simply teaching proficiency in the use of diagnostic, therapeutic, and research tools requires little emotional investment on our part while cultivating

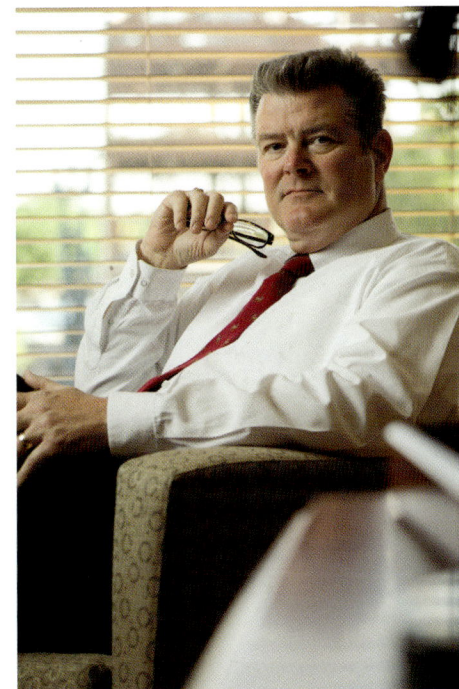

President Tedd Mitchell, MD, reflecting on the future of TTUHSC

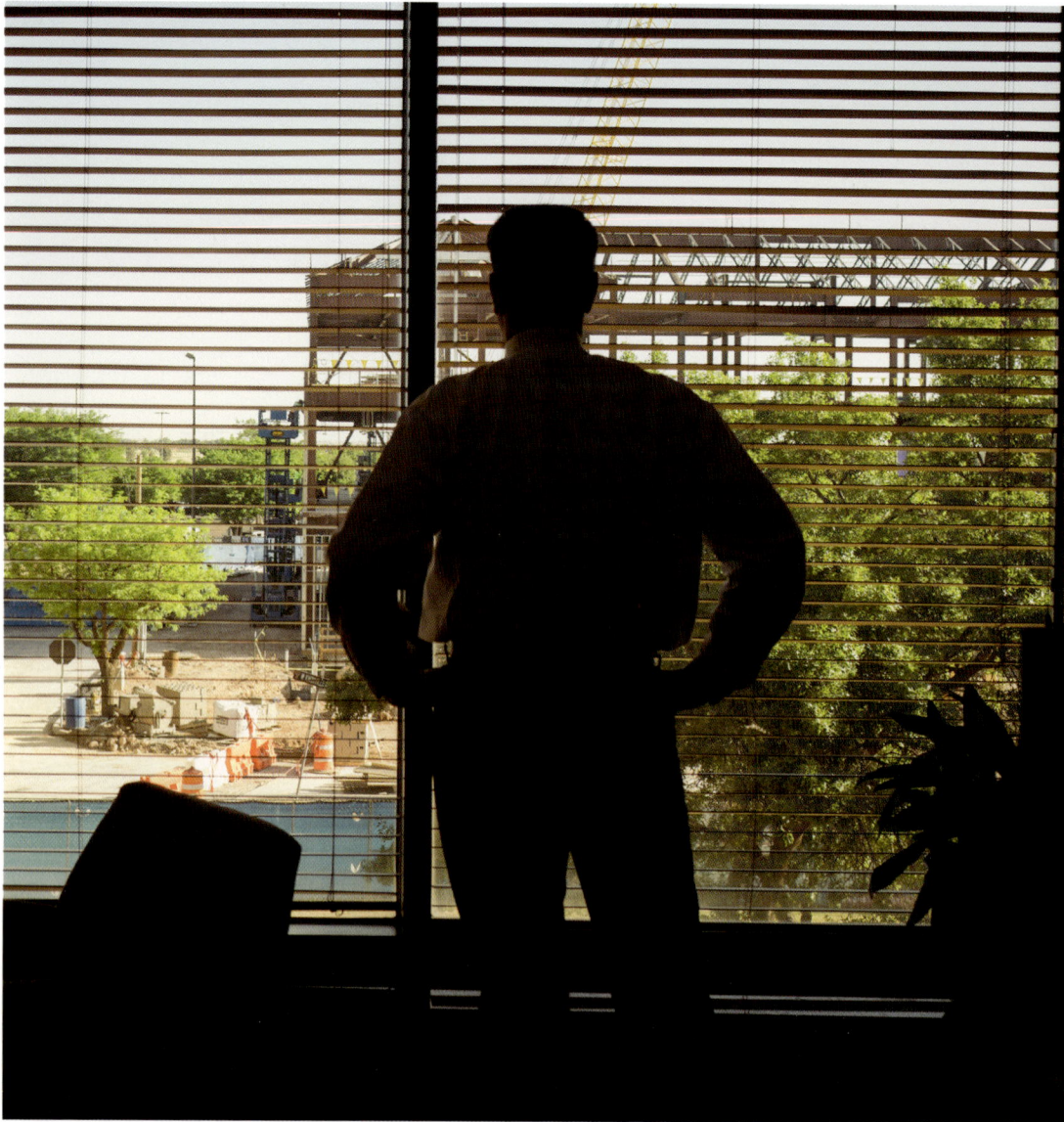

President Tedd Mitchell, MD, viewing
construction projects

a sense of altruism and selflessness in students requires a great deal of engagement from faculty and staff. But it is this understanding—that competency and compassion are two sides of the same coin—that will differentiate us from our peers and best serve future generations of Texans.

Sir William Osler said, "The good physician treats the disease; the great physician treats the patient who has the disease." Such a sentiment is important for all of our folks in all of our schools to reflect upon, because it underscores the immense importance of the human interaction, whether in a hospital, clinic, office, or research laboratory. In a world that has become increasingly mechanized, many have neglected this aspect of their development. If, as a health university we can nurture this essential part of the experience, we will have prepared for our region, our state, our nation, and our world generations of healers and scientists trained to use any technology the future brings to improve the lives of those they will serve. In doing so, we will have fulfilled our mission and our future will be as wide open and bright as the West Texas skies.

Tedd L. Mitchell, MD
President, TTUHSC, and Chancellor, TTU System

APPENDICES

CELEBRATORY LETTERS AND OFFICIAL PROCLAMATIONS

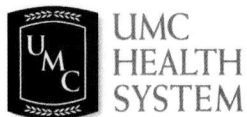

UMC HEALTH SYSTEM

Tedd Mitchell, M.D.
President
Texas Tech University Health Sciences Center
3601 4th Street
Lubbock, TX 79430

Dear Dr. Mitchell,

On behalf of University Medical Center, we extend congratulations to our strong partner, Texas Tech University Health Sciences Center, on this auspicious occasion of your 50th anniversary. Through the years, the reach and impact of the Health Sciences Center has been immense. West Texas enjoys a strong and varied medical community, due to the vision and leadership of the academic programs at Texas Tech. The schools can be proud and gratified that they have remained steadfast to their original intent to train tomorrow's medical professionals for the West Texas communities.

Former Governor Preston Smith and the legislators of the late 1960's cast a vision for what the Health Sciences Center could achieve. The leadership of Texas Tech has delivered mightily on that vision. In 2017, Texas Tech became the most productive health sciences center in Texas, producing more graduates than any other. Today, hospitals and health care entities across the region owe a debt of gratitude to the faculty and staff of the Health Sciences Center for the wonderful healthcare professionals produced over the years.

The entire UMC Health System wishes the Health Sciences Center heartfelt congratulations on its 50th anniversary. As we celebrate our 40 years of service in 2018, we are very proud of all the accomplishments you have achieved and the legacy of learning you have established. The mark left on the region is indelible. Truly, the citizens of West Texas have been well served. President Mitchell, faculty and staff, we congratulate you all on your first 50 years. We look forward with gratitude and admiration to the next 50!

Sincerely,

Mark Funderburk
President and Chief Executive Officer

Wendell Davis
Chair, Board of Managers

Service • Teamwork • Leadership

University Medical Center Letter
Courtesy University Medical Center,
Lubbock, Texas

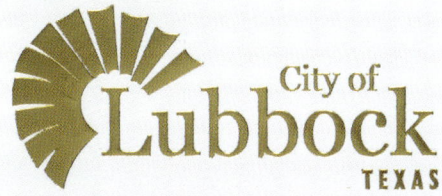

City of Lubbock, TEXAS

Special Recognition

WHEREAS: Texas Tech University Health Sciences Center was established in 1969, and serves the healthcare needs of more than two million people living in more than 100 counties, stretching from the Texas Panhandle, south to the Permian Basin and West Texas into El Paso and eastern New Mexico; and,

WHEREAS: Texas Tech University Health Sciences Center, being nationally recognized for innovative programs, academic achievement, licensure pass rates, and cutting-edge research, educates and trains highly qualified health professionals through its schools of medicine, nursing, pharmacy, health professions, and biomedical sciences; and,

WHEREAS: Texas Tech University Health Sciences Center has a continual trajectory of advancement and growth, graduating more healthcare professionals and researchers each year than any other health related university in the state of Texas, with over 28,000 graduates to date; and,

WHEREAS: Texas Tech University Health Sciences Center provides quality, affordable education and supports the development of academic, research, patient care, and community service programs throughout its regional campuses in Lubbock, Abilene, Amarillo, Dallas, and the Permian Basin, with the El Paso campus having transitioned into a full-fledged, standalone health sciences center university; and,

WHEREAS: Texas Tech University Health Sciences Center, through its commitment to provide substantial and meaningful contributions to support West Texas populations, has reduced the shortage of primary care providers in the region by more than half; and,

WHEREAS: It is appropriate to recognize Texas Tech University Health Sciences Center for excellence in healthcare, education, and research as they celebrate an important historical milestone,

NOW, THEREFORE, we the Mayor and City Council of the great City of Lubbock do hereby recognize

Texas Tech University Health Sciences Center's 50th Anniversary

and call upon all citizens to celebrate this important institution, headquartered in Lubbock, as they begin a new half century of achievement, excellence, and quality healthcare.

Dated this 1st day of January, 2019

Daniel M. Pope
Mayor

Jeff Griffith
Mayor Pro Tem

Juan A. Chadis
Council member

Shelia Patterson Harris
Council member

Steve Massengale
Council member

Randy Christian
Council member

Latrelle Joy
Council member

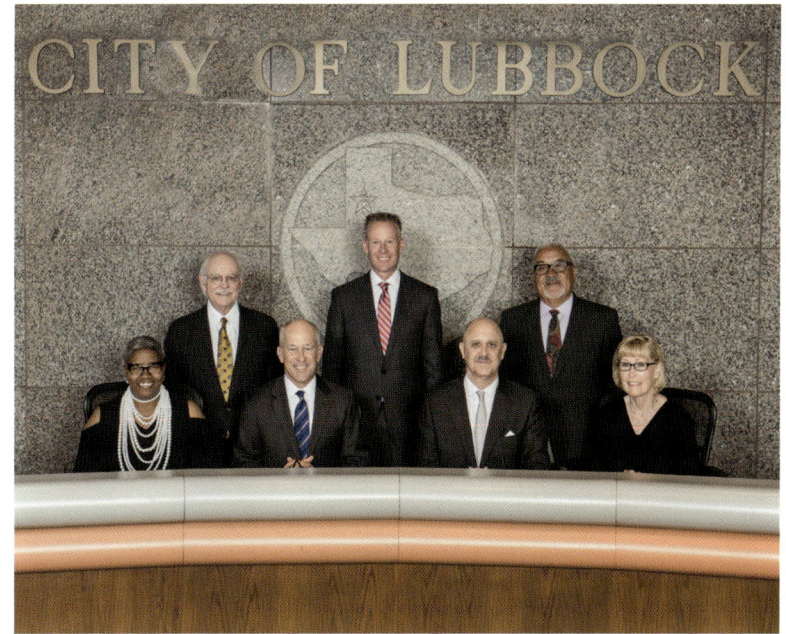

(ABOVE) Mayor and city council members, 2019
Courtesy City of Lubbock, Texas, Mayor's Office

(LEFT) Lubbock City Proclamation

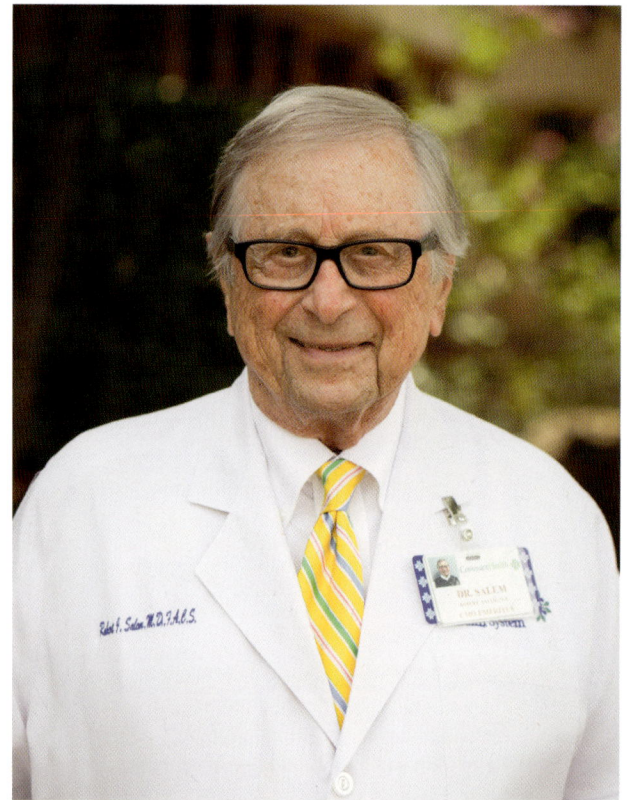

(RIGHT) Robert Salem, MD, founding regional vice dean for Covenant Branch Medical Education Programs,

(BELOW) Robert Salem, MD, with faculty and some students from Covenant branch

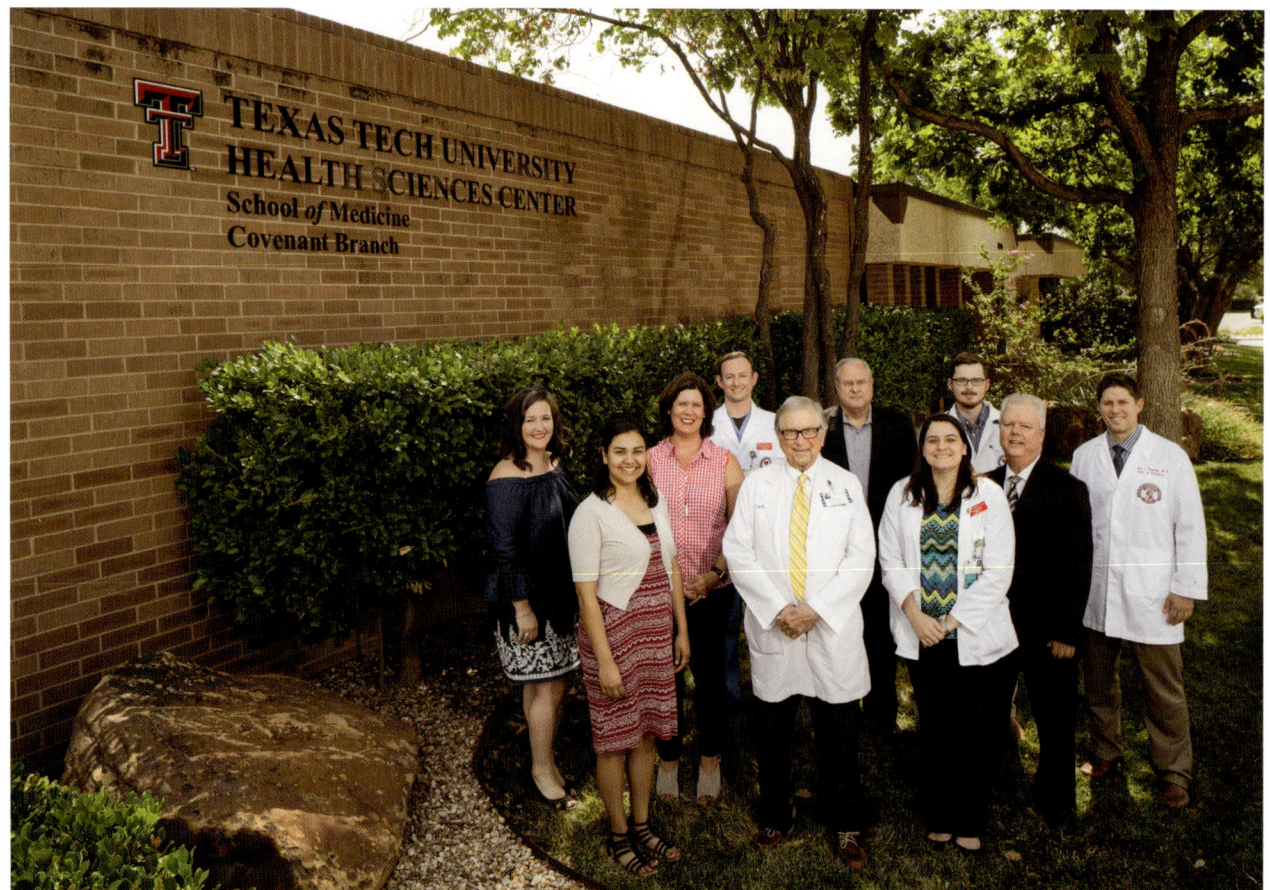

CovenantHealth

Richard Parks, FACHE
COVENANT HEALTH | Chief Executive Officer
PROVIDENCE ST. JOSEPH HEALTH | Regional Chief Executive
Tel: 806.725.0447 | Email: richard.parks@covhs.org

Tedd L. Mitchell, MD
President
Texas Tech University Health Science Center

Covenant Health – or more accurately its predecessors – helped birth Texas Tech University Health Sciences Center and 50 years later the relationship has never been stronger.

Robert Salem, Covenant Health's Chief Medical Officer Emeritus, helped then-Texas Technological College sell the idea of a Lubbock-based medical school to state officials in Austin in the 1960s. Once the school was approved, Dr. Salem served on the search committee selecting the first dean. He also served as the Chief of Staff at then-Methodist Hospital when he asked doctors to serve as clinical physicians at the new school and 77 helped.

A lot of the early success of the new school was thanks to local doctors who taught during the school's fledgling years. Shortly before the school opened in 1972, the dean asked Dr. Salem to lead the Department of Surgery. He was reluctant because he had a busy private practice, but wanted the new school to succeed, after all, he was a Red Raider. Dr. Salem's partners said they'd help and he told the school he'd do it for a few months until they found someone permanent. That few months turned into three years.

Until the county-operated hospital opened in 1978, Methodist and St. Mary hospitals – merged in the late 1990s to form Covenant Health – served as the primary teaching hospitals. The connections continued. In the early 1980s, Craig Rhyne, MD became the first School of Medicine resident to rotate at Methodist Hospital – under Dr. Salem. Dr. Rhyne is now our Regional Chief Medical Officer.

When it was hard to recruit neurologists to the region, Covenant and Dr. Salem helped develop the neurological residency program at TTUHSC. It's one example of many where Covenant Health collaborated with the school to address a medical deficiency in Lubbock and the region.

Five years ago, School of Medicine Dean Steven Berk approached Covenant again this time to help expand their class size from 150 to 180 students. Again, Dr. Salem was involved and became the founding dean. In July of 2016, Covenant was officially designated as the TTUHSC School of Medicine Covenant Branch offering a wide variety of subspecialty experiences for medical students. We opened with 30 third-year students in July of 2016 and expanded the following year adding fourth-year students. Students do their rotations with Covenant Health doctors or doctors with Covenant Health ties. In 2018 we graduated our first class.

The relationship of physicians training at Texas Tech and practicing at Covenant is strong. Today, more than half of Covenant's physicians did some form of training at TTUHSC. More than 125 Covenant Health physicians have been appointed as clinical practitioners at TTUHSC as we continue to step up to the plate to provide medical education.

3615 19th Street • Lubbock, TX 79410
T: (806) 725-0000

www.covenanthealth.org

CovenantHealth

Tedd L. Mitchell, MD
Texas Tech University Health Science Center
Page Two (2)

Last year Covenant entered its second century of service. As TTUHSC enters the second half of its first century we congratulate the leadership of the medical school and health science center on its fifty-years of service. We also celebrate a mutually beneficial relationship that continues a legacy of providing medical students with unique learning opportunities with the faith that many of these bright, young physicians will stay and work our West Texas communities in the future.

Sincerely,

Richard Parks

3615 19th Street • Lubbock, TX 79410
T: (806) 725-0000

www.covenanthealth.org

Covenant Health System Letter
Courtesy Covenant Health, Lubbock, Texas

THE STATE OF TEXAS

GOVERNOR

To all to whom these presents shall come, Greetings: Know ye that this official recognition is presented to the:

Texas Tech University Health Sciences Center

on the occasion of its

50th Anniversary

Across the Lone Star State, institutions of higher learning offer invaluable opportunities, fostering the foundation of excellence on which we are building the future. Unrelenting in your focus and commitment to providing a rigorous, well-rounded education, you have established a legacy of success — a legacy that will long highlight the best of our great state.

To all the men and women who have helped build this fine institution, I applaud you. Your successes will be mirrored in the achievements of your students for generations to come.

First Lady Cecilia Abbott joins me in sending best wishes for a joyous and memorable celebration.

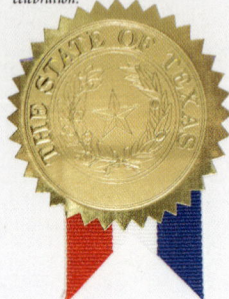

In testimony whereof, I have signed my name and caused the Seal of the State of Texas to be affixed at the City of Austin, this the 3rd day of December, 2018.

Greg Abbott
Governor of Texas

Proclamation from the Texas Governor

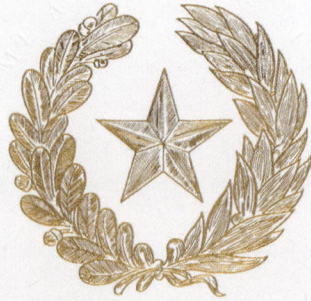

STATE OF TEXAS
OFFICE OF THE GOVERNOR

Greetings to the:

Texas Tech University Health Sciences Center

Congratulations to your esteemed institution of higher learning for achieving a significant milestone in celebrating 50 years of providing the people of West Texas with world class patient care as well as developing the next generation of physicians and health care professionals.

In 1969, 23 of the western-most counties in Texas had no hospital, 19 had no physician, and the area had only one-half the national ratio of physicians-to-patients. In May of that year, the 61st Texas Legislature and Governor Preston Smith took action and created the Texas Tech University School of Medicine as a multi-campus institution with campuses in Amarillo, El Paso, Lubbock, and Odessa.

Ten years later, the state expanded the charter to form the Texas Tech University Health Sciences Center. Through the years, TTUHSC has expanded to include schools of Health Professions, Nursing, Pharmacy, and a Graduate School of Biomedical Sciences as well as added campuses in Abilene and Dallas-Fort Worth. In May 2013, the El Paso campus was established as its own independent institution.

Today, TTUHSC serves almost 5,000 students across the nation and boasts almost 25,000 alumni, 24 percent of whom remain in the university's 108-county service area. The health care landscape is much different now thanks to the visionary leadership of those who saw a need not only for a medical school in West Texas, but also a full-fledged Health Sciences Center.

First Lady Cecilia Abbott joins me in sending best wishes and congratulations to the faculty, staff, students and alumni of the Texas Tech University Health Sciences Center in achieving 50 years of excellence.

Sincerely,

Greg Abbott
Governor

Grover Elmer Murray, PhD
1st President, Texas Tech University
School of Medicine
1969–1976

In 1969 Grover Murray, North Carolina native, internationally known geologist and member of the National Science Board, was instrumental in getting legislative, coordinating board, and local approval for a medical school to serve West Texas. The school opened in 1972 when the first students were enrolled. During Murray's tenure, the medical school established centers in Amarillo and El Paso, graduated its first class in 1974, and gained coordinating board approval for schools of veterinary medicine, allied health, pharmacy, and nursing. Construction of the health sciences center building, the largest in West Texas, was initiated.

Maurice Cecil Mackey Jr., PhD
2nd President, Texas Tech University
Health Sciences Center
1976–1979

Cecil Mackey, a native of Alabama, economist, and lawyer, received doctoral and law degrees from the University of Illinois. He coordinated the growth and development of the fledgling school of medicine. During his presidency the first phase of construction of the Health Sciences Center building was completed and phase II begun. The academic Health Center in El Paso was dedicated and new construction was initiated to house the growing program in El Paso. Signifying the expansion of the medical school's operation, the state legislature in 1979 changed the school's name to the Texas Tech University Health Sciences Center.

Lauro F. Cavazos Jr., PhD
3rd President, Texas Tech University
Health Sciences Center
1980–1988

Lauro Cavazos, fifth-generation Texan and first-generation Texas Tech alumnus to serve as president, led the Health Sciences Center from infancy to maturity. He guided the expansion that nearly doubled the operating budget and oversaw more than $27 million in facilities development at all four campuses. The School of Nursing and Allied Health joined the School of Medicine to create the Texas Tech University Health Sciences Center during Cavazos's tenure. He resigned to become U.S. secretary of education, serving under presidents Reagan and Bush.

Robert William Lawless, PhD
4th President, Texas Tech University
Health Sciences Center
1989–1996

Robert William Lawless became the fourth president of Texas Tech University Health Sciences Center on July 1, 1989. Previously, he served as executive vice president and chief operating officer for Southwest Airlines and held numerous academic and administrative positions at the University of Houston.

Dr. Lawless initiated the presidential endowed scholarship program for the Health Sciences Center. Under his leadership the Graduate School of Biomedical Sciences was established in 1991 and the School of Pharmacy was established in 1993. Dr. Lawless was the last president to serve in the dual role of president over both Texas Tech University Health Sciences Center and Texas Tech University.

David Robert Smith, MD
5th President, TTUHSC
1996–2002

David R. Smith, MD, a board-certified pediatrician and former commissioner of health for the State of Texas, became the fifth president of Texas Tech University Health Sciences Center in September 1996 and served through May 2002. Dr. Smith was the first president to serve solely in this role under the newly created Texas Tech University System. Through his efforts at the state, national, and private levels, the largest endowment in the history of Texas Tech to that point in time was established in the amount of $98 million. Additionally, he oversaw the largest facilities expansion represented by significant investments in Lubbock, Amarillo, Dallas, El Paso, Midland, and Odessa. Two significant programmatic expansions and endowments were established for a geriatric program, teaching nursing home, and the Office of Rural and Community Health.

M. Roy Wilson, MD
6th President, TTUHSC
2003–2006

Born in Yokohama, Japan, M. Roy Wilson, MD, a board-certified ophthalmologist, became the sixth president of Texas Tech University Health Sciences Center in 2003. He received his medical doctorate from Harvard Medical School in 1980. He earned his master of science in epidemiology at the University of California at Los Angeles in 1990. As an internationally renowned scholar, his research focused on glaucoma and blindness in populations from the Caribbean to West Africa. Under his leadership, Texas Tech University Health Sciences Center El Paso Medical Education Building was constructed. The F. Marie Hall Institute for Rural and Community Health was established in February 2006 as an interdisciplinary institute to synthesize the medical needs of the region. Wilson was elected as a lifetime member of the National Academy of Medicine in 2003.

John C. Baldwin, MD
7th President, TTUHSC
2007–2009

John C. Baldwin, MD, a native Texan, became the seventh president of Texas Tech University Health Sciences Center in 2007. He received his medical doctorate from Stanford School of Medicine and completed his cardiothoracic surgery residency at Stanford Medical School in 1983. The Paul L. Foster School of Medicine at Texas Tech University Health Sciences Center El Paso received its accreditation as a four-year medical school in 2008 during his tenure. As chief of cardiothoracic surgery at Yale University School of Medicine, Baldwin performed the first successful heart-lung transplant on the East Coast. He served on the board of directors of the Robert F. Kennedy Foundation and received a 2011 presidential appointment to the U.S. Defense Health Board.

Tedd L. Mitchell, MD
8th President, TTUHSC
2010–Present

Tedd L. Mitchell became the eighth president of the Texas Tech University Health Sciences Center on May 17, 2010. As its longest-serving president, Mitchell has successfully led a period of record growth in enrollment, academic excellence, and physical expansion on all campuses. Dr. Mitchell is an Ashbel Smith Distinguished Alumnus of the University of Texas Medical Branch, where he received his doctor of medicine degree in 1987. After graduation he pursued training in internal medicine. In 2012, Dr. Mitchell was honored as a distinguished alumnus of the Department of Internal Medicine. He is a fellow of the American College of Physicians and the American College of Sports Medicine. From 1988 to 1996, he served as a captain in the U.S. Army Reserves (Medical Corps). Prior to coming to Texas Tech University Health Sciences Center, Mitchell served as president and chief executive officer of the Cooper Clinic in Dallas, an internationally recognized center of excellence in preventive and sports medicine. Dr. Mitchell is a member of the faculty. His research interest is focused on the effects of activity and lifestyle on health, and he has authored or coauthored dozens of scientific papers, abstracts, and book chapters. He is a frequent lecturer, both nationally and internationally, on the physiology of exercise and the effects of exercise on aging, fitness, and overall quality of life. As health editor and a weekly columnist for *USA Weekend* from 1998 to 2010, Dr. Mitchell has published more than 600 articles. He received the 2006 Clarion Award and the 2008 Walter C. Alvarez Award for Excellence in Medical Communication from the American Medical Writers Association. His writings led to collaborative efforts with other health experts, culminating in the publication of the books *Fit to Lead* (2004, St. Martin's Press), *Move Yourself* (2008, Wiley Press), and *Fit to Lead 2*

(2012). In 2002, Dr. Mitchell was appointed by President George W. Bush to the President's Council for Physical Fitness and Sports and served until 2009. During his term, he was engaged in efforts that changed the president's test from one that was fitness based to one that is health based.

The Texas Tech University Board of Regents appointed Dr. Mitchell the fifth chancellor of the Texas Tech University System on October 25, 2018. He will continue his role as president of Texas Tech University Health Sciences Center while serving as chancellor of the Texas Tech University System.

TEXAS TECH UNIVERSITY HEALTH SCIENCES CENTER: PRESIDENTS AND DEANS

Presidents or Chief Administrative Officers

1969–1976	Grover Elmer Murray, PhD, first president, Texas Tech University
1970–1974	John Buesseler, MD, founding vice president, Texas Tech University School of Medicine
1974–1976	Richard A. Lockwood, MD, vice president, Health Sciences Center
1976–1980	M. Cecil Mackey, PhD, president, Texas Tech University and the TTU School of Medicine
1980–1989	Lauro F. Cavazos, PhD, president, TTU and TTUHSC
1989–1996	Robert Lawless, PhD, president, TTU and TTUHSC
1996–2003	David R. Smith, MD, president, TTUHSC
2003–2007	M. Roy Wilson, MD, president, TTUHSC
2007–2009	John C. Baldwin, MD, president, TTUHSC
2009–2010	Elmo M. Cavin, MBA, acting president, TTUHSC
2010–	Tedd Mitchell, MD, president, TTUHSC

Deans of the School of Medicine

1970–1974	John Buesseler, MD, founding dean, TTU School of Medicine
1974–1981	George S. Tyner, MD, dean, TTU School of Medicine
1981–1982	J. Ted Hartman, MD, interim dean, TTUHSC School of Medicine
1982–1988	J. Ted Hartman, MD, dean, TTUHSC School of Medicine
1988–1990	Bernhard Mittemeyer, MD, interim dean, TTUHSC School of Medicine
1990–1995	Darryl Williams, MD, dean, TTUHSC School of Medicine
1995–1996	Bernhard Mittemeyer, MD, interim dean, TTUHSC School of Medicine
1996–1997	David R. Smith, MD, interim dean, TTUHSC School of Medicine
1997–2001	Joel Kupersmith, MD, dean, TTUHSC School of Medicine
2001–2005	Richard Van Ness Homan, MD, dean, TTUHSC School of Medicine
2005–2006	Bernhard Mittemeyer, MD, interim dean, TTUHSC School of Medicine
2006–	Steven L. Berk, MD, dean, TTUHSC School of Medicine (and 2010– executive vice president and provost)

Deans of the School of Nursing

1979–1991	Teddy Langford Jones, PhD, FNP, founding dean, School of Nursing
1991–1993	Patricia S. Yoder-Wise, EdD, RN, interim dean, School of Nursing
1993–2000	Patricia S. Yoder-Wise, EdD, RN, dean, School of Nursing
2000–2010	Alexia Green, PhD, RN, dean, School of Nursing
2010–2012	Yondell Masten, PhD, RN, WHNP—BC, interim dean, School of Nursing
2010–	Michael L. Evans, PhD, RN, dean, School of Nursing

Deans of the School of Pharmacy

1994–2012	Arthur A. Nelson Jr., RPh, PhD, founding dean, School of Pharmacy
2012–	Quentin Smith, PhD, dean, School of Pharmacy

Deans of the School of Health Professions

1983–1985	Robert Cornesky, ScD, founding dean, School of Allied Health
1985–1987	Lawrence Peake, OTR, interim dean
1987–1998	Shirley McManigal, PhD, MT(ASCP), dean, School of Allied Health
1998–2012	Paul P. Brooks, PhD, dean, School of Allied Health
2012–2016	Robin Satterwhite, MBA, EdD, dean, School of Health Professions
2016–2017	Hal Larsen, PhD, MT(ASCP), interim dean, School of Health Professions
2017–	Lori Rice-Spearman, PhD, MT(ASCP), dean, School of Health Professions

Deans of the Graduate School of Biomedical Sciences

1994–1996	Kenneth L. Barker, PhD, vice president for Research, interim dean, Graduate School of Biomedical Sciences
1996–1997	David J. Hentges, PhD, interim dean, Graduate School of Biomedical Sciences
1997–2000	Joel Kupersmith, MD, dean, Graduate School of Biomedical Sciences
2001–2005	Richard Van Ness Homan, MD, dean, Graduate School of Biomedical Sciences
2005–2007	Roderick Nairn, PhD, dean, Graduate School of Biomedical Sciences, Executive Vice President, Academic Affairs
2007–2008	Douglas M. Stocco, PhD, interim dean, Graduate School of Biomedical Sciences
2008–2010	Luis Reuss, MD, dean, Graduate School of Biomedical Sciences
2010–2011	Thomas Pressley, PhD, interim dean, Graduate School of Biomedical Sciences
2011–2012	Douglas M. Stocco, PhD, dean, Graduate School of Biomedical Sciences
2013–	Brandt L. Schneider, PhD, dean, Graduate School of Biomedical Sciences

INDEX

Page number in *italics* refer to images.